WELLNESS
AND PHYSICAL THERAPY

SHARON ELAYNE FAIR, PT, MS, PhD
President of The Wellness Society

JONES AND BARTLETT PUBLISHERS
Sudbury, Massachusetts
BOSTON   TORONTO   LONDON   SINGAPORE

World Headquarters

Jones and Bartlett Publishers	Jones and Bartlett Publishers	Jones and Bartlett Publishers
40 Tall Pine Drive	Canada	International
Sudbury, MA 01776	6339 Ormindale Way	Barb House, Barb Mews
978-443-5000	Mississauga, Ontario L5V 1J2	London W6 7PA
info@jbpub.com	Canada	United Kingdom
www.jbpub.com		

Jones and Bartlett's books and products are available through most bookstores and online booksellers. To contact Jones and Bartlett Publishers directly, call 800-832-0034, fax 978-443-8000, or visit our website, www.jbpub.com.

Substantial discounts on bulk quantities of Jones and Bartlett's publications are available to corporations, professional associations, and other qualified organizations. For details and specific discount information, contact the special sales department at Jones and Bartlett via the above contact information or send an email to specialsales@jbpub.com.

The author, editor, and publisher have made every effort to provide accurate information. However, they are not responsible for errors, omissions, or for any outcomes related to the use of the contents of this book and take no responsibility for the use of the products and procedures described. Treatments and side effects described in this book may not be applicable to all people; likewise, some people may require a dose or experience a side effect that is not described herein. Drugs and medical devices are discussed that may have limited availability controlled by the Food and Drug Administration (FDA) for use only in a research study or clinical trial. Research, clinical practice, and government regulations often change the accepted standard in this field. When consideration is being given to use of any drug in the clinical setting, the health care provider or reader is responsible for determining FDA status of the drug, reading the package insert, and reviewing prescribing information for the most up-to-date recommendations on dose, precautions, and contraindications, and determining the appropriate usage for the product. This is especially important in the case of drugs that are new or seldom used.

Production Credits

Publisher: David Cella	Composition: Arlene Apone
Associate Editor: Maro Gartside	Cover and Title Page Design:
Production Director: Amy Rose	Kristin E. Parker
Associate Production Editor: Julia Waugaman	Cover and Title Page Image:
Marketing Manager: Grace Richards	© Inga Ivanova/Dreamstime.com
Manufacturing and Inventory Control	Printing and Binding: Malloy Incorporated
Supervisor: Amy Bacus	Cover Printing: Malloy Incorporated

Library of Congress Cataloging-in-Publication Data
Fair, Sharon Elayne, 1960-
  Wellness and physical therapy / by Sharon Elayne Fair.
    p. ; cm.
  Includes bibliographical references and index.
  ISBN-13: 978-0-7637-5821-9 (pbk.)
  ISBN-10: 0-7637-5821-3 (pbk.)
  1. Physical therapy. 2. Physical fitness. 3. Health. I. Title.
  [DNLM: 1. Physical Therapy Modalities. 2. Health Behavior. 3. Health Promotion. WB 460 F163w 2010]
  RM700.F35 2010
  615.8'2—dc22
                                          2008055384
6048

Printed in the United States of America
13 12 11 10 09   10 9 8 7 6 5 4 3 2 1

Dedication

I dedicate this book to my daughter, Embury Elayne Fair-Russell, whom I love more than the universe is big and always will, and my brother, Michael James Fair, who sacrificed his life for our country and whom I continue to love and miss every single day.

Contents

Preface

Two roads diverged in a wood, and I—
I took the one less traveled by,
And that has made all the difference.

━ ━ ━ ━ ━ ━ ━

Robert Frost

PHYSICAL THERAPY EDUCATORS

This book was designed to meet or exceed the educational objectives related to wellness outlined in *A Normative Model of Physical Therapist Professional Education: Version 2004*. Accordingly, this textbook can be utilized, and it is indeed suggested that it be adopted, as a (required) textbook in the wellness courses offered by the entry-level physical therapy programs accredited by the Commission on Accreditation in Physical Therapy Education (CAPTE).

Some entry-level physical therapy programs require two courses related to wellness: an introductory course and a more advanced course. For example: "Wellness I" and "Wellness II"; or "Health Promotion and Wellness for Physical Therapy Practice I" and "Health Promotion and Wellness for Physical Therapy Practice II." This two-tier model mirrors the multistep model deemed appropriate and employed for other core subject matters and specialties, such as musculoskeletal and neuromuscular curricula and research. (Note: I believe the two-tier system is the best model for wellness pedagogy.) In those cases in which this textbook is adopted for use in a two-tier model of wellness pedagogy, the contents of the book may be readily divided as indicated by the number of credit hours per course and at the discretion of the professor.

Many physical therapy programs offer a single course related to wellness. These courses are known by a variety of names, such as "Health and Wellness," "Prevention and Wellness," "Physical Therapy Constructs of Health and Wellness," "Health Promotion and Disease Prevention," or simply "Wellness." In some cases, the course is offered early in the curriculum (e.g., term two); in other cases, it is offered relatively late in the curriculum (e.g., term seven). Placement of the wellness course will be a factor in how to best utilize this textbook to meet or exceed the objectives of *A Normative Model of Physical Therapist Professional Education: Version 2004*. For example, if the wellness course is offered early in the curriculum, perhaps a mock, rather than an authentic, community wellness project might be appropriate. However, if the wellness course is offered later in the curriculum, a genuine community wellness project might be indicated and of substantial benefit.

Some physical therapy programs do not offer a "wellness" course, and instead integrate topics related to wellness into another course or courses. In these cases, the contents of this book may be integrated into the program's classes/modules/labs related to wellness. If the wellness content is divided into two or more courses, it may be a challenge for the professors to integrate the information from the textbook into their respective courses. However, these challenges can be overcome with communication and coordination among the involved faculty. One suggestion is for involved faculty to agree upon which chapter will be examined in which course.

Indeed, the task of serving as one of the required textbooks (if not the only textbook) in a wellness course(s) in a physical therapy program is daunting. The reasons include, but are not necessarily limited to (1) the relationship between physical therapy and wellness has not been clearly delineated (Culver, 2007); (2) compared to subject matter that has traditionally been offered in physical therapy curricula and is often considered to be "core coursework" (such as musculoskeletal and neuromuscular curricula), wellness is a relatively new concept; and (3) compared to traditional specialties (such as gerontology and women's health), wellness is an emerging forte. Few physical therapists or physical therapist faculty members possess an "expertise" in wellness. Accordingly, it can be speculated that fewer physical therapy programs appreciate the uniqueness of wellness and recognize the value of a multitier model of wellness pedagogy and the necessity of requiring a wellness-related textbook. The challenges that face a textbook relating physical therapy and wellness may be exemplified by comparing the number of physical therapy textbooks dedicated to traditional subject matters to the number of physical therapy textbooks related to wellness. This textbook is a first step in a largely unchartered territory to elucidate the provision of wellness by physical therapists.

PHYSICAL THERAPY STUDENTS

This textbook is designed to serve as an educational tool for you to learn about wellness and its relationship to the provision of physical therapy. This is the first textbook with this long-overdue goal.

As you should be aware, *A Normative Model of Physical Therapist Professional Education: Version 2004* includes educational objectives related to wellness, just as it includes educational objectives related to such areas as orthopedics and neurology. The contents of this book are designed to meet or exceed CAPTE's educational objectives related to wellness and are poised to meet the wellness-related educational objectives in the next edition of *A Normative Model of Physical Therapist Professional Education.*

Historically, the focus of physical therapy has been restorative care (Moffat, 1996). This means that physical therapists primarily provided rehabilitative care to patients who had a disease (e.g., Parkinson's disease) or had been injured (e.g., presented status post sprain or fracture). While current-day physical therapists still provide this type of care, more and more are learning about and providing wellness-related care.

The three dimensions of wellness are physical, mental, and social wellness, and each of these is linked to the provision of physical therapy. Of the three dimensions of wellness, physicals therapists are best educated and trained to provide certain types of physical wellness, particularly body composition and fitness wellness. While physical therapists can directly provide these aspects of physical wellness (e.g., by teaching a patient/client about aerobic capacity and facilitating an improvement in her/his exercise regimen), they can and should also integrate wellness into their restorative care. For example, a physical therapist might utilize her or his knowledge related to mental wellness to motivate a patient/client to adhere to the home program the physical therapist has designed.

I am confident that your exploration of this textbook will provide a solid foundation to provide direct wellness services as well as to integrate wellness into your restorative practice. I wish you the best!

Acknowledgments

Although this book is dedicated to my daughter, Embury Fair-Russell, and my brother, Michael Fair, I also wish to acknowledge the unique contributions these two wondrous individuals have made to my life, which, among other things, propelled me to fulfill my childhood dream of becoming a writer.

I also acknowledge other family members who have contributed to the completion of this book in one form or another, including my dad, Donald Fair, and my late paternal grandfather, Joseph Fair. In particular, I thank my mom, Perena Cianelli-Fair. When I attempted to express myself through poetry, she gifted me Robert Frost's *The Book of Poetry* and closed her inscription with "To my creative writer." And during the seemingly eternal process of writing this book, she offered continuous encouragement.

Professionally, I acknowledge those colleagues who have supported my interest and expertise in wellness, including, but not limited to, former University of St. Augustine for Health Sciences faculty members Emily Fox, PT, MA; Patricia (Trish) King, PT, MA, MTC; and David Lehman, PT, PhD. I am especially grateful to Dr. Fox for her support of my pursuit of the triad of wellness. I also value the criticisms received from certain colleagues in response to my attempts to catechize others, including them, that wellness mirrors the World Health Organization's (1947; 2009) unwavering definition of health, and that consequently wellness consists of three and only three dimensions of wellness (i.e., physical, mental, and social). In part, it was their insistence upon what might be described as a "pre-Copernican" perception of wellness that has propelled me, and will continue to propel me, to educate myself and others about the enlightened concept of the triad of wellness.

If a flower is of a fair seed, its roots are embedded in hardy soil,
and there is adequate sunshine,
Even a dreary rain from a murky cloud helps that flower to blossom.

■ ■ ■ ■ ■ ■

Tamar Fair

Last but not least, I acknowledge my physical therapy wellness clients and my physical therapy "restorative" patients. My wellness patients and clients have inspired me to share with others, including current and future colleagues, my understanding of the relationship between wellness and physical therapy. As I teach and help my patients and clients, they teach and help me. As they thank me, I thank them. As I bring well-being into their lives, they bring well-being into mine.

Introduction by the Series Editor

Enhancing and restoring physical fitness and wellness by way of specific exercise instruction and education with regard to exercise and healthy living habits has been a cornerstone of physical therapy from the inception of the profession. In fact, it was the concern about declining levels of physical fitness in new military recruits that directly contributed to the emergence of physical education in the 18th century and the subsequent development of physical therapy in the early and mid-19th century in various Northern and Western European countries, including Sweden, Germany, and the Netherlands (Ottoson, 2005; Terlouw, 2007).

Over time, however, and perhaps related to the limited number of physical therapists available, limited societal resources were allotted to fund physical therapy services. At the time, greater societal recognition was for those working and with the sick and disabled, and the emphasis shifted from therapists also providing wellness, preventative, and maintenance services to the profession of physical therapy almost exclusively associated with restorative services. Physical therapy came to be synonymous with treatment to address impairments and associated limitations in activities and restrictions in participation resulting from congenital, degenerative, trauma-related, post-surgical, disease-related, and other causes.

In the first half of the 20th century, increasing standards of living, especially in the developed world, led to a resurging recognition of the importance of wellness and fitness with regard to health and well-being. This demand for services related to enhancing and restoring wellness and fitness was initially filled by alternative healthcare providers working from unsubstantiated and often implausible underlying theoretical models (Whorton, 1988). However, the recognition of the role of wellness and fitness again increasingly gained ground in mainstream medicine as reflected in the World Health Organization view of health as a triad of physical, mental, and social well-being. Health was thus defined as not merely the absence of disease but rather as a state of complete physical, mental, and social well-being (WHO, 1947).

Undoubtedly driven by more down-to-earth motives of seeking alternate avenues of generating revenue in the face of diminishing reimbursement for restorative physical therapy services, and also by more lofty motives related to a recognition of the importance of wellness in attaining optimal results when providing restorative services and in the growing understanding of the crucial and natural leadership role physical therapy has in promoting health and well-being in individuals and society as a whole, therapists are once again increasingly engaging in providing wellness services outside and within the traditional restorative service model. In fact, *A Normative Model of Physical Therapist Professional Education* (CAPTE, 2004) has required entry-level physical therapy students to be educated in wellness since 2004. The 2004 edition further elaborated on requirements with regard to wellness in the physical therapy entry-level curriculum (CAPTE, 2004). The American Physical Therapy Association, in *The Guide to Physical Therapist Practice*, has also included a discussion of wellness, defining wellness as the "concepts that embrace positive health behaviors that promote a state of physical and mental balance and fitness" (APTA, 2001b).

When comparing the World Health Organization definition with the definition proposed in *The Guide to Physical Therapist Practice* above, it becomes evident that the latter definition overtly excludes the social realm of the wellness triad. Dr. Sharon Fair is eminently qualified with degrees in physical therapy, exercise science, psychology, and education. She has professional experience as a personal trainer, physical therapist, and educator, and has a body of publications including a doctoral dissertation on the topic of wellness and physical therapy. In this book she proposes and constructs a comprehensive approach to wellness in physical therapy based on her more inclusive definition of wellness as a lifestyle that promotes physical, mental, and social health in the cognitive, psychomotor, and affective domains, both internally and externally (Fair, 2002b).

Following the five-element approach to patient management discussed in *The Guide to Physical Therapist Practice*, Dr. Fair discusses examination, evaluation, diagnosis, prognosis and plan of care, and interventions in the context of nutritional wellness, fitness wellness, body composition wellness, and mental and social wellness. Examination sections include sufficient detail for immediate clinical application discussion of screening, history, and tests and measures. The author introduces both validated history and physical examination items and tools developed as part of her original research and doctoral work in the area of wellness. All information is supported by up-to-date and relevant references from the peer-reviewed literature. Didactic elements in each chapter include learning objectives and definitions of basic terms and concepts. The author also makes the link to ICD codes and Preferred Practice Patterns discussed in *The Guide to Physical Therapist Practice*. Data on the "typical client" and athlete allow for comparison of findings to normative data. An eight-step community wellness project and an in-depth wellness case example will help the reader to apply the concepts introduced in the text.

In this book, Dr. Fair provides readers with the information on knowledge and skills that will allow physical therapists to truly align with the portion of the APTA *Vision Statement for Physical Therapy 2020* that proposes physical therapists as the practitioners of choice in the area of wellness. Her comprehensive and at times passionate discussion of the topic is certain to appeal to both entry-level physical therapy students and experienced clinicians.

Peter A. Huijbregts, PT, MSc, MHSc, DPT, OCS, FAAOMPT, FCAMT
Series Editor, Contemporary Issues in
Physical Therapy and Rehabilitation Medicine
Victoria, British Columbia, Canada

chapter one

The Basics of Wellness

*Health is a state of complete physical, mental and social well-being;
and not merely the absence of disease or infirmity.*

▪ ▪

World Health Organization (1947, 2009)

OBJECTIVES

Upon the completion of this chapter, you should be able to:

1. Define the terms *health, health promotion, prevention*, and *wellness*.
2. Discuss the impact of the World Health Organization's definition of health as it applies to wellness.
3. Discuss the Healthy People initiative, particularly *Healthy People 2010*.
4. Compare the definitions of health and wellness.
5. Critique the definitions of wellness.
6. Differentiate between primary prevention, secondary prevention, and tertiary prevention.
7. Discuss the concept of the triad of wellness and list its components.
8. Differentiate between the six models of wellness.
9. Discuss the dimensions and sub-dimensions of the humanistic model of wellness.

10. Provide a rationale for the secondary dimension of the humanistic model of wellness and determine if it is best classified as a component of the physical, mental, or social aspects of the definition of wellness.
11. Discuss the stages of wellness and apply them to yourself and others.
12. Differentiate between a lapse and relapse as well as maintenance and permanent maintenance. Apply these definitions to yourself and others.
13. Given a scenario, identify and provide a rationale for the stage of wellness in an evaluation of a patient/client.
14. Compare the use of surveys and direct examination as methods to assess wellness.

SECTION 1: HEALTH AND WELLNESS

Health

In its constitution, the World Health Organization (WHO) defines health as "Not merely the absence of disease . . . a state of complete physical, mental and social well-being" (1947, p. 7; 2009, para. 2). Thus, the WHO views health as a triad of the physical, the mental, and the social states of being. It is logical to apply the concept of health as a triad when assessing wellness and health models, if not also medical models (**Figure 1-1**).

Health Promotion

"Health promotion is the science and art of helping people change their lifestyle to move toward a state of optimal health. Optimal health is defined as a balance of physical, emotional, social, spiritual, and intellectual health. Lifestyle change can be facilitated through a combination of efforts to enhance awareness, change behavior and create environments that support good health practices. Of the three, supportive environments will probably have the greatest impact in producing lasting change" (O'Donnell, 1986, p.1). According to the "Health Promotion" Web page of the Centers for Disease Control and Prevention (CDC), "Adopting healthy behaviors such as eating nutritious foods, being physically active, and avoiding tobacco can prevent or control the devastating effects of many diseases. The CDC is committed to programs that reduce the health and economic consequences of the leading causes of death and disability and ensure a long, productive, healthy life for all people" (2009a, para. 1).

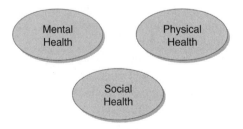

Figure 1-1 The World Health Organization's Triad of Health

Health promotion can be described simply as purposeful activities designed to enhance the health of oneself and/or others.

Wellness

Countless definitions of wellness exist. Halbert Dunn (1896–1975), considered by many as the "founding parent of wellness," defined it as "An integrated method of functioning which is oriented toward maximizing the potential of which the individual is capable, within the environment in which [she or] he is functioning" (1961, p. 4). Dunn served as a public health physician and was the first nationally recognized U.S. medical doctor to explore the concept of wellness.

A current leader in the arena of wellness is Don Ardell (1938–), PhD. Ardell, who wrote the first mass-market wellness book entitled *High Level Wellness*, offered several definitions of wellness. In 1985, he stated that wellness is a "dynamic or ever-changing, fluctuating state of being" (p. 5). In 1986, Ardell added that wellness is "giving care to the physical self, using the mind constructively, channeling stress energies positively, expressing emotions effectively, becoming creatively involved with others, and staying in touch with the environment." In 1999, Ardell stated that "Wellness is about perspective, about balance and about the big picture. It is a lifestyle and a personalized approach to living your life in such a way that you enjoy maximum freedom, including freedom from illness/disability and premature death to the extent possible, and freedom to experience life, liberty and the pursuit of happiness. It is a declaration of independence for becoming the best kind of person that your potentials, circumstances and fate will allow" (p. 1).

The American Physical Therapy Association (APTA), in its *Guide to Physical Therapist Practice*, defined wellness as the "concepts that embrace positive health behaviors that promote a state of physical and mental balance and fitness" (2001b, p. 691). Because this definition excludes the social realm of the wellness triad, I consider it narrow in scope and therefore flawed.

A number of physical therapists who possess an expertise in wellness have provided more comprehensive definitions of wellness. For example, Janet Bezner, who currently serves as the APTA's Senior Vice President of Education, proposed that, "wellness is an individualistic concept that is multidimensional and more than just physical health habits . . . . Wellness is about positive health actions . . . . Said best, wellness is a lifestyle process that never ends . . ." (personal communication, September 22, 2004). This description of wellness is strong in several aspects. Most importantly, it recognizes and emphasizes that wellness is individualistic, multidimensional, and dynamic in nature.

As many regard me as an expert in the field of wellness as it relates to physical therapy, the following is my definition of wellness: "A lifestyle that promotes physical, mental, and social health in the cognitive, psychomotor, and affective domains, both internally and externally" (Fair, 2000b). This definition is based upon the following terminology and concepts:

- Lifestyle: Wellness is a process (Ardell, 1986b; Dunn, 1961; Jonas, 2000)
- Physical, mental, and social health: "a state of complete physical, mental and social well-being" (WHO, 1947, p. 29; 2009, para. 2)

- Cognitive: Knowledge or mental skills (Bloom, 1956, 1984) (i.e., knowledge about wellness as demonstrated by words and or actions)
- Psychomotor: Physical actions or skills (Simpson, 1972) (i.e., wellness-related behaviors and practices)
- Affective: Feelings (Krathwohl, Bloom, & Bertram, 1973) (i.e., the commitment to a lifestyle that promotes wellness)
- Internal: Individual or self-wellness (APTA, 2001b; Ardell, 1986b; CDC, 2007b; Dunn, 1961; Jonas, 2000)
- External: Those aspects of wellness that are "outside" of the individual, such as family wellness (Ardell, 1986b; Dunn, 1961)
- Community wellness (APTA, 2001b; Dunn, 1961; Jonas, 2000)
- Environmental wellness (Ardell, 1986b; Dunn, 1961; Jonas, 2000)

My definition of wellness proposes that if a person possesses a satisfactory level of an aspect of wellness, then that individual is aware of specific activities promoting that aspect of wellness, is committed to that aspect of wellness, and participates in activities that promote that aspect of wellness. For example, if Jane 1) knows about a number of activities that promote fitness, 2) participates in those activities, and 3) is committed to a lifestyle that promotes a satisfactory level of fitness wellness, then she has a satisfactory level of fitness wellness. In contrast, if Jane is 1) unaware of how to be fit, 2) does not engage in activities that promote fitness wellness, and/or 3) does not care about her personal fitness, then Jane has an unsatisfactory level of fitness wellness. Of course, one may have a satisfactory level of wellness in one dimension of wellness (e.g., aerobic capacity wellness or nutritional wellness) but have an unsatisfactory level in another aspect of wellness (e.g., flexibility wellness or mental wellness). It is important to reiterate that an individual is defined as having a satisfactory level of wellness only if she or he possesses each of three domains—cognitive, psychomotor, and affective—but an individual has an unsatisfactory level of wellness if she or he is missing one or more of the three domains.

Health Versus Wellness

Some professional organizations have adopted the WHO definition of health based upon the physical, mental, and social triad. The American Occupational Therapy Association (AOTA) supports the notion that health is "the absence of illness, but not necessarily disability, a balance of physical, mental and social well-being attained through socially valued and individually meaningful occupation; enhancement of capacities and opportunity to strive for individual potential; community cohesion and opportunity; and social integration, support and justice, all within and as part of a sustainable ecology" (Wilcock, as cited in AOTA, 2000, p. 656). Other professional organizations, including the APTA (as previously discussed), have not adopted WHO's paradigm.

While components of health are measured at a specific point in time (e.g., a blood pressure reading or a Beck Depression Inventory score), wellness is an active process that consists of habits and practices (National Wellness Institute, n.d.). Accordingly, in contrast to health, which is static; wellness is dynamic. An individual does not have to be healthy to be well. Individuals with acute or chronic medical disorders, including a terminal disease such as some forms of cancer, can be well as long as they are practicing a healthy lifestyle. Likewise, an individual does not have to be well to be healthy. For example, a person may be considered healthy if she or he does not exhibit any signs or symptoms of illness or disease; but that individual nonetheless may be engaging in unhealthy behaviors, such as excessive consumption of "junk foods."

Summary: Health and Wellness

The World Health Organization defines health as "Not merely the absence of disease . . . a state of complete physical, mental and social well-being" (1947, p. 29; 2009, para. 2). "Health promotion is the science and art of helping people change their lifestyle to move toward a state of optimal health . . ." (O'Donnell, 1986, p. 1). The APTA (2001b) divides prevention into three categories: primary, secondary, and tertiary. Numerous definitions of wellness exist. My definition is "A lifestyle that promotes—both internally and externally—the physical, mental, and social health in the cognitive, psychomotor, and affective domains" (Fair, 2000b, p. 2). Health is static and is measured at a specific point in time. In contrast, wellness is dynamic and consists of an individual's health-related habits and practices over time.

SECTION 2: PREVENTION

Although the emphasis of physical therapy is restorative care (Moffat, 1996), it is within the scope of physical therapists to provide preventative care. Prevention services that medical professionals, including but not limited to physical therapists, medical doctors, and nurses, provide can be categorized into three types: primary prevention, secondary prevention, and tertiary prevention.

Primary Prevention

According to the APTA (2001b), primary prevention is defined as "Prevention of disease in a susceptible population or potentially susceptible population through specific measures such as general health promotion efforts" (p. 32). In the medical community, one definition of primary prevention is "Stopping disease before it starts"; for example, immunization programs (Jonas, 2000, p. 9). Related healthcare professionals define primary prevention similarly. For example, the AOTA (2000, p. 657) defines primary prevention as "Education or health promotion strategies designed to help people avoid the onset of unhealthy conditions, diseases, or injuries." Compared to secondary prevention and tertiary prevention, a concise description of primary prevention is "pure prevention." An example of a physical therapist providing primary prevention would be she or he performing lower back screenings at a community health fair.

Secondary Prevention

According to the APTA (2001b), secondary prevention is "Efforts to decrease duration of illness, severity of disease, and sequelae through early diagnosis and prompt intervention" (p. 32). In the medical community, one definition of secondary prevention is "Early detection of existing disease before it becomes clinically apparent" (Jonas, 2000, p. 9). An example is screening for hypertension.

Related healthcare professionals define primary prevention similarly. For example, the AOTA (2000, p. 658) states that it "includes the early detection and treatment designed to prevent or disrupt the disabling process." Compared to primary and tertiary prevention, a concise description of secondary prevention is "early diagnosis and intervention." Physical therapists integrate secondary prevention into their practice when they perform a systems review (as per APTA, 2001b) and refer to another expert as indicated. If the newly diagnosed problem is within their area of practice, they can (in direct access states) directly manage the problem. Physical therapists also provide tertiary prevention or wellness to those with a chronic or irreversible medical condition.

Tertiary Prevention

According to the APTA, tertiary prevention is described as "Efforts to decrease the degree of disability and promote rehabilitation and restoration of function in patients with chronic and irreversible diseases" (2001b, p. 32). The medical community defines it as "Optimum management of clinically apparent disease so as to prevent or least minimize the development of future complications" (Jonas, 2000, p. 9). An example would be the control of blood sugar level in people with diabetes. Related healthcare professionals define tertiary prevention similarly. For example, the AOTA defines it as "Treatment and services designed to arrest the progression of a condition, prevent further disability, and promote social community" (2000, p. 659). A concise description of tertiary prevention is "wellness for those with a chronic condition." An example of a tertiary prevention is physical therapist providing maintenance group exercise classes for the residents of a skilled nursing facility.

Prevention: Present and Future

Currently, physical therapists provide primary, secondary, and tertiary preventative care. In the future, the provision of prevention services will expand as more physical therapy students and practitioners become educated in prevention strategies. This provision of preventative care by physical therapists should include the integration of prevention measures in restorative care and direct prevention services. **Figure 1-2** and **Figure 1-3** illustrate my conception of the current and future relationship between prevention and physical therapy, respectively.

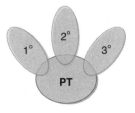

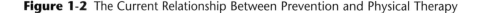

Figure 1-2 The Current Relationship Between Prevention and Physical Therapy

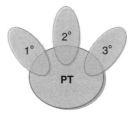

Figure 1-3 Proposed Future Relationship Between Prevention and Physical Therapy

Summary: Prevention

The APTA divides prevention into three categories: 1) primary prevention (i.e., pure prevention); 2) secondary prevention (early diagnosis and intervention); and 3) tertiary prevention (wellness for those with a chronic or irreversible condition). Physical therapists should continue to expand their knowledge of new strategies to improve preventative care measures in their patients/clients.

SECTION 3: HEALTHY PEOPLE

Healthy People is a federal initiative managed by the United States Department of Health and Human Services (DHHS) to quantify and describe the health status, develop health-related goals, and assess changes in the health of the U.S. population. The Healthy People initiatives are updated every decade. The first initiative, *Healthy People 2000*, was established in 1990. *Healthy People 2010* was established in 2000, and by 2010, *Healthy People 2020* will be published. *Healthy People 2010* is relevant to all professions, including physical therapists.

> Healthy People 2010 builds on initiatives pursued over the past two decades. The 1979 *Surgeon General's Report, Healthy People, and Healthy People 2000: National Health Promotion and Disease Prevention Objectives* both established national health objectives and served as the basis for the development of State and community plans. Like its predecessors, Healthy People 2010 was developed through a broad consultation process, built on the best scientific knowledge and designed to measure programs over time. Healthy People 2010 is a set of health objectives for the Nation to achieve over the first decade of the new century. It can be used by many different people, States, communities, professional organizations, and others to help them develop programs to improve health (U.S. DHHS, 2000, para.1)

According to *Healthy People 2010*, the determinants of health are biology, behaviors, social environment, physical environment, and policies. Physical therapists need to consider the patients' biology (i.e., an individual's physical/physiologic status) when they examine, evaluate, diagnose, determine a prognosis and plan of care that includes goals, and provide treatment. The goal is to facilitate the improvement of her or his patients' biology. Additionally, physical therapists must consider and improve their patients' behaviors, social environment, and physical environment. Physical therapists also can have a marked influence on state and national policies that affect the profession and patients; these include governmental and other insurance policies; policies of the APTA, and policies of the clinic at which they are employed.

Healthy People 2010 is designed to achieve two overarching goals. The first goal "is to help individuals of all ages increase life expectancy and improve their quality of life [and] the second goal of *Healthy People 2010* is to eliminate health disparities among different segments of the population" (U.S. DHHS, 2000, para.1). *Healthy People 2010* is particularly concerned about disparities due to gender, race/ethnicity, education/income, disability, living in rural localities, and sexual orientation.

According to *Healthy People 2010*, there are 10 leading health indicators: 1) physical activity; 2) overweight and obesity; 3) tobacco use; 4) substance abuse; 5) responsible sexual behavior; 6) mental health; 7) injury and violence; 8) environmental quality; 9) immunization; and 10) access to health care. While physical therapists may not play a large role in indicators such as immunization, except perhaps to refer as necessary, we are involved in physical activity and injury and also are involved in obesity and smoking cessation (Rea, Marshak, Neish, & Davis, 2004). I propose that it is appropriate for physical therapists to specialize in obesity and body composition. More information about *Healthy People 2010* is on the Internet (http://www.healthypeople.gov/).

Summary: Healthy People

Healthy People is a federal initiative managed by the U.S. Department of Health and Human Services to quantify and describe the health status, develop health-related goals, and assess changes in the health of the U.S. population. Of the *Healthy People 2010's* determinants of health (biology, behaviors, social environment, physical environment, and policies), physical therapists must recognize that they can help their patients/clients to improve upon these factors as they apply to their lives. *Healthy People 2010* is designed to achieve two overarching goals: 1) increase quality and years of healthy life and 2) eliminate health disparities. While physical therapists may be involved in a variety of *Healthy People 2010's* leading health indicators, the most relevant are physical activity, injury, and obesity. I propose that it is appropriate for some physical therapists to specialize in obesity and body composition.

SECTION 4: WELLNESS MODELS AND SURVEYS

While there are many definitions of the term *wellness*, because every health promoter has either created her or his own or adopted an established definition, only a few wellness models exist (Ardell, 2009b). The reason is "in part because they take more time to construct and in part, perhaps, because they do not seem as essential to the non-theoreticians of the wellness idea" (Ardell, 2009b, para. 2).

While there are likely more wellness models in existence, six are discussed in this section: 1) Travis' illness/wellness continuum; 2) Ardell's model; 3) Hettler's six-dimensional model; 4) Witmer and Sweeney's holistic model for wellness and prevention over the life span; 5) Adams, Bezner, and Steinhardt's perceived wellness model, and 6) my humanistic model of wellness (HMW). The illness/wellness continuum is included because it is perhaps the oldest of the ones in use today. Ardell's and Hettler's models are included because they are widely recognized (Ardell, 2009b). To my knowledge, the perceived wellness and the HWM models are the only wellness models in which a physical therapist was involved in its development.

To date, the APTA has not created or adopted a model of wellness. I believe that the wellness model that the association publishes should be in compliance with the World Health Organization's (1947; 2009) stance that there are three components of well-being (i.e., physical, mental, and social) and that additional aspects of wellness should be classified as sub-dimensions. I also contend that the wellness model should be directly applicable to the profession and practice of physical therapy.

Illness–Wellness Continuum

John Travis, MD, developed the "illness–wellness continuum" in 1972 (Ardell, 2009b). Unlike future models, the symbol for this model is a two-way arrow. The extreme right is high-level wellness and the extreme left is premature death. Movement toward high-level wellness includes awareness, education, and growth; while movement toward premature death includes signs, symptoms, and disability (Wellness Associates, 2009).

Ardell's Models of Wellness

Don Ardell, PhD, has developed a series of wellness models. The first appeared in the book *High Level Wellness* (1977) and was illustrated as a simple circle with five dimensions: 1) self-responsibility, 2) physical fitness, 3) stress management, 4) environmental sensitivity, and 5) nutritional awareness. His next model appeared in the book entitled *14 Days to High Level Wellness* (1982). This illustration was a circle with five different dimensions: 1) self-responsibility, 2) relationship dynamics, 3) meaning and purpose, 4) nutritional awareness and physical fitness, and 5) emotional intelligence. His most recent model consists of three domains and 14 skill areas, as follows: 1) the physical domain that consists of exercise and fitness, nutrition, appearance, adaptations/challenges, and lifestyle habits; 2) the mental domain that consists of emotional intelligence, effective decisions, stress management, factual knowledge, and mental health; and 3) the meaning and purpose domain, which consists of meaning and purpose, relationships, humor, and play (Ardell, 2009b).

Although the foundation of Ardell's most recent model is a triad, only two of the three components are consistent with the WHO triad. Of interest, Ardell's meaning and purpose component includes relationships, humor, and play; which I suggest are linked to social wellness.

The Six-Dimensional Model of Wellness

In 1979, William Hettler, PhD, cofounder and current president of the board of directors at the National Wellness Institute (NWI, Stevens Point, Wisconsin), authored an article that showcased what some now recognize as the "six-dimensional model of wellness." In his model, Hettler (1979) declared that the dimensions of wellness are emotional, intellectual, occupational, physical, social, and spiritual. According to Jonas (2000), Hettler's model of wellness is linked to Ardell's (1977) previous conceptualization of wellness. The

NWI suggests that the physical component goals are "good exercise and eating habits while discounting the use of tobacco, drugs and excessive alcohol consumption"; social component goals are "contributing to one's environment and community"; emotional component goals are "to be aware of and accept one's feelings and to feel positive and enthusiastic about oneself and life"; occupational component goals are to "contribute one's unique gifts, skills and talents to work that is both personally meaningful and rewarding"; and intellectual goals are "to expand knowledge and skills while discovering the potential for sharing one's gifts with others" (NWI, n.d., para. 7).

Hettler's six-dimensional model of wellness was expanded into what some consider the "eight-dimensional model of wellness" by Wiener, Mastroianni, and their colleagues at the State University of New York at Stony Brook (Jonas, 2000). The eight-dimensional model of wellness includes the emotional, intellectual, occupational, physical, social, and spiritual dimensions as identified by Hettler, as well as environmental and cultural dimensions. The environmental element emphasizes the pursuit of harmony with the surroundings and the world; including regular contact with nature, balance, and self-preservation (Jonas, 2000). The cultural component emphasizes "an awareness, acceptance, and appreciation for diverse cultures and backgrounds as well as understanding and valuing one's own culture" (Jonas, 2000, p. 23). More recently, creativity was added as a ninth dimension to the "component-based" conception of wellness (Jonas, 2000). This model has been referred to as the "nine-dimensional model of wellness." According to Jonas, the creative dimension of wellness draws upon feelings and intelligence and may include building or the arts (e.g., acting, drawing, painting, or sculpting).

Although Hettler's wellness model is perhaps the most widely recognized of all wellness models, it does not mirror the WHO's concept of the triage of well-being and consists of dimensions of wellness that should, in my opinion, be classified as sub-dimensions. For example, the emotional, intellectual, and spiritual components should be identified as sub-dimensions of mental wellness.

Holistic Model for Wellness and Prevention Over the Life Span

Witmer and Sweeney presented the "holistic model for wellness and prevention over the life span" in 1992. Myers, Sweeney, and Witmer presented a revised version in 2000. In contrast to its predecessors, this model is rooted in what the creators concluded are the five life tasks: spirituality, self-regulation, work, friendship, and love. Within the spiritual domain, there are two components: 1) inner life and oneness; and 2) values, optimism, and purposiveness. Witmer and Sweeney's (1992) self-regulation life task is composed of seven components: 1) the sense of personal worth; 2) the sense of personal control; 3) realistic beliefs; 4) emotional responsiveness and spontaneity; 5) intellectual stimulation, creativity, and problem solving; 6) a sense of humor; and 7) health habits and physical fitness. The self-regulation life task consists of items related to both physical and mental wellness and is expansive. It shares elements with Dunn's (1973) concept of individual wellness and Ardell's (1977) dimension of self-responsibility. Within Witmer and Sweeney's (1992) life task of work, which includes but is not limited to gainful employment, homemaking, child-rearing, educational endeavors, and volunteer services, are two components: 1) occupation as a lifespan task; and 2) the economic, psychological, and social benefits of work.

The third life task therefore builds upon concepts proposed by Dunn (1973) and Ardell (1977), and is analogous to Hettler's (1979) occupational dimension of wellness. Their life task of friendship emphasizes connectedness and social interest and thus mirrors the social dimension described by Hettler and writings by Dunn. Witmer and Sweeney's (1992) life task of love speaks to the bond between close friends, family members, and spouses, and includes sexual satisfaction. Witmer and Sweeney's life task of love is in alignment with Dunn's discussions of family, community, and social wellness, and overlaps Hettler's social dimension.

Witmer and Sweeney's wellness model includes the central concepts espoused by other wellness models and can be viewed as a five-component model of wellness: spirituality, self-regulation, work, friendship, and love. Myers et al. (2000) applied this model to the discipline of counseling, but to my knowledge it has not been applied to the profession of physical therapy. Moreover, it is not in alignment with the WHO's triad of well-being. In my opinion, it consists of dimensions of wellness that should be classified as sub-dimensions of wellness and other sub-dimensions of wellness that should be classified as (primary) dimensions (e.g., health habits and physical fitness).

The assessment tool for the holistic model for wellness and prevention over the life span is the Wellness Evaluation Lifestyle (WEL). The purpose of the WEL is to operationalize the model. "The instrument consists of 131 items generated as self-statements to which respondents reply using a five-point Likert scale" (Myers, et al., 2005, para. 1). While the WEL contains 121 items related to mental and social wellness, only 10 questions relate to physical wellness (i.e., three questions related to exercise, three questions related to nutrition, and four questions related to medical self-care). In my opinion, physical therapists might opt to use the WEL to survey the mental wellness of patients/clients, but it is not an appropriate tool to assess physical wellness.

Perceived Wellness Model

Adams, Bezner, and Steinhardt (1997) developed the "perceived wellness model," which contains six dimensions of wellness: physical, social, psychological, emotional, spiritual, and intellectual. Although a physical therapist (Bezner) was involved in creating this model, the emphasis of it is the mental dimension of wellness. I believe that this is a weakness, not only in terms of its applicability to the profession of physical therapy but also in the implication that there are four distinct dimensions related to mental well-being (i.e., psychological, emotional, spiritual, and intellectual), rather than recognizing that each is subcomponent of the dimension of mental wellness. My view was recently supported in an empirical study by Harari, Waehler, and Rogers, who investigated the model and found that there was "no psychometric evidence for the existence of separate [mental] subscale dimensions" (2005, p. 251).

The assessment tool for the model of perceived wellness is the Perceived Wellness Survey (PWS). Its purpose is to operationalize the perceived wellness model. While the 36-item PWS contains five items related to physical wellness (e.g., item number 28; "I expect to always be physically healthy"), they are not directly related to fitness, body composition, or nutritional wellness. Moreover, the majority of the items relate to mental wellness. In my opinion, physical therapists might wish to use the PWS to survey the mental and social wellness of their patient/clients, but it is not an appropriate tool to assess physical wellness.

Humanistic Model of Wellness

In response to the lack of a wellness model that adhered to the WHO's position on the triad of well-being and regulated secondary aspects of wellness to a sub-dimension status, I created the "humanistic model of wellness" (HMW) (Fair, 2002b).

The HMW elevates and expands my definition of wellness (i.e., a lifestyle that both internally and externally promotes physical, mental, and social health in the cognitive, psychomotor, and affective domains). Specifically, it recognizes the importance of the cognitive knowledge of, the affective commitment to, and the psychomotor behaviors associated with the physical, mental, and social dimensions of wellness. The relevance of the learning domains is supported in APTA's *A Normative Model of Physical Therapist Professional Education: 2004 Version.* The model also appreciates that wellness can be applied to oneself (i.e., the internal) and/or to another person (i.e., the external).

The sub-dimensions of the physical dimension of wellness are diseases and medical conditions (that are not primarily mental in nature); drugs; nutrition; aerobic capacity; muscular fitness; flexibility; and body composition. (These sub-dimensions are discussed in Chapters 4 through 7.) The sub-dimensions of the mental aspect of wellness are diseases and conditions that are primarily mental in nature; intellectual stimulation; emotions; behavior-type pattern; locus of control; hardiness; stress; happiness; and purpose of life. (Mental sub-dimensions are discussed in Chapter 8.) The sub-dimensions of the social aspect of wellness are ethics, the family, the community, the environment, the provision of physical therapy, and occupational wellness. (These sub-dimensions are discussed in Chapter 8.)

It is important to recognize that a sub-dimension of one dimension of wellness can overlap the sub-dimension of another. For example, occupational wellness often overlaps several domains of mental wellness, such as intellectual stimulation, stress, and happiness. This overlapping supports the holistic concept of the mind–body connection. Traditional physical therapy as well as complementary alternative medicine (CAM) can enhance one or more sub-dimensions and positively affect overall wellness. As physical therapists, we can improve patient outcomes and satisfaction if we enhance one or more sub-dimensions and address the disease or medical condition that prompted the episode of care. For example, the patient/client might be introduced to the Tai Chi system of exercising to enhance balance and reduce stress.

The assessment tool for the HMW is the Self-Wellness Survey (SWS). (Figures 5-1 to 5-4 in Chapter 5, Figures 6-1 to 6-3 in Chapter 6, Figures 7-1 to 7-3 in Chapter 7, and Figures 8-1 to 8-3 in Chapter 8 are used in the SWS assessment.) The purpose of the survey is to operationalize the HMW. The SWS contains 250 items: 100 are related to nutritional wellness, 72 relate to fitness wellness, 27 are about body composition wellness, and 51 are about mental and social wellness. The instrument is designed to be utilized by a physical therapist as part of the tests and measures section of a physical therapy examination.

Summary: Wellness Models

The APTA has not yet established a model of wellness. The World Health Organization's (1947; 2009) stance is that there are three components of well-being: physical, mental, and social. I propose that a better model of wellness consists of the three primary dimensions of WHO and secondary aspects of wellness (emotional wellness, spiritual wellness, and fitness wellness) classified as sub-dimensions.

Travis's model, developed in 1972, is a continuum between high-level wellness and premature death. Ardell (1977, 1986, 1990) developed a series of dimensional models, the most recent of which has three domains (physical, mental, and meaning and purpose) and 14 skill areas. Hettler's (1979) model of wellness consists of six dimensions: emotional, intellectual, occupational, physical, social, and spiritual. This model may extend to include occupational, environmental, and creativity components (Jonas, 2000). Witmer and Sweeney's (1992) holistic model of wellness and prevention over the lifespan includes five life tasks: spirituality, self-regulation, work, friendship, and love. Ardell's (1997) model of perceived wellness contains six dimensions of wellness: physical, social, psychological, emotional, spiritual, and intellectual. My humanistic model of wellness (HMW) consists of the three dimensions of well-being as advanced by the WHO (1947; 2009) (physical, mental, and social) and recognizes the three domains of learning (cognitive, psychomotor, and affective), as supported in APTA's *A Normative Model of Physical Therapist Professional Education: 2004 Version.* Of the models discussed, several have corresponding assessment instruments. The SWS, the instrument to operationalize the HMW, is specifically designed to be utilized by a physical therapist as part of the tests and measures section of a physical therapy examination.

SECTION 5: STAGES OF WELLNESS: EXAMINATION, EVALUATION, PLAN OF CARE, AND INTERVENTIONS

When examining a patient's/client's aspect of wellness (e.g., nutritional wellness, aerobic capacity wellness), you must also identify her or his stage of wellness as it relates to that aspect of physical, mental, or social wellness. During the evaluation stage of the session, you must evaluate the findings of your examination. Your evaluation then is used to design your wellness plan of care.

The seven stages of wellness are primordial, pre-contemplation, contemplation, preparation, action, maintenance, and permanent maintenance. As a group, they are an integration and modification of the change models discussed by Dunn (1961), Ardell (1977), and Jonas (2000). Attention to the stages of wellness is critical for physical therapists to successfully enhance the wellness of her or his patient/client. The following sections take a closer look at each stage.

Primordial Stage

A patient/client in the primordial stage is not aware that she or he has a health-related problem and/or that she or he is unknowingly engaging in a behavior that is unhealthy. In other words, the person does not even recognize that a health-related problem exists (Jonas, 2000).

For example, in terms of flexibility, this would be a man who has decreased muscle length in his hamstrings but isn't aware of the impairment. A patient/client in the primordial stage in terms of alcohol abuse consumes three or more alcoholic drinks per day (which exceeds Harvard's School of Public Health [2009a] recommendation of no more than one drink per day for women and no more than one to two drinks per day for men), but considers her or his alcohol habits to be perfectly normal and harmless.

It is extremely difficult to facilitate change in a patient/client who is in the primordial stage. This is because behavioral change can only occur after an awareness that a problem exists; once that occurs, the patient/client moves to the pre-contemplation, preparation stage, and then on to the action stage. Certainly, patient education is critical. Psychological and interpersonal skills are required also. If the integration of psychological skills is insufficient, the physical therapist should refer the patient/client to a mental health counselor because the provision of direct psychological counseling is outside the scope of physical therapy.

Pre-Contemplation Stage

A patient/client in the pre-contemplation stage has not yet embraced the notion that there is a health-related problem and/or she or he is engaging in unhealthy behaviors, but has begun to recognize that she or he may have a health-related problem and/or poor health habits. In other words, the person accepts her or his current health status but as yet does not have the intention to make a health-related change (Jonas, 2000).

An example of a patient/client in the pre-contemplation stage in terms of flexibility is a man who has decreased muscle length in his hamstrings, and notices that sometimes the back of his thighs are tight. Perhaps he has transiently considered that one day he may need to address the matter, but he has not given it serious consideration. Another example of a patient/client in the pre-contemplation stage is a woman who smokes cigarettes and generally knows that smoking increases the risk of certain medical problems (e.g., cancer) but has not applied that knowledge of these health risks to herself and has not seriously contemplated quitting.

Contemplation Stage

A patient/client in the contemplation stage recognizes that she or he is engaging in a behavior that is linked to a health problem and may begin to investigate that behavior, including its pros and cons, but remains ambivalent about what to do about the situation, if anything (Jonas, 2000).

People move into the contemplation stage at different speeds. Think of this stage as a light bulb being turned on, where sometimes the light brightens slowly as the dimmer switch is slowly raised; in other cases, the light suddenly illuminates a dark room. An example of an abrupt move from the pre-contemplation stage to the contemplation stage would be an obese woman who appreciates that she is perhaps a little overweight, but after looking at a recent photograph of herself recognizes for the first time that she is indeed obese. Another example is a man playing basketball with his teenage children who suddenly becomes so exhausted that he has to sit down. His heart is racing and he thinks, "Wow, I had no idea I was so out of shape!"

Preparation Stage

During the preparation stage, a patient/client has made the choice to change the unhealthy behavior. Her or his unhealthy behavior is either self-assessed or assessed by a professional and a plan of care is developed (modification of Jonas, 2000). For example, a woman moves from the contemplation stage to the preparation stage when she not only recognizes that she is obese, but makes a conscious decision that she is going to "lose weight" to enhance her body composition. To complete the preparation stage, the woman self-assesses her weight and develops a plan. Better yet, she hires a professional to assess her body composition, alimentation, and exercise habits, and together they develop a plan of care.

An example of fitness wellness assessment is the Fitness Wellness Survey (see Figure 6-3 in Chapter 6). An example of a body composition goal is to reduce the percent of body fat from 32% to between 25% and 28% within 6 months via a healthy 1500 calorie per day diet (e.g., high complex carbohydrate, high fiber, adequate protein, adequate healthy fat, low saturated fat, zero trans fat) and an appropriate exercise regime. This might include aerobic strength training 4 days per week at 30 minutes per session, and brisk walking 1 to 2 days per week for 20 to 30 minutes per session.

Action Stage

When a patient/client enters the action stage, she or he initiates a change in her or his behaviors (Jonas, 2000). For example, a woman who has decided that she will stop smoking discards all of her cigarettes and then buys and applies an over-the-counter nicotine medication.

It is imperative that a person *not* advance directly from the contemplation stage to the action stage. The interim step helps to prepare adequately for the contemplated changes. Skipping the preparation stage increases the risk for failure and may incur an adverse side effect (e.g., a physical injury if the goal involves exercise).

Maintenance

During the maintenance stage, the patient/client is regularly practicing the new behavior (modification of Jonas, 2000). If the problem was smoking cigarettes, the patient/client no longer smokes; if the person was obese, she or he has begun a diet and exercise program; if the problem was stress, the patient/client is now practicing stress-reduction techniques on a regular basis. During the maintenance stage, a lapse or a relapse may occur. A comparison of a lapse and a relapse follows.

Lapse

A lapse is a cessation of a healthy behavior, but the cessation is temporary and does not produce significant adverse effects (modification of Jonas, 2000). A lapse may occur during the maintenance or the permanent maintenance stages. A lapse can be defined as major or minor. A major lapse is one in which the cessation is or was complete or nearly complete. A minor lapse is one in which cessation is or was brief. The case scenarios illustrate the difference between a major and minor lapse.

Case Scenarios

Case 1. Four weeks ago, John established a goal to exercise three times per week. John met his goal for 3 weeks, but during the current week he has exercised only once. This week's transgression is a major lapse. (Note: Had John been compliant with his exercise program for a few months and returned to it immediately, this week's transgression would be considered a minor lapse.)

Case 2. One week ago, Rachel established a goal to consume about 1500 calories per day and since that time, she has met her daily goal. Today, however, she consumes about 2800 calories. Rachel's diet today constitutes a major lapse. (Note: If Rachel's maintenance caloric intake was 2000 calories per day and she had consumed 2300 calories today, she would have committed a minor, rather than a major, lapse.)

Case 3. Two years ago, Susan established a goal to exercise four times per week. Since then she has met her goal for most weeks, but on occasion (e.g., once every 6 months) she exercises only twice per week. Last month Susan didn't exercise at all because her relatives from out of town were visiting. As soon as her relatives departed, Susan returned to exercising four times per week. When Susan exercises only twice per week, she commits a minor lapse. However, Susan committed a major lapse when she didn't exercise for a full month. (Note: Susan's month-long transgression is not considered a relapse [discussed below] because she had a very long history of consistent exercise, and suspended her exercise regime for a specific reason and immediately resumed it as soon as her relatives left town.)

Relapse

A relapse is a cessation of a healthy behavior that it is longer than temporary and produces significant adverse affects (modification of Jonas, 2000). Like a lapse, a relapse can be defined as major or minor. A major relapse is one in which the cessation is or was complete (or nearly complete). On example is a patient/client who completely stopped exercising after following a regimen for several months. A minor relapse is one in which cessation is or was not complete (or nearly complete). For example, a woman's goal was to exercise 4 days per week, and while she did exercise 4 days per week for a month, during the second month she has exercised only 2 days per week.

A relapse can occur for a variety of reasons, including but not limited to unrealistic goals, decreased motivation, and a change in circumstances (Jonas, 2000). If a relapse occurs, one should return to the preparation stage (Jonas, 2000). A relapse may occur during the maintenance stage but cannot occur if an individual has truly reached the permanent stage. If a relapse occurs during the permanent maintenance stage, the individual just thought she or he was in the permanent stage, but was actually in the maintenance stage.

Case Scenarios:

Case 1. Two weeks ago, John established a goal to exercise three times per week for 30 minutes per session, but he exercised only once in the first week and did not exercise at all during his second week. John's transgression is significant and should be considered a relapse. John transgression during the first week should be considered a minor relapse and during the second week should be considered a major relapse.

Case 2. Three weeks ago, Rachel established a goal to consume approximately 1500 calories per day in order to reduce her body fat. (Rachel is aware that if she consumes approximately 2000 calories per day, she will maintain her current body fat level.) She met her goal during the first 2 weeks and for the first 3 days of the third week. During the third week, however, Rachel consumed 2000 calories on day four, 2800 calories on day five, 2500 calories on day six, and 2700 calories on day seven. Day four's intake of that third week would not be considered a lapse because she did not consume more than her maintenance caloric input of 2000 calories. On day five of that third week, however, Rachel suffered a minor lapse. Day five's minor lapse evolved into a major lapse or perhaps even a minor relapse by day six. Rachel's relapse from day seven on is considered major because her caloric intake on days five through seven is significantly above her goal as well as significantly above her maintenance caloric intake.

Case 3. Two years ago, Karen established a goal to practice stress-reduction exercises 6 days per week. Karen has met her goal for the past 2 years, but has only practiced stress-reduction exercises once a week for the past 8 weeks. During the first week of her transgression, Karen suffered a minor lapse. (Note: It is considered a minor rather than a major lapse because Karen had been compliant for a significantly extended time frame.) During the second week of her transgression, Karen's minor lapse rose to the status of a major lapse. Her reduction in exercise became a minor relapse during the third week and a major relapse during the fourth weeks of the transgression.

Lapse versus Relapse

It is important to appreciate that a specific transgression (e.g., 1 week of no exercise) in some cases is defined as a lapse and in other cases as a relapse. Generally speaking, if a patient/client has been practicing a healthy behavior for a longer period of time (e.g., many months to years), then she or he is allowed more leeway before a transgression is considered a relapse rather than a simple lapse. For example, if I've been exercising four times per week for 20 years, and I only exercise twice this week, I definitely consider my transgression a minor lapse. However, if I had been sedentary for years and 1 week ago developed a new goal to exercise four times per week; but then only exercised two times this week, I'd consider my transgression a minor relapse.

Consider another example: If Karen is limiting her caloric consumption by avoiding sweets and has a piece of cake at a social gathering, it would be entirely appropriate to consider the offense a minor lapse. However, if Karen ate an inordinate amount of sweets day after day, very soon it would be considered a minor and then a major relapse.

Cessation of a healthy activity should be categorized a lapse (rather than a relapse) if the transgression is secondary to a medical contraindication. For example, if John cannot stretch his right hamstring for 6 weeks because it is in a cast secondary to a femoral fracture, John's extended period of not stretching that hamstring is not a relapse, but a lapse secondary to a medical contraindication. However, John's medical contraindication secondary to a femoral fracture does not extend to noninvolved body parts, such as the stretching of his pectorals.

Case Scenarios:

Case 1. Sharon did not exercise for 10 weeks because she is pregnant. During her initial office visit, her obstetrician told her to not return to exercise until the 13th week of her pregnancy. Prior to her pregnancy, Sharon had been exercising five times per week (with occasional lapses) for her entire adult life. At the beginning of her 13th week of pregnancy, Sharon returned to an exercise protocol that was equal in frequency but slightly decreased in intensity to her pre-pregnancy exercise regime. Now she is 30 weeks into pregnancy and has been exercising in accordance with her protocol since week 13. The 12-week period in which Sharon did not exercise is considered a lapse secondary to a medical contraindication.

Case 2. Jon has a history of abusing alcohol. A month ago, he decided to limit his alcohol consumption to no more than two drinks per day and a maximum of three drinks per week. During the first week, Jon consumed one drink on Friday and two drinks on Saturday. The second week, he consumed two drinks on Friday and two drinks on Saturday. The third week, he consumed three drinks on Friday and four drinks on Saturday. Jon had a minor lapse during week two and a major relapse during week three.

Permanent Maintenance Stage

When an individual has reached the permanent maintenance stage of a behavior, the behavior itself is reinforcing and the person is intrinsically motivated to continue the healthy behavior. Most of us have reached the permanent stage for several health behaviors. A notable behavior is brushing our teeth. If we do not brush our teeth at least once, if not more often per day, then we feel an overwhelming urge to do so. We "just don't feel right" and will make concerted efforts to perform the activity. Of course, if you are unable to brush your teeth due to circumstances beyond your control (e.g., you are a contestant on the hit reality show *Survivor*), you should not consider it a relapse.

Although a person may experience a lapse in the permanent maintenance stage, she or he is beyond the risk of relapse (modification of Jonas, 2000). If a person experiences a relapse, it is appropriate to state in the evaluation that the person only thought she or he was in the permanent maintenance stage but actually is still in the maintenance stage.

It may take months, if not years, to truly reach the permanent maintenance stage. In some cases, a person never advances to the permanent maintenance stage, and the best she or he can do is remain perpetually in the maintenance stage. An example is an alcoholic who chooses not to imbibe. Another example is a woman who recognizes the importance of eating four servings of vegetables each day, and manages to do so most days but is not intrinsically motivated and believes that it is a burden rather than a pleasure.

Summary: Stages of Wellness

When assessing an aspect of a patient's/client's wellness, you must determine her or his stage of wellness as it relates to that aspect. During the evaluation portion of the physical therapy session, you must list the findings and evaluate them. This evaluation can be used to design a wellness plan of care.

The seven stages of wellness are primordial, pre-contemplation, contemplation, preparation, action, maintenance, and permanent maintenance. If a patient/client is completely unaware of a personal health issue, then she or he is in the primordial stage. When a patient/client has glimmers of recognition of personal health issues, she or he is in the pre-contemplation stage. A patient/client who knows that she or he has personal health issues is in the contemplation stage. When a patient/client makes the choice to change his or her unhealthy behavior, the health issue is either self-assessed or assessed by a professional, and a plan of care is developed, then she or he is in the preparation stage. A patient/client who actually initiates a change in his or her health behavior is in the action stage. One who regularly practices a new health behavior is in the maintenance stage. When a healthy behavior has become a genuine habit, the patient/client has progressed to the permanent stage. A lapse (i.e., temporary cessation of a healthy behavior without significant adverse effects) may occur during the maintenance or permanent stage. A relapse (a longer cessation of a healthy behavior that produces significant adverse affects) can occur during the maintenance stage but not during the permanent stage. If a relapse occurs during the permanent maintenance stage, then the patient/client just thought she or he was in the permanent stage but was actually in the maintenance stage. A lapse and relapse can be defined as major or minor.

SECTION 6: SURVEYS TO ASSESS WELLNESS

An aspect of health can be examined either directly; for example, by using a skinfold caliper to measure body composition, or indirectly through a survey, such as the Beck Depression Inventory to measure the emotions of a patient/client). To directly examine an aspect of wellness, the examiner directly observes a patient's/client's habits and practices related to that aspect of wellness. This time-consuming and rigorous observation would be required because wellness is, by definition, comprised of an individual's habits and practices. To avoid countless hours of direct observation, it is usually appropriate to use a survey to discover information about each aspect of wellness.

The debate about the credibility of survey research began in 1941 when the National Opinion Research Center was established (Raymond, 1991). Noelle-Neumann (1996) reported that because of the early successes of survey research—particularly the election research of Gallup, Crossley, and Roper—a belief emerged that the validity of surveys need not be explored. Despite the lack of quality criteria for validation, Presser (1984) claimed that survey research matured in the early 1980s when the first handbook on survey research was published.

While survey results are subject to the limitations associated with self-reported data, information obtained within it may explain unique variance data not otherwise accounted for in more objective measurements of health (Nunnally, 1978). In fact, self-report variability can be viewed as additional information rather than an error to be controlled (Nunnally, 1978). However, to minimize the limitations of a survey, the questions should be developed in accordance with survey guidelines. Surveys should include clear and succinct instructions (Andrews, 1984; Best & Kahn, 1989; Gall, Gall, & Borg, 2003; van Dalen, 1979) that are of medium length, 16 to 64 words according to Andrews (1984), should be neither too short (Andrews, 1984) nor too long (Gall et al., 2003), and the items should be numbered and organized into a logical sequence (Gall et al., 2003; van Dalen, 1979). Medium and longer length items (16–24 words or ≥25 words, respectively) should be prefaced by a medium-length introduction. Long introductions followed by shorter or longer items should be avoided (Andrews, 1984). Items should encourage a complete response (Best & Kahn, 1979; van Dalen, 1979). For example, subordinate items or an exhaustive list of alternative choices should be provided (van Dalen, 1979). Complex terms and jargon that prospective respondents might not understand should be avoided (Gall et al., 2003; van Dalen, 1979). Items that might be misunderstood should be defined (Gall et al., 2003) or linked to an example (Best & Kahn, 1979). "Double-barreled" items that require the respondent to respond to more than one idea in single response should be avoided. Avoid the use of double negatives (Best & Kahn, 1979; Gall et al., 2003) and leading or biased items (Gall et al., 2003). Descriptive adverbs and adjectives that have vague meanings (e.g., *rarely*, *seldom*, and *occasionally*) should be used with caution (Best & Kahn, 1979) or avoided (Gall et al., 2003). Emphasized words should be underlined (Best & Kahn, 1979). A reference point should be provided for a comparison or rating (Best & Kahn, 1979). Items should be phrased so that they are applicable to all prospective respondents (Best & Kahn, 1979). Surveys should begin with non-threatening items (Gall et al., 2003; van Dalen, 1979). Emotionally difficult and threatening items (e.g., those related to smoking or use of anabolic steroids) should be placed near the end of the survey (Mirabella, 2003a). Important items should not be placed at the end of the survey (Gall et al., 2003).

According to Mirabella (2003a), a survey item can assess attitude, knowledge, or behavior. Attitude (affective) items assess satisfaction or agreement. An example of an attitude question is "How important do you think it is to engage in exercise at least 30 minutes at least five times per week?" Knowledge (cognitive) items assess the respondent's understanding of a specific issue. An example of a knowledge question is "Which of the following describes the *Healthy People 2010* guidelines regarding the recommended frequency and duration of exercise?" A behavior (psychomotor) item assesses the variables (e.g., when, how often, how much) of a selected behavior. An example of a behavioral item is "Of the following, which best describes your level of exercise during the past week?"

In my chapters about the various aspects of wellness (e.g., nutritional wellness, mental wellness), I introduce wellness surveys that I have developed during my discussion of the respective Examination section. The rationale for the content within each of these surveys was based upon research related to the topic and to survey research. For example, my fitness wellness surveys were based, in part, upon the *ACSM's Guidelines for Exercise Testing and Prescription* (American College of Sports Medicine, 2006), the United States Department of Health and Human Services' (2000) *Healthy People 2010*, relevant publications of the APTA including the *Guide to Physical Therapist Practice* (APTA, 2001b), and survey research.

Summary: Surveys to Assess Wellness

An aspect of health can be examined directly (e.g., a skinfold caliper) or indirectly through a survey (e.g., the Beck Depression Inventory). It is cost- and time-efficient to examine an aspect of wellness indirectly through a survey. In the chapters about the various aspects of wellness, I introduce wellness surveys developed during my discussion of the respective Examination section.

chapter two

The Application of Wellness to Physical Therapy

The concept of total wellness recognizes that our every thought,
word, and behavior affects our greater health and well-being.

■ ■ ■ ■ ■ ■

G. Anderson

OBJECTIVES

Upon the completion of this chapter, you should be able to:

1. Define the disciplines that contribute to and impact wellness.
2. Differentiate between the credentials of wellness practitioners and medical professionals.
3. Differentiate between medical providers with and without an expertise in wellness.
4. Differentiate between the terms *restorative physical therapy, maintenance physical therapy, prevention physical therapy*, and *wellness physical therapy*.
5. Discuss the issues of standards of care and malpractice as they relate to the practice of wellness by physical therapists.
6. Identify why physical therapists need to possess an operational knowledge of wellness.
7. Discuss the entry-level physical therapy accreditation requirements related to wellness.

8. Describe how a patient's wellness can affect her or his health and ability to engage in and benefit from physical therapy.
9. Explore how physical therapists answer patients' questions about wellness.
10. Discuss physical therapists as wellness role models.

SECTION 1: WELLNESS PRACTITIONERS

Disciplines That Contribute To and Impact Wellness

Many disciplines contribute to public wellness and health promotion. Medical disciplines that contribute to wellness include, but are not limited to, athletic trainers, chiropractors, dentists, dieticians, exercise physiologists, healthcare administrators, medical physicians, mental health counselors, nurses, occupational therapists, physical therapists, podiatrists, psychologists, recreation therapists, social workers, and speech and language pathologists. Scientists who contribute to wellness include, but are not limited to, biologists, chemists, epidemiologists, and statisticians. Other disciplines that contribute to wellness include, but are not limited to, accountants, architects, economists, educators, entrepreneurs, financial planners, insurance personnel, managers, marketing personnel, and politicians. Obviously, a wide array of disciplines contribute to and impact wellness, and physical therapy is only one of these disciplines.

Credentials

Generally speaking, the hierarchy of credentials from most to least prestigious is licensure, registration, and certification. Unregulated practice is not on this list at all. When the physical therapy profession was initially established in the early 20th century, it was unregulated. During World War I, certification was established. Some years thereafter, physical therapists were required by most states to be registered. Eventually, everyone in the physical therapy profession was required to be state licensed.

Credentials and accreditation of medical and healthcare practitioners varies from discipline to discipline and from state to state. For example, every U.S. state requires medical doctors and physical therapists to be licensed, but not all of them require occupational therapists and athletic trainers to be licensed. Only a few states require a massage therapist to be licensed and only Louisiana requires an exercise physiologist to be licensed (Salzman, 2001a). Additionally, while occupational therapists must be registered in all states, physical therapist assistants must be licensed in certain states and registered or certified in others; they are completely unregulated in still others (APTA, 2008c).

Credentials of medical and healthcare practitioners are often linked to their educational requirements. Physical therapy programs, occupational therapy programs, and medical programs each must be accredited by a specific entity. These include the Commission on the Accreditation of Physical Therapy Education (CAPTE), the Accreditation Commission of Occupational Therapy Education (ACOTE), and the American Medical Association (AMA), respectively. A more generalized accreditation entity, the Commission on Accreditation of Allied Health Education Programs (CAAHEP) certifies many other healthcare educational programs (Salzman, 2001b). Not surprisingly, it is generally accepted that the AMA, CAPTE, and the ACOTE are more prestigious than the CAAHEP accreditation.

Unlike all other medical and healthcare practitioners, with the notable exception of exercise physiologists, there is no regulation of wellness practitioners. There are no minimal educational requirements and no state license or registration is needed by anyone providing wellness services. While several organizations offer a certification in the fitness aspect of wellness (e.g., APTA and the American College of Sport Medicine [ACSM]), proof of education or certification in wellness is not required for someone to offer wellness programs.

Provider Expertise

A physical therapy clinic employs physical therapists and support personnel (e.g., physical therapist assistants, aides, office employees) to provide *restorative* (i.e., medically indicated) physical therapy to patients. Only those providers with the appropriate expertise should provide skilled services. While it should be obvious that an aide does not possess the expertise of a physical therapist, it is worthwhile to note that most insurance companies do not recognize or differentiate between the expertise of an athletic trainer, exercise physiologist, and many other healthcare providers. The bottom line is that most insurance companies place these healthcare providers in the same category as aides and do not reimburse for their services.

In contrast to a physical therapy clinic, a wellness clinic does not provide medically indicated physical therapy services. Instead, a wellness clinic provides wellness therapy. In some cases, a wellness facility also may provide prevention and/or maintenance services. Typically, wellness clinics do not employ physical therapists but instead employ healthcare providers whose salary requirements are less than that of a physical therapist. These providers include an athletic trainer, exercise physiologist, or a so-called "fitness trainer." While athletic trainers are well educated and licensed in an increasing number of states, and exercise physiologists are well educated and licensed in Louisiana, "fitness trainers" may or may not have completed a series of courses or specific education in fitness and wellness, and may not even be certified.

Summary: Wellness Practitioners

Physical therapy is just one among a wide variety of medical professional and nonmedical practitioner disciplines that contribute to and impact the wellness of others. Unlike physical therapists, wellness practitioners are unregulated and usually not certified. Physical therapy clinics employ physical therapists and similar medical professionals as well as support personnel to provide restorative therapy to patients; wellness clinics tend to provide nonmedically indicated therapy.

SECTION 2: PHYSICAL THERAPY SERVICES: RESTORATIVE, MAINTENANCE, PREVENTION, AND WELLNESS

While in many (if not most) cases physical therapists provide restorative physical therapy, they also provide maintenance physical therapy. There is increasing evidence that they are providing preventative and wellness physical therapy. Accordingly, physical therapists must understand the difference between restorative, maintenance, prevention, and wellness physical therapy. Independent of the type of physical therapy a physical therapist provides, she or he must maintain high standards of care and not commit malpractice.

Although the APTA (2001b) states that individuals receiving physical therapy may be referred to as a "patient" or as a "client," I believe that it is more appropriate to define an individual as a *patient* if she or he is receiving restorative physical therapy and as a *client* if she or he is receiving wellness services. I do not condone the label of "customer" under any circumstances, even if the individual is purchasing a physical therapy or wellness product from a physical therapist or a physical therapy clinic.

Restorative Physical Therapy

Restorative physical therapy is also referred to as *medically indicated, skilled,* or *traditional therapy*. To be medically indicated, physical therapy must be 1) necessary; that is, there must have been a change in condition that warrants a new episode of care; 2) reasonable in terms of frequency, duration, and type; 3) anticipated to provide significant benefit, especially in terms of functional gains; and 4) provided by an individual with the appropriate credentials, such as a physical therapist or in some cases a physical therapist assistant (Miller, 2002).

Restorative therapy is typically provided to clients in a rehabilitative setting, such as a medical center, skilled nursing home, or outpatient center. It also can be provided in the patient's home (also termed *home health*). Restorative physical therapy often is provided one-on-one; however, group therapy is an option for patients who present with a similar diagnosis. Typically, restorative physical therapy is largely, if not totally, reimbursed by a third-party payer, which most likely is the patient's health insurance company.

Maintenance Physical Therapy

The primary goal of *maintenance* physical therapy is to maintain the current level of function and/or other medical status (e.g., safe blood pressure levels). In contrast to restorative therapy, it is not medically indicated. Specifically, there is no change in condition that warrants restorative physical therapy and/or it is not anticipated that the patient/client will obtain a significant benefit from this therapy. In fact, the patient's function and/or other medical status may decline secondary to disease progression and/or advancing age over the course of the maintenance therapy. The instructor of a maintenance session may require an expertise but not necessarily the knowledge of a physical therapist. An example of maintenance therapy is a walking exercise program for residents in a skilled nursing facility.

Maintenance therapy typically is provided to patients/clients by a sponsoring organization, such as a skilled nursing facility or an assisted living facility. The sponsoring organization may provide the maintenance free of charge or charge a fee to participants. Maintenance therapy can be provided to a group of clients or to an individual. One example is a physical therapist who provided maintenance therapy to a gentleman who had chronic functional deficits secondary to a cerebral vascular accident (stroke) sustained years earlier. Both the physical therapist and the patient recognized that the therapist's interventions would not enhance the patient's function, but they were successful in delaying his decline in function. This physical therapist had been providing maintenance to the patient twice per week for well over 5 years and the client was happy to self-pay for the therapy.

Prevention Physical Therapy

Prevention physical therapy is provided to clients to avoid or delay onset of a disease (primary prevention), provide an early diagnosis and prompt intervention to at-risk clients (secondary prevention), and provide interventions to prevent a regression of a chronic or irreversible condition (APTA, 2001b). Like maintenance therapy, it is not anticipated that clients will obtain significant functional benefit from prevention therapy. However, it can enhance a client's function and quality of life. Prevention physical therapy is often sponsored by an organization, such as a health club, a company, or a skilled nursing facility. It also can be offered by an agency such as a county health department. Prevention therapy is not typically reimbursed by insurance companies but may be provided free of charge to participants.

Wellness Physical Therapy

The primary goal of *wellness* physical therapy is to maintain or enhance the wellness practices of an individual or group. Wellness practices can be related to the physical, mental, and/or social domains.

In contrast to restorative therapy, it is not medically indicated. Specifically, there has been no change in condition that warrants restorative physical therapy. Wellness therapy will enhance one or more aspects of a client's overall wellness (e.g., aerobic capacity wellness or mental wellness). While the client may derive much benefit from the wellness therapy (e.g., a woman reducing her body fat from 35% to 28%), the benefit is not considered significant in the medical community.

The instructor of a wellness session may require expertise but not necessarily the depth of knowledge of a physical therapist. An example of wellness therapy is an exercise and nutrition program to reduce body fat. (Note: If the client is obese, this type of therapy might be considered restorative. However, if the client is simply over-fat, and there is no medical/rehab diagnosis; it can be defined as wellness therapy, if not also prevention therapy.)

Wellness therapy is typically provided to clients by a sponsoring organization such as a company or health club. The sponsoring organization may provide the wellness free of charge or charge a fee. Wellness therapy can be provided to a group of clients (e.g., a healthy cooking class at a wellness center) or to an individual (e.g., personal training). Typically, wellness therapy is not reimbursed by insurance companies.

I have been hired by organizations and individual people to provide wellness services. Examples of these wellness services include, but are not limited to develop a wellness program for the employees of the Sheppard Pratt Medical Center (Baltimore, Maryland); present a private seminar about fitness and body composition wellness to small groups; present an 8-hour wellness seminar to Kaiser Permanente physical therapists; assess and provide recommendations to single individuals or those in small groups.

Standards of Care and Malpractice

Standards of care can be defined as the "ways and means by which services should be delivered to give reasonable assurance that desired outcomes will be achieved in a safe manner" (ACSM, 2000, p. 264). Organizations that influence the standards of care of medical and healthcare practitioners include federal and state statutes (e.g., Medicare statutes and state practice legislations), professional organizations (e.g., the APTA and the ACSM), third-party payers (e.g., Medicare as well as the policies of other insurance companies, such as Blue Cross and Blue Shield), and medical corporations and agencies (e.g., the rehabilitation company for which you might be employed). It is important that you examine the physical therapy practice legislation and related statutes of the state in which you seek employment as a physical therapist. It is also important that before you accept employment, you ascertain and consider the standards of care of the prospective employer to ensure that they are compatible with your personal convictions.

If an individual is *negligent*, defined as one who fails to comply with a standard of care, that individual has engaged in a type of civil wrong called a *tort*. Negligence acts by a medical provider is specifically referred to as *malpractice*. Because physical therapists are licensed medical professionals, any act of negligence is malpractice. Because wellness practitioners are unregulated, acts of negligence are not considered malpractice. However, if a physical therapist or another medical practitioner provides wellness services, she or he can be liable for malpractice secondary to his or her credentials as a physical therapist. In addition, the physical therapist's licensure may be jeopardized.

Summary: Physical Therapy Services

Physical therapists provide four different types of therapeutic services: restorative, maintenance, preventative, and wellness. Restorative physical therapy is the traditional type of therapy and is known also as medically-indicated therapy. Maintenance physical therapy, prevention physical therapy, and wellness physical therapy are not medically indicated but nonetheless may provide much benefit to the participants. While restorative therapy is generally reimbursed by a patient's insurance company, the other types of therapy are not.

Standards of care define how skilled therapy should be provided. A physical therapist practicing wellness may be sued for malpractice and/or be subject to licensure infractions.

SECTION 3: PHYSICAL THERAPY EDUCATION

Students in physical therapy programs should endeavor to possess an operational knowledge of wellness because *A Normative Model of Physical Therapist Professional Education* has required entry-level students to be educated in wellness since 2001. *A Normative Model of Physical Therapist Professional Education* is published periodically by the Commission on the Accreditation of Physical Therapy Programs (CAPTE), an affiliate of the American Physical Therapy Association. The version used by entry-level physical therapy programs until 2004 was the *Normative Model of Physical Therapist Professional Education: Version 2000*, including the *Supplement to a Normative Model of Physical Therapist Professional Education: Version 2000*, which consisted of information related to wellness. *A Normative Model of Physical Therapist Professional Education: Version 2004* became effective in June 2004 (publications representative for the APTA; personal communication; August 24, 2004).

A Supplement to a Normative Model of Physical Therapist Professional Education: Version 2000 contained three sections related to wellness: exercise science, exercise physiology, and nutrition. In the 2004 version, the exercise science section was expanded and the exercise physiology and nutrition sections were combined, but enhanced. The 2004 version also introduced two new wellness sections: 1) a practice management section dedicated to prevention, fitness, health promotion, and wellness, and 2) a section related to wellness in the Foundational Sciences Matrix.

The exercise science content within *A Normative Model of Physical Therapist Professional Education: Version 2004* is verbatim to the exercise science content in the *Supplement to a Normative Model of Physical Therapist Professional Education: Version 2000*. The exercise science content continued to consist of exercise prescription, implementation, and modeling of strength training; power training; aerobic and anaerobic conditioning; coordination, agility, and balance; and stress management and relaxation. In *A Normative Model of Physical Therapist Professional Education: Version 2004*, the terminal and instructional objectives for exercise science content requires students to be able to analyze and implement programs to enhance strength, aerobic capacity, flexibility, relaxation, and balance and coordination.

The exercise physiology content identified in *A Supplement to a Normative Model of Physical Therapist Professional Education: Version 2000* included the thermoregulatory system, including effects of the environment; skeletal muscle cell anatomy and physiology, including fiber types and cellular changes and fiber type adaptations in response to exercise; adipocyte anatomy and physiology, including changes with diet and exercise, and cardiac muscle adaptations. The sole terminal objective related to exercise physiology was to "discuss mechanisms to exercise an individual to their maximum capacity" (p. 6). Compared to the exercise physiology information presented in the 2000 supplement, the exercise physiology content in the 2004 version was significantly enhanced. For example, there are behavioral and terminal objectives related to neuromuscular, musculoskeletal, and cardiopulmonary responses during progressive exercise; the principles of exercise testing and prescription; and the assessment and analysis of body composition.

The definition of wellness provided in *The Normative Model of Physical Therapist Professional Education: Version 2004* is "[a]n active process of becoming aware of and making choices toward a more successful existence" (p. 69). Educational outcomes related to wellness in the 2004 version include assessment and screenings, referrals, evidenced-based interventions, patient education, patient compliance, and reevaluation. Expectations related to prevention, fitness, health promotion, and wellness in the 2004 version are

> Provide culturally competent physical therapy services for prevention, health promotion, fitness and wellness to individuals, groups, and communities;
>
> Promote health and quality of life by providing information on health promotion, fitness, wellness, disease, impairment, functional limitation, disability, and health risks related to age, gender, culture, and lifestyle within the scope of physical therapist practice;
>
> Apply principles of prevention [health promotion, fitness, and wellness] to specific populations. (pp. 63–64)

Unlike its earlier editions, *The Normative Model of Physical Therapist Professional Education: Version 2004* includes an entire practice management section dedicated to prevention, fitness, health promotion, and wellness. Within this section is the Health Promotion, Fitness, and Wellness Matrix that includes the primary content areas and examples of terminal objectives and instructional objectives related to those content areas. The Prevention, Health Promotion, Fitness, and Wellness Matrix consists of four content areas: "Foundational and clinical sciences; Cost-benefit analysis; Community information health and wellness; public-sector and private sector resources . . . ; [and] prevention, health promotion, fitness and wellness programs" (p. 80).

A Normative Model of Physical Therapist Professional Education: Version 2004 also discusses wellness in the Foundational Sciences Matrix. In this section, wellness theories and models, including the change model, are discussed. Sample terminal objectives related to wellness theories and models are expansive. For example, a sample terminal objective is to "promote health, exercise, fitness, and wellness to all populations, including those with a disease or condition that may lead to impairments, functional limitations, or disabilities" (p. 101). The sample instructional objectives also require clinical expertise. For example, a sample instructional objective is related to developing strategies to address modifiable cardiac risk factors.

A Normative Model of Physical Therapist Professional Education: Version 2004 also includes content related to psychological, social, ethical, and intellectual wellness; however, it does not overtly identify these as being related to the wellness. In the psychosocial realm, the 2004 version identifies the awareness of self and others, teamwork and group dynamics, cultural competence, health behavior change theories and models, emotional and psychological responses to functional limitations and diseases, physical and emotional abuse, faith and religion, sexuality, and holistic health. In the social realm, the 2004 version identifies professional roles and recognition, the sociology of health professions, and professional organizations. In the ethical realm, it identifies patient rights, values education, the role of virtue in the profession, and advocacy. In the intellectual realm, it identifies teaching methods and learning theory. Within the management sciences content, it identifies time management. Effective time management is directly related to wellness because it is linked to stress management and psychological wellness.

Physical therapists who possess an enhanced understanding of wellness may find that their ability to provide restorative therapy is improved. Of the various dimensions of wellness, physical therapists are likely to possess a basic competence in fitness and nutritional wellness, because these aspects apply best to the needs of most patients/clients. (The ability to engage in and benefit from physical therapy is discussed in Section 4 in this chapter.) Competence in applicable aspects of psychological wellness will benefit the physical therapist when she or he addresses patient compliance, both in the clinical setting as well as in terms of a patient's home exercise program. (Mental wellness is discussed in Chapter 8.) Physical therapists who possess a competence, if not an expertise, in wellness also may find that their marketability is greater. Those who did not explore wellness in their entry-level curriculum and/or in post-professional seminars or courses should endeavor to obtain at least a basic competence knowledge of wellness.

Summary: Physical Therapy Education

A Normative Model of Physical Therapist Professional Education: Version 2004, which is utilized in the accreditation of entry-level physical therapy curriculums, includes numerous sections related to wellness. Some of these sections utilize the term *wellness* and other sections do not. In comparison to its earlier versions, the wellness requirements in the 2004 version are significantly expanded. Physical therapists who did not explore wellness in their entry-level curriculum should gain a competence in wellness so they can enhance their marketability and improve patient/client care.

SECTION 4: WHY SHOULD PHYSICAL THERAPISTS POSSESS AN OPERATIONAL KNOWLEDGE OF WELLNESS?

Wellness is important in the provision of physical therapy. Wellness directly affects the patient's/client's health, which in turn can decrease her or his ability to engage in and benefit from physical therapy. Impaired wellness also can negatively impact those with chronic condition. Stuifbergen, Becker, Blozis, Timmerman, & Kullberg (2003) found that a wellness intervention improved health-promoting behaviors, self-efficacy for health behaviors, mental health scales, and pain scales in women with multiple sclerosis. In addition, decreased body composition wellness negatively impacts the exercise capacity of those with type 2 diabetes (Ribisl et al., 2007) and also negatively impacts those with osteoporosis (Zhao et al., 2007).

Independent of a patient's physical health and medical (including physical therapy) diagnoses, a patient's wellness affects her or his ability to engage in and benefit from physical therapy. For example, if a patient's aerobic capacity wellness is poor and/or she or he presents with a comorbidity (i.e., in addition to her or his primary diagnosis), she or he may only be able to tolerate a more conservative treatment plan. Patients who are only able to engage in a conservative treatment plan may require an extended duration of rehabilitation and/or not be able to achieve the maximum benefits from the physical therapy program.

Because wellness is global and pervasive in scope, it is likely that most if not all of your patients/clients will present with an impaired level of wellness. In fact, in many cases, a particular patient/client will present with a deficiency in more than one dimension of wellness. For example, one patient may present with deficiencies in the financial, family, and environmental dimensions of wellness; another patient may present with deficiencies in psychological, fitness, and nutritional dimensions of wellness. While it is beyond the scope of a physical therapist to comprehensively address all types of wellness deficiencies, we should perform a wellness systems review (similar to that described in the *Guide to Physical Therapist Practice* [APTA, 2001b]) for each (restorative) patient and refer her or him to appropriate professionals as indicated. Further, we should examine, evaluate, diagnose, define prognoses, and treat those dimensions of wellness that are medically indicated and within our scope of expertise.

If a patient is deficient in one or more dimensions of wellness, her or his ability to engage in and/or benefit from physical therapy may be impaired. For example, I once provided physical therapy to an 80-year-old female patient who was anorexic. She weighed about 80 pounds. She did not eat an appropriate amount of calories, protein, and carbohydrates; her consumption of certain vitamins and minerals was also deficient. The patient presented with muscular weakness and atrophy, the physician's order was for strengthening. It would not have been appropriate for me to engage the patient in strength training exercises until her nutritional intake was properly addressed. Forcing her to engage in strengthening exercises without first having her diet improved might have caused her body to engage in an unhealthy even life-threatening level of muscle degradation for gluconeogenesis.

Another example is financial wellness. Certainly, if a patient is financially impoverished, her or his ability to engage in physical therapy can be significantly impaired if not prohibited. A further example involves mental wellness. A patient's mental wellness, including but not limited to interest in the rehabilitation process, awareness, and importance of self-selected functional goals, self-image, and motivation can significantly affect a patient's ability and willingness to engage in and indeed benefit from physical therapy.

Patient Questions Related to Wellness

Patients and clients ask physical therapists all kinds of questions related to their wellness. We should provide advice that is evidence based rather than only anecdotal data. People tend to respect information provided by physical therapist because we are credentialed medical professionals. Many are perhaps more likely to query those of us who possess a doctorate.

Physical therapists should possess a basic knowledge of those dimensions of wellness that their patients/clients are likely to present. Perhaps more importantly, physical therapists should possess the ability and willingness to critically analyze the published wellness information to ensure that it is valid before applying it to the therapeutic realm or sharing it with their patient. As with other types of physical therapy, wellness therapy always should be evidence based.

If a physical therapist does not possess the knowledge to appropriately answer a patient's question, a personal opinion and/or anecdotal information should not be offered because it may be flawed. Erroneous advice may give the patient false hope and possibly cause the patient harm. If the question is outside of the professional scope, the physical therapist should advise the patient to consult with another medical professional. In certain cases, it may be appropriate for the physical therapist to seek out additional information and then decide if she or he should answer the patient's question or refer the patient to an appropriate specialist.

Physical Therapists Are Wellness Role Models

Diverse nonphysical therapy medical professionals, including physicians (Hash, 2002), nurses (Fuimano, 2004; Pierson, 2000; Resnick, Magaziner, Orwig, & Zimmerman, 2002; Somerset-Butler, 2004), psychologists (McLoughlin & Kubick, 2004), and counselors (Myers, Mobley, & Booth, 2003), recognize and support their status as wellness role models. Of all of the medical disciplines, nursing appears to most strongly embrace their function as role models. According to Fenton (2004), nurses need to be role models to each other and to other health professional colleagues. Nursing practitioners have even hypothesized that positive role modeling can enhance patient compliance (Resnick et al., 2002). A succinct definition of a role model is one who is "walking the talk" (Yancey et al., 2004). A more detailed description of the concept is provided by Fuimano:

> Being a model means that you consciously decide to act in a way that others will want to emulate. . . . [It] demonstrates a commitment to yourself and others as you "walk your talk" . . . . It means you care about yourself and how you present yourself to the world. . . . It says that you take yourself . . . seriously. Modeling for others doesn't mean that you

expect others to be like you; you can only model your personal best. But when you model a way of being; others can learn to adopt those qualities they find most . . . (2004, p. 16)

Like all other medical providers, physical therapists are wellness role models. Until recently, however, there has been little affirmation of this position in the literature. Preliminary studies of the wellness of physical therapy students suggested that physical therapists do and should serve as wellness role models (Fair, 2003, 2004b). In an article published in the *Magazine of Physical Therapy*, Landry (2004) discussed the role of physical therapists as wellness role models. However, because the APTA's (2001b) *Guide to Physical Therapist Practice* and *A Normative Model of Physical Therapist Professional Education: Version 2004* emphasize the physical fitness aspects of wellness, physical therapists should focus their attention on themselves as fitness wellness role models. In my own study comparing the aerobic capacity wellness of a group of female and male physical therapist members of the APTA, I concluded that "[Physical therapists] PTs should prioritize fitness self-wellness and role model fitness wellness. Similar to other [medical] professionals, the APTA should advocate that PTs [physical therapists] lead by example in the area of fitness wellness" (Fair, 2007, p. 10).

Even if a physical therapist is capable of properly educating a patient/client about a specific wellness issue, the patient/client may consciously or unconsciously model the therapist's behaviors even if these actions contradict that wellness education. A hypothetical (yet all too often actual) case is the medical doctor who smokes cigarettes but tells his patients that they should not smoke. Another example is the parent who consumes great quantities of alcohol and demands that the children not imbibe. How much credibility do you demonstrate if you tell your patients/clients that they should or should not do something to be well, and you are a poor wellness role model?

Despite our value as wellness role models, particularly fitness wellness role models, there is no evidence that physical therapists actually are well in terms of their fitness wellness. In fact, my own research suggests that physical therapists are deficient in fitness wellness and mirror the typical American rather than other groups of medical professionals (Fair, 2005, 2007).

Summary: Why Should Physical Therapists Possess an Operational Knowledge of Wellness?

Physical therapists must possess an operational knowledge of wellness because a patient's/client's wellness directly affects her or his health as well as the ability to engage in and benefit from physical therapy. Because wellness is global in nature, many of our patients/clients will present with an impaired level of wellness. While it is beyond the scope of a physical therapist to comprehensively address all types of wellness deficiencies, we should perform a wellness systems review of each (restorative) patient and, as indicated, make referrals to appropriate professionals. Further, we should examine, evaluate, diagnose, define prognostics, and treat those dimensions of wellness that are medically indicated and within our expertise.

Patients ask physical therapists about wellness. Patients assume that physical therapists are experts about all aspects of wellness and trust their opinions. Physical therapists should provide evidence-based information rather than anecdotal advice, and refer questions that are outside of their expertise to an appropriate practitioner. Physical therapists should not provide information that may mislead or cause harm to the patient.

A succinct definition of a role model is one who is "walking the talk" (Yancey et al., 2004). Many medical professionals do embrace their value as wellness role models. Like all other medical practitioners, physical therapists are wellness role models (Fair, 2004b; Landry, 2004). Patients and clients model the behaviors of their physical therapist even if the therapist's actions contradict the wellness advice provided.

chapter three

Physical Therapy and Wellness: Past, Present, and Future

The doctor of the future will give no medicine, but will educate
[her or] his patients in the care of the human frame, in diet,
and in the cause and prevention of disease.

■ ■ ■ ■ ■ ■ ■ ■ ■ ■ ■ ■ ■ ■

Thomas A. Edison (1847–1931)
Inventor

OBJECTIVES

Upon the completion of this chapter, you should be able to:

1. Summarize the history of the physical therapy profession and wellness, including dualism and the development of the medical profession.
2. Provide an overview of the evolution of U.S. medicine and medical training, including the integration of wellness.
3. Compare the biomedical and biopsychosocial models.
4. Summarize the progression of the physical therapy profession.
5. Examine research relating physical therapy and wellness.
6. Critically analyze my wellness-related goals for the physical therapy profession.

SECTION 1: ROOTS OF PHYSICAL THERAPY AND WELLNESS

The development of physical therapy, including the conceptualization and integration of wellness, is rooted and intertwined with the advancements of medicine through the ages. From the dawn of humans, societies have held beliefs about health, disease, and cures (Jayne, 1925). Neolithic tribes located in what is now Europe believed that illness was caused by mystical forces and surgeons engaged in sophisticated medicinal surgeries such as trephination, a process in which coin-size holes were made in the skull to release evil spirits (Sarafino, 2008; Trephination, *Ancient Surgery*, n.d.).

Medicine in 6th century BCE (before the common era) was a mere branch of philosophy and doctors believed that reflections and argument were superior to experimentation and practice (McDaniel & Hammond, 1997c). Alcmaeon (of Croton), writing sometime between 500 and 450 BCE, stated that the brain was the seat of feeling and thought (McDaniel & Hammond, 1997c, para. 3).

Alcmaeon "was probably the first physician to formulate the doctrine of health as a balance among the powers of the body" (McDaniel & Hammond, 1997c).

Hippocrates (of Kos, 460–370 BCE), known as the "father of medicine," separated medicine from philosophy by disproving the notion that disease was a punishment for sin (McDaniel & Hammond, 1997d). Hippocrates also developed the humoral system of medicine and reportedly created the Hippocratic Oath, which pertains to the ethical practice of medicine and is taken in revised form by Western physicians to this day (McDaniel & Hammond, 1997).

In the 4th century BC, Herophilos (of Chalcedon, 280 BCE) dissected cadavers and contributed to the advancement of medicine in many ways, including the diagnostic value of the pulse (McDaniel & Hammond, 1997). Erasistratos (of Alexandria) described the brain even more accurately than Herophilos, and distinguished the cerebrum from the cerebellum, determined the brain was the origin for all nerves, and distinguished motor and sensory nerves (McDaniel & Hammond, 1997a).

The biomedical and biopsychosocial models of health and disease are also rooted in Ancient Greece. Like most of their contemporaries, these physicians worshipped the God of Medicine (Asklepios) and/or the Goddess of Health (Hygenia) (Jayne, 1925). Those who followed Asklepios focused on diseases and miracle cures and those worshipping Hygenia based medical therapies on equilibrium (Jonas, 2000). The tenants of Asklepios and Hygenia were the precursors to the contemporary biomedical and biopsychosocial models, respectively. The *biomedical model* is reductionist, meaning that illness is defined only by biological factors without consideration of psychological processes. A central component of the biomedical model is dualism, which emphasises the separation of the mind and body (Sarafino, 2008). In contrast to the medical model, the *biopsychosocial model* is holistic and emphasizes the interrelationship of the mind and the body (Sarafino, 2008).

Although medical advancement slowed during the first centuries of the common era (CE), some advances did occur. For example, Vienna Disoscuride, a Roman physician during the 1st century, wrote a compendium of then known medicine that included descriptions of some 600 plants and their possible medical cures (McDaniel & Hammond, 1997b). In the

2nd century in Rome, during the time when the biomedical model of medicine was flourishing, Galen (131–201 CE) combined Hippocrates' writing about pathology and humors with the extensive anatomical works of the Alexandrians (National Institutes of Health, 2009). He dissected animals, declared that illness can be localized and different diseases can cause different effects, and argued against dualism (Kings College London, 2005). His experimental physiological research using careful observation and reasoning became lost to history for centuries. Because Galen's anatomical knowledge remained limited and there were few cures, physicians were only able to address minor ailments and soothe chronic conditions. They were defenseless in the spread of epidemic diseases (Sarafino, 2008). The origin of the hospital as an independent institution for the care and treatment of the sick can be dated to the third quarter of the 4th century CE (McDaniel & Hammond, 1997b).

During the Middle Ages, the Catholic Church significantly slowed the advancement of all aspects of medicine by prohibiting such practices as dissection and resurrecting the notion that illness was a punishment from God (Sarafino, 2008). In fact, priests were called upon to torture the body to drive out evil spirits (Sarafino, 2008) and trepanation was still used to treat such conditions as skull fractures and seizures (Jayne, 1925). The Christian theologian Thomas Aquinas (1225–1274) argued that disease and healing processes are mediated by the patterns of His causality in the world (Aquinas, n.d.).

During the Renaissance (14th through 17th centuries), new discoveries facilitated the progression of medical science, and physicians were "able to rely on science and not exclusively on healing methods derived from ancient Greek, Chinese, Indian and other systems" (Ardell, 2009a, para. 1). During this time frame, it was discovered that illness can be caused from cellular pathology (Hardinge & Shroyck, 1991). Between the 14th and 15th centuries, physicians regained their place as healers of the body; philosophers were relegated to the mind (Sarafino, 2008). In the 17th century, although René Descartes argued in the defense of dualism (Serendip, 1996), the Catholic Church agreed to dissection of cadavers based upon the rationale that the human soul leaves the body at death and animals have no soul (Sarafino, 2008).

Although it is impossible to trace the origins of the term *wellness*, the term was coined in the year 1654. Some believe that Epicurus (of Samos, 341 BC) first coined the term in his hedonistic philosophy. Others point to the word *wealness* that appeared in a 1654 dairy entry of the Scotts physician, Sir A. Johnson. However, the term was not popularized in the United States until the 20th century.

Summary: Roots of Physical Therapy and Wellness

The development of physical therapy, including the integration of wellness, parallels the evolution of Western medicine. Medical technology and practice was advanced in Ancient Greece, slowed during the Middle Ages, and revived during the European Renaissance. Certain religious beliefs (e.g., the cause of illness is evil) and treatments (e.g., trepanation) persisted throughout history. Despite their flaws, dualism and the biomedical model have been mainstays in the philosophy of medicine. The origin of the term *wellness* cannot be determined precisely, but may have been coined toward the close of the Renaissance.

SECTION 2: PRECURSORS OF WELLNESS AND PHYSICAL THERAPY IN THE UNITED STATES

Most Native American cultures, although lacking many of the technological advancements of the European invaders, supported the mind–body connection of health and disease. Along with herbal and/or surgical remedies to treat a condition would be a spiritual ceremony led by a healer with family and friends praying for help and health. The ability to *walk in balance* with all aspects of life remains a prized virtue to this day. A Navajo belief was: "[When there is a] balance between the individual and his total physical and social environment, as well as . . . balance between the supernatural and man . . . good health is the result; an upset in this equilibrium causes disease" (Jonas, 2000, pp. 13, 14). In contrast to these holistic views, American colonists adhered to the medical beliefs and practices of their European contemporaries (Hardinge & Shroyck, 1991).

During the early colonial days through the 1800s, the apprenticeship model was used to train physicians in their profession by (Hardinge & Shroyck, 1991; Harvard College, 2007). A man (or in very rare instances a woman) who may or may not have gained a high school education served as an apprentice to a physician for up to 3 years. Menial chores were done along with observation of treatments. When the physician–educator believed it was appropriate, the tasks progressed to assisting the mentor on house calls (Hardinge & Shroyck, 1991). Upon completion of apprenticeship, the proctoring physician awarded the new "doctor" a signed certificate, enabling her or him to practice on her or his own. The first medical school was established in 1765 at the University of Pennsylvania. Although Harvard College began to offer medical seminars in 1782, there were no prerequisites and students attended lectures for only a semester or two; proficiency was not examined (Harvard College, 2007). Like their predecessors, these students were required to complete several years of apprenticeship after attending these lectures (Harvard College, 2007). Sometime in the early 1800s, physicians established schools usually associated with a hospital to educate prospective physicians in the sciences before beginning their apprenticeship (Hardinge & Shroyck, 1991).

Through most of the 1800s, physicians classified diseases by symptoms (e.g., pain, fever, stool, headaches) and believed that an imbalance of "humors" caused disease (Hardinge & Shroyck, 1991). As in the Greek and Roman eras, it was often thought that illness was the curse of God or the devil or due to fate. While herbal medicines were used, dosage was imprecise and the general attitude was, "If one doesn't work, another will" (Hardinge & Shroyck, 1991, p. 25). In addition to a lack of knowledge about pharmacologic toxicity, treatments such as dehydration, purging and vomiting, and draining blood ("blood letting" using leeches) were standard procedures (Hardinge & Shroyck, 1991). Moreover, surgeons wore street clothes and wiped instruments "clean" before moving on to the next surgery (Hardinge & Shroyck, 1991). Because nearly 20% of the surgeries during this period were amputations, it is not surprising that nearly one-half of the amputees died from infection. Sadly, "Even laity observed that if the doctor failed to arrive, the patient's chance of recovery was improved" (Hardinge & Shroyck, 1991, p. 25).

Despite the comparatively primitive state of medical practice in colonial America advances in chemistry, laboratory equipment and techniques, bacteriology, and use of previously discovered concepts during the 19th century in Europe gradually revolutionized medicine (Jayne, 1925). For example, although Robert Hooke invented the microscope in 1665 and first proposed the theory of cellular life, it was Anton Van Leeuwenhoek who first described bacteria a few years later (Bellis, 2008). Microscopes were rare and not widely incorporated into medical practice until the late 1800s (Hardinge & Shroyck, 1991). Despite the research findings, however, most physicians scoffed at the idea of bacteria-causing infections until well after the 1870s when the germ theory was proven. The use of the microscope enabled scientists and physicians to understand that microorganisms produce diseases, which prompted the development of antiseptic techniques (Sarafino, 2008). Furthermore, through research, tools, and reasoning, scientists and physicians developed cures for a variety of endemic infectious diseases (Jayne, 1925). Medical advancements made during the 19th century caused the long-held humoral theory to be replaced by the biomedical model of medicine (Sarafino, 2008). This model emphasized the biological process of illness, and alleviating symptoms and curing diseases with pharmaceutical and surgical interventions. Although the biopsychosocial model of medicine was still in its infancy, it is worth noting that many attributed the decline in the most lethal cases to improvements in public health and nutrition rather than medicine.

In 1847, the American Medical Association (AMA) was established. By 1849, the AMA sent a formal letter urging medical schools to increase the length of classes to 6 months (Hardinge & Shroyck, 1991). In the 1870s, Harvard and other medical schools eliminated the apprenticeship system, raised admission standards, required written exams and passing grades on those written exams, introduced a 3-year curriculum, and established departments in the basic and clinical sciences (Harvard College, 2007). The medical school became a professional school of Harvard University, setting the U.S. standard for the organization of medical education within a university (Harvard College, 2007). By 1885, most other U.S. medical schools included a 2-year curriculum, with the second year being a clinical experience at a hospital, rather than an apprenticeship with a private physician (Hardinge & Shroyck, 1991).

During the late 19th century, as the country experienced prosperity and a middle class began to emerge, the newly prosperous public had the time and resources to pursue wellness and other forms of self-improvement. Although the biomedical model did not support the concept of wellness, capitalism did. In fact, many early consumer products, from processed breakfast cereals to mouthwash, derived from or exploited this emerging interest in health and wellness . It was also during this time that Sigmund Freud (1856–1939), an Austrian neurologist and the founder of psychoanalysis, investigated what was then known as *hysteria* (extreme fear and emotional excess) and is now termed *conversion syndrome*. His studies demonstrated that some patients have symptoms, including paralysis, blindness, and deafness, without an organic disorder (Bass, 2007). The popularization of wellness and the enhanced understanding of psychological disorders contributed to the growth of the biopsychosocial model of medicine and health.

Summary: Precursors of Wellness and Physical Therapy in the United States

Native Americans' holistic views of health and disease contrasted with those of the U.S. colonists, whose practice of medicine reflected the philosophies and technologies of their European contemporaries. Harvard University played a significant role in the development of the medical profession. The rise in prosperity during the late 1800s led to a larger middle class of people with the leisure and resources to invest in self-improvement and wellness.

SECTION 3: THE FIRST HALF OF THE 20TH CENTURY: BIRTH OF THE PHYSICAL THERAPY PROFESSION

By the early 1900s, most medical schools required a high school diploma and offered a 4-year curriculum (Hardinge & Shroyck, 1991). About this same time, the apprenticeship model of medical training had markedly declined (Hardinge & Shroyck, 1991) and the discipline of physical therapy was born (Moffat, 1996).

Physical therapy came into existence around 1914 to help address the functional deficits of some of the 200,000 Americans wounded in World War I as well as victims of the devastating poliomyelitis epidemic (Guccione, 1999; Moffat, 1996). The foundation of physical therapy is in restorative care (Moffat, 1996). These early physical therapists, known as *reconstruction aides*, received orders from physicians but did not evaluate patients, determine diagnoses and prognoses, or create plans of care. In many ways, reconstruction aides were similar to present-day physical therapy aides. Unlike the tasks undertaken by today's physical therapy aides, all reconstruction (restoration) aides were certified (Moffat, 1996; Murphy, 1995). Furthermore, some aides were graduates of physical education or nursing programs, such as the nursing program at Walter Reed Hospital, Washington, D.C. (Moffat, 1996; Murphy, 1995).

During the early to mid-1900s, great advances were made in medicine, including major breakthroughs in surgery and pharmacology. As the reputation of medicine flourished, so too did the biomedical model of medicine (Sarafino, 2008). Similarly, as technology and practice patterns expanded in the medical profession, the role of the physical therapist progressively increased "from that of a technician to that of a professional practitioner" (Moffat, 1996, p. 3). To meet the enhanced practice challenges in physical therapy, for the first time physical therapists were required to pass a professional competency examination. Moreover, in an increasing number of states, physical therapists were required to become licensed rather than certified. During this time period, many physical therapists rehabilitated patients with polio and soldiers injured in World War II (Moffat, 1996; Murphy, 1995).

In 1947, the World Health Organization's (WHO) constitution defined *health* as not merely the absence of disease, but a state of complete mental, social, and physical well-being. However, while the medical community was beginning to consider the benefits of prevention and a holistic framework, physical therapy remained focused on the restorative care of those who were diseased or crippled, particularly post-polio patients and those soldiers who had been injured in the Korean War (Moffat, 1996; Murphy, 1995). *Physiotherapists*, as the reconstruction aides were now called, were primarily employed by the U.S. military and hospitals. Their duties were quite similar to those accomplished by present-day physical therapy assistants. For example, physiotherapists documented only subjective and objective findings and modified treatment plans, but they received all orders and plans of care from medical doctors (Moffat, 1996). As the duties and responsibilities of the physiotherapists increased, the physical therapy educational training increased from certificate programs to university-based baccalaureate degree (Moffat, 1996; Murphy, 1995). The increased educational rigor in physical therapy complemented the progression in medical school curricula, which by the 1950s adopted the model that continues to the present day: prerequisite college courses in the sciences, 4-year medical curriculum, 1-year internship, and 3-year residency (Hardinge & Shroyck, 1991).

During the 1950s, physiotherapists were increasingly recognized as *physical therapists*. Insurance and market changes enhanced the viability of independent physical therapy practice (Moffat, 1996). Although the Self-Employment Section of the APTA was founded in 1955 (Moffat, 1996) and more physical therapists gradually began to move from the institutionalized setting to the outpatient clinic (Moffat, 1996; Murphy, 1995), physical therapists who established private practices throughout the 1950s were considered to be charlatans and were largely ostracized by the physical therapy profession (G. Gorniak, PhD, PT, personal communication, March 28, 2003).

Summary: The First Half of the 20th Century: Birth of the Physical Therapy Profession

By the early 1900s, medical school had an established 4-year curriculum of study, series of examinations, and hospital residency program before a student could become certified as a physician. The profession of physical therapy was born in the early 1900s, and its evolution mirrored the technological advances and needs of the medical profession. Precursors to present-day physical therapists were reconstruction aides, who helped to alleviate the suffering of soldiers from World War I, II, and the Korean War as well as those stricken with polio. The profession continued to enhance their education, credentials, and skills. As their responsibilities increased, they became known as physiotherapists. In 1947, the WHO defined health as not merely the absence of disease, but a state of complete mental, social, and physical well-being. By the 1950s, physiotherapists were known as physical therapists and were eligible to receive insurance premiums.

SECTION 4: THE SECOND HALF OF THE 20TH CENTURY: PHYSICAL THERAPY AND WELLNESS

The 1960s Through the 1980s

To meet the ever-increasing demands in the clinical setting, the first graduate entry-level physical therapy program was initiated in 1960 (Moffat, 1996; Murphy, 1995). Despite the move to a graduate-level education, entry-level physical therapy programs continued to focus on restorative care and the biomedical model. In contrast, the medical community began to discuss the merits of preventive care and wellness.

Halbert Dunn (1896–1975), a medical doctor with a doctorate of philosophy, is regarded as the "father of the wellness movement." Dr. Dunn introduced the concept of high-level wellness in a series of 13 lectures he gave at the Unitarian Church in Arlington County, Virginia, in the late 1950s. Those lectures provided the basis for his 1961 book, *High Level Wellness*. Dr. Dunn proposed that because environments differ, wellness is unique to each individual. Dunn also identified the five domains of wellness:

1. Individual (including basic human needs, growth, aging, and the inner and outer worlds)
2. Family
3. Community
4. Society
5. Environment

Although Dunn's book was reissued in a number of editions, initially it had little impact. It did, however, come into the hands of a number of the future leaders of the wellness movement. More than a decade later these leaders included Don B. Ardell (doctorate of philosophy), Elizabeth Neilson, Robert Russell, and John Travis. Three events in 1977 broadened the impact of Dunn's ideas. First, Don Ardell published a book using Dunn's title and giving Dunn due credit for his origination of the title and concept. Second, Elizabeth Neilson founded the journal, *Health Values: Achieving High Level Wellness* (Nielson, 1988) (renamed the *American Journal of Health Promotion* in 1996), which was dedicated to Dunn and reprinted one of his papers in its first edition. Third, the publisher of *Health Values* published a reprint edition of Dunn's *High Level Wellness*, which achieved a wider distribution and impact.

The profession of physical therapy at first did not embrace or perhaps even understand the concept of wellness. Nonetheless, the physical therapy profession continued to expand during the 1960s. This expansion was fueled by the inclusion of physical therapists in the Medicare health insurance program and Health Professions Education Act by President Kennedy's administration (Moffat, 1996). Physical therapists actively served overseas in the Vietnam War (Moffat, 1996; Murphy, 1995), and medical developments during the early 1970s prompted an enhancement of the practice expertise and reputation of physical therapists throughout the next two decades (Moffat, 1996; Murphy, 1995).

For example, in the early 1970s, physical therapists expanded their clinical knowledge of and ability to manage orthopedic and neurologic patients in response to the advent of the positron-emission tomography scanner, x-ray computed tomography, and joint replacements (Moffat, 1996). To meet the needs posed by the development of open-heart surgery, the role of physical therapy in preoperative and postoperative units was expanded and the physical therapy specialty of cardiopulmonary was founded (Moffat, 1996). Despite these advances, restorative care continued to be the focus of physical therapy (Moffat, 1996) and wellness was not commonly considered.

Although those in the medical professions, including physical therapy, were entrenched in the biomedical model, the biopsychosocial model was refurbished by George Engel, a psychiatrist (Engel, 1977). The biopsychosocial model, as proposed by Engel (1977), declared that physical, mental, and social factors all play significant roles in human functioning in the context of disease or illness. A significant strength of the biopsychosocial model is that it adheres to the WHO's triad of health. The biopsychosocial model also rejected dualism and supported the mind–body connection (Jayne, 1925).

In the same year that Engel's biopsychosocial model was published, Ardell (1977) proposed a model of wellness composed of self-responsibility, nutritional awareness, stress management, physical fitness, and environmental sensitivity. During these early days of the development of the wellness philosophy, an increasing number of physical therapists moved from hospital-based to private-based practice as a result of federal government's adoption of a policy that physical therapy "practice independent of practitioner referral is not unethical as long as it is legal . . ." (Moffat, 1996, para. 36). While the move from institutionalized to private practice settings might have helped to prompt an interest in a more holistic approach to physical therapy, the profession continued to embrace the biomedical model and "high tech" became commonplace in many aspects of physical therapy practice (Moffat, 1996).

The 1990s

The increasing number of wellness publications, including Sheridan and Radmacher's 1991 urgent appeal for the medical profession to move from the biomedical model to a biopsychosocial model, prompted pockets of the medical community to begin to relinquish their reliance solely upon the biomedical model. The physical therapy profession began to formally move into the wellness arena in the early 1990s. The earliest policy, position, or guideline related to wellness by the APTA was the "Health Promotion and Wellness by Physical Therapists and Physical Therapist Assistants," issued in June of 1993 as a position statement. According to the APTA, a position is "[a] firmly held point of view that APTA members are expected to support" (2004d, para. 2). The definition of a position is weaker than a policy, which is a requirement that obligates the actions of members and directs decisions on similar matters; but stronger than a guideline, which is an approved, but non-binding statement of advice. The APTA's 1993 position declared:

> The American Physical Therapy Association recognizes that physical therapists are uniquely qualified to assume leadership positions in efforts to prevent injury and disability, and fully supports the positive roles that physical therapists and physical therapist assistants play in the promotion of healthy lifestyles, wellness and injury prevention. (para. 1)

Many, but proportionally few, physical therapists possessed at least some knowledge of wellness and some of these therapists integrated wellness into their practice. For example, since 1981, I had owned and operated a fitness wellness sole proprietorship. After becoming licensed as a physical therapist in 1993, I applied my wellness knowledge to enhance the care provided to my patients, most of whom were receiving restorative care with the rest receiving maintenance care. I integrated body composition wellness and aerobic capacity wellness into my restorative care therapy and continued to provide fitness wellness services to organizations and individual clients on a fee-for-service basis. I also began to educate other physical therapists on how to provide wellness care. While the grassroots efforts of diverse physical therapists can have a positive influence on the evolution of physical therapy and wellness, our professional association's acknowledgement and involvement in the philosophy can impact its progress more significantly.

Perhaps the earliest article in an APTA publication that spoke to the relationship between physical therapy and wellness was entitled, "Three unique PTs and their specialized fitness programs," which appeared in the May 1994 issue of the *Magazine of Physical Therapy*. Two years later, the Commission on Accreditation of Physical Therapist Education (CAPTE, 1996) published *A Normative Model of Physical Therapist Professional Education*, stating that wellness objectives were compulsory in entry-level physical therapy curricula. *A Normative Model of Physical Therapist Professional Education* stipulated two wellness-related objectives:

1. Physical therapists must be able to formulate and implement a personal wellness plan based upon self-assessment and feedback from others. (Section 3.8.3.14)
2. Physical therapists must be able to "identify and assess the health needs of individuals, groups, and communities, including . . . wellness programs that are appropriate to physical therapy [and] promote optimal health by providing information on wellness . . . related to age, gender, culture, and lifestyle." (Sections 3.8.33–3.834).

Also in 1996, the *Magazine of Physical Therapy* published an article by Gersh and Echternach that discussed the integration of wellness concepts into the physical therapy treatment of patients with chronic pain. The authors recommended instruction in 1) an exercise program within the patient's capabilities; 2) somatic relaxation, such as imagery, self-hypnosis, biofeedback, for other cognitive means; 3) increased recreational and vocational activity; 4) increased socialization time; and 5) dietary modifications. Although the article did include a bibliography that identified research related to pain, the concepts within the article, including the recommendations related to wellness, were not referenced.

In 1997, in their initial publication of the *Guide to Physical Therapist Practice*, the APTA declared that physical therapists are and should be involved in the practice of wellness and prevention. The *Guide* defined wellness as "the concepts that embrace positive health behaviors (e.g., exercise, nutrition, stress reduction)" (Appendix 1-5, column 2, para. 4). This publication also provided multiple examples of health, fitness, and wellness promotion programs that physical therapists could offer. These included programs to manage and prevent lumbar pain and job-related disabilities; decrease the risk and progression of osteoporosis; decrease the risk of falls and fractures and the incidence of cardiovascular and pulmonary diseases; enhance the functional ability of those with cardiopulmonary disorders; and prevent various problems, including head injuries, dysfunction in women who are pregnant, and the development of secondary problems in individuals with chronic conditions.

Also in 1977, Adams et al. proposed the *perceived model of wellness*. This model is of particular significance to the profession of physical therapy because one of its creators, Janet Bezner, PhD, is a physical therapist and is well-recognized in the APTA. At the time the perceived model of wellness was published, Dr. Bezner was the Vice President of the APTA; she currently serves as the APTA's Senior Vice President of Education.

An increasing number of articles that linked physical therapy to wellness were published in the late 1990s. In 1999, for example, *Disease Management Health Outcomes* published "Health promotion for individuals with disabilities: The need for a transitional model in service delivery" (Rimmer, 1999). Rimmer's article overviewed health promotion, including health education, exercise, and diet, for individuals with disabilities. The emphasis of Rimmer's model was the provision of instructional guidance in a transitional setting that would facilitate participation in the community.

Summary: The Second Half of the 20th Century: Physical Therapy and Wellness

Halburt Dunn, MD, PhD, introduced the concept of high-level wellness just prior to 1960. Initially, the physical therapy profession did not embrace the concept of wellness. Although the medical professions continued to rely solely upon the biomedical model, a few began to consider the biopsychosocial model as advanced by the psychiatrist George Engel. In 1993, the APTA published their first position related to wellness that stated they fully support the positive role physical therapists play in wellness. In 1996, the CAPTE published *A Normative Model of Physical Therapist Professional Education*. A year later, the APTA published the first edition of the *Guide to Physical Therapist Practice*, which spoke briefly to the relationship between physical therapists and wellness.

SECTION 5: PHYSICAL THERAPY'S EXPANSION OF WELLNESS IN THE NEW CENTURY

The Years 2000 Through 2004

To offer physical therapists a means to enhance their education about wellness and fitness, the APTA initiated the Fitness and Wellness Consultation course in 2001. This two day, 14.25-hour course was designed "for physical therapists who wished to sharpen their knowledge of the physical therapy components of fitness and wellness consultation" (APTA, 2001a, para. 2). As the primary objective implies, the course emphasized the physical aspects of wellness, particularly physical fitness. Of the topics itemized in the outline, 7 hours were devoted to concepts directly related to exercise and fitness, such as the principles of training, physiologic adaptations to exercise, development of training plans, and exercise equipment; 1 hour focused on nutrition; and 1 hour discussing the psychological concepts including motivation. The Fitness and Wellness Consultation course was discontinued in 2003 (M. Phillips, Director of Professional Development, APTA; personal communication; June 15, 2004). Reportedly, there was a lack of sufficient interest in wellness to sustain or revamp the course.

In 2002, I created the humanistic model of wellness (HMW) in accordance with my definition of wellness (i.e., a lifestyle that both internally and externally promotes physical, mental, and social health in the cognitive, psychomotor, and affective domains). To my knowledge, this is the first model to incorporate well-being as defined by the WHO's triad. It consists of three primary dimensions: physical, mental, and social. It is also the first model to discuss wellness in terms of the affective, cognitive, and behavioral domains; the importance of which was later supported in *A Normative Model of Physical Therapist Professional Education: Version 2004*. (The humanistic model of wellness is detailed in Chapter 1.)

During 2003, several articles relating physical therapy and wellness were published. For example, "Improving the health status of U.S. working adults with type 2 diabetes mellitus" was published in *Disease Management Health Outcomes* (Akinci, Healy, & Coyne; 2003). *Archives of Physical Medicine Rehabilitation* published an investigation of the effects of a "wellness intervention for women with multiple sclerosis [and found that it improved] the time effect for self-efficacy for health behaviors, health-promoting behaviors, and the mental health and pain scales on the [36-Item Short-Form Health Survey] SF-36" (Stuifbergen et al., 2003, p. 467).

The year 2003 was particularly important in the history of physical therapy and wellness. The APTA published a goal stating that physical therapists should be universally recognized as the wellness practitioners of choice. I provided feedback to the APTA that the definition of wellness is too broad in scope for one discipline to be the practitioner of choice, and recommended the goal be modified to state that physical therapists should be universally recognized as the fitness wellness practitioners of choice (S. Fair, unpublished letter, 2004). The goal was amended to read, "Physical therapists are universally recognized and promoted as providers of fitness, health promotion, wellness, and risk reduction programs to enhance quality of life for persons across the life-span" (APTA, 2004a, para. 2). This modified wellness goal is similar in ambition to their initial goal published in 1993 but in my opinion fails to appreciate the leading role that physical therapists can and should obtain in fitness wellness.

In 2004, several articles relating physical therapy and wellness were published. An important meta-analysis appeared in *Sports Medicine*: "Exercise and multiple sclerosis" (White & Dressendorfer, 2004). The authors concluded that exercise enhances lifestyle activity, enhances quality of life, and reduces risk of secondary disorders in patients with multiple sclerosis.

Also in 2004, the *Journal of the Section on Women's Health* (Fair, 2004b) published an article entitled, "A comparison of the self-wellness of female and male students in one entry-level physical therapy program," which was my first published article related to physical therapy and wellness. My study found that both female and male physical therapy students scored a moderate level in total wellness and certain subscales, but low in fitness/nutrition, medical self-care, and environmental wellness. Women also scored low in intellectual wellness. Compared to men, women scored higher in fitness/nutrition, but lower in emotional and intellectual wellness. Three terms were differentiated: *fitness* (i.e., status of body composition, aerobic capacity, muscular fitness, and flexibility), *wellness* (habits and practices that promote physical, mental, and social well-being), and *fitness wellness* (habits and practices that promote fitness). Periodically, the APTA has offered a part or full-day course related to fitness wellness. I presented two platform presentations related to wellness at the Preview 2020 Conference in Las Vegas, Nevada, in November 2004. The first seminar was entitled "Health Promotion and Physical Therapy: The Fitness and Nutritional Dimensions of Wellness"; the second seminar was "Health Promotion and Physical Therapy: The Psychological Dimension of Wellness and Literature Relating PT and Wellness."

Perhaps the most important article linking physical therapy and wellness published in 2004 (if not the entire decade) appeared in *Physical Therapy*. Rea et al. investigated the physical and psychological components of wellness utilizing the term *health promotion behaviors* rather than *wellness*. The objectives of the study were to: "1) investigate perceptions of practice patterns in four focus areas of *Healthy People 2010* (disability and secondary conditions by assessing psychological well-being, nutrition and overweight, physical activity and fitness, and tobacco use) and 2) identify related self-efficacy and outcome expectations in California, New York, and Tennessee." The results indicated that "health promotion behavior most commonly thought to be practiced by physical therapists was assisting patients to increase physical activity (54%), followed by psychological well-being (41%), nutrition and overweight issues (19%), and smoking cessation (17%)" (p. 510). The researchers concluded that "physical therapists believe they are addressing health promotion topics with patients, although in varying degrees and in lower than desirable percentages based on *Healthy People 2010* goals. This study demonstrated that the confidence of a physical therapist to perform a behavior (self-efficacy) was the best predictor of perceptions of practice patterns and is an area to target in future interventions" (p. 510).

Although the APTA has considered reengineering the *Fitness and Wellness Consultation* course (Marilyn Phillips, Director of Professional Development, APTA, personal communication; August 24, 2004; Janet Bezner, Vice President of the Education Section of the APTA, personal communication, June 23, 2006), such a course (as of this date) has not been offered.

The Years 2005 Through 2008

In 2005, the APTA's Board of Directors "recognized the need for a more complete description of the role of the physical therapist in the promotion of health, wellness, and fitness, and for a well-articulated message to be communicated to a variety of audiences." To that end, a plan was adopted at the November 2005 Board of Directors meeting. The goals of the plan are

1. Clarify the language used in APTA communications to distinguish among populations served, services provided, and states of being influenced in the areas of health, wellness, and fitness.
2. Catalog current activities and initiatives relative to physical therapist services that improve physical fitness in the targeted populations.
3. Promote the physical therapist's role and increase recognition among all stakeholders of the value of services provided by physical therapists that improve physical fitness in the targeted populations.
4. Increase member expertise in providing services that improve physical fitness for patients and clients of all acuity levels.
5. Increase recognition of services that improve physical fitness when integrated into a physical therapist plan of care, including patients with identified risk of impairments, functional limitations, or disabilities and promote self-pay/first party payment for non-covered services . . . (Culver, 2007, para. 7).

In 2005, my investigation of the fitness wellness of a random sample of physical therapist members of the APTA was published. A majority of physical therapist subjects possessed unsatisfactory levels of flexibility wellness (~93%), muscular fitness wellness (~75%), aerobic capacity wellness (~75%), and physical fitness wellness (~97%). These statistics mirrored the typical U.S. population levels rather than data from certain other medical professionals who had been studied previously (Fair, 2005). The results also suggested that many physical therapists did not demonstrate a working knowledge of the concepts and terminology related to wellness and physical fitness. For example, approximately one-third of the subjects did not know how to define and/or apply the term *body composition*.

In April 2006, the *Education Strategic Plan* of the APTA was published. Goal number 8 was to "Enhance the physical therapist's perception, knowledge, and skills in contemporary and emerging health trends" (2006a, para. 10), and included the bullet: "PTs' role as exercise experts" (para. 10). The suggestion that physical therapists should be "the exercise experts" is of critical importance to the future relationship of fitness wellness and the physical therapy profession because "the content of the Education Strategic Plan represents the specific initiatives the [APTA] deems critical to the realization of Vision 2020" (Wojciechowski, 2006b, para. 1). Also in 2006, the *Magazine of Physical Therapy* included an article, "Improving women's health across the lifespan" (Ries), which provided a distinction between fitness wellness and wellness (although the term *fitness wellness* was not used).

In 2007, the *American Physical Therapy Association: Journal of the Section on Women's Health* published my article entitled, "A comparison of the aerobic capacity wellness of female and male physical therapy members of the American Physical Therapy Association." Results showed that both genders of physical therapists are equally "unwell" in terms of aerobic capacity wellness. In contrast to data on U.S. women, who possess less aerobic capacity wellness than men, the women in my study did not.

In 2008, the seminar entitled, "Cash Practice: Strategies for Integrating Rehabilitation, Health Promotion, and Fitness" was offered at the APTA Annual Conference in San Antonio, Texas. According to Gamboa and White (2008), the course included:

1. A detailed timeline and plan for successful implementation of the integration of cash practice related to health promotion, fitness, and wellness services.
2. The rationale and business model for a full-spectrum cash-based musculoskeletal health, wellness, and rehabilitation clinic.
3. Specific strategies for overcoming roadblocks, as well as designing, marketing, and implementing health promotion, fitness, and wellness services.

Summary: Physical Therapy's Expansion of Wellness in the New Century

While the APTA initiated the *Fitness and Wellness Consultation* course in 2001, those in the profession lacked sufficient interest in wellness to sustain the course. I created the humanistic model of wellness in 2002, which adapted the WHO triad of physical, mental, and social well-being, and discuss wellness in terms of the affective, cognitive, and behavioral domains. Several articles relating physical therapy and wellness were published in 2003 and 2004. My research suggested that physical therapy students are "unwell" in numerous domains, including fitness wellness (Fair, 2004b). Rea et al.'s (2004) study found that physical therapists are addressing patient wellness, but less than what is desirable. These authors concluded that self-efficacy was the best predictor of perception of practice patterns related to mental well-being, nutrition and overweight, physical fitness, and tobacco use. In 2005, APTA's Board of Directors adopted a plan to better articulate the role of the physical therapist in the promotion of health, wellness, and fitness (Culver, 2007). My 2005 study found that a majority of physical therapist members of the APTA did not understand the term *body composition* and possessed an unsatisfactory level of fitness wellness, which mirrored the U.S. population rather than certain other medical professionals who had been studied previously (Fair, 2005). The APTA's Education Strategic Plan of 2006 mentioned "PTs' role as exercise experts" (2006a, para. 10). My 2007 study found that APTA physical therapist members were "unwell" in terms of aerobic capacity wellness.

SECTION 6: FUTURE RELATIONSHIP BETWEEN PHYSICAL THERAPY AND (FITNESS) WELLNESS

The APTA states in their *Education Strategic Plan for Vision 2020* (2007a) that physical therapists should have a role as exercise experts. I agree. I believe APTA should appoint a Wellness Task Force comprised of physical therapists who possess an expertise in wellness, particularly fitness wellness, to facilitate the achievement of five wellness-related goals.

The first goal is to create or adopt both a definition and a model of wellness that are congruent with the WHO's (1947, 2009) triad conceptualization of wellness tailored to the profession of physical therapy. Developers of the physical therapy wellness model should consider the known wellness models, but critically evaluate each for its applicability to all of humankind and tease out any personal biases. For example, while the definition of mental wellness includes a purpose of life (e.g., Adams et al., 1997; Bailey & Nava, 1989; Fehring, Brennan, & Keller, 1987), which some refer to as spiritual wellness; being "well" does not mandate a belief in a unifying force (Adams et al., 1997), which others contend is equivalent spiritual wellness. To ensure that the wellness model does not focus on a minority or even a majority of the populace rather than all humankind, I suggest the model mimic the WHO's appreciation of global diversity.

The second goal is to revise and expand areas related to wellness, particularly fitness wellness, in the next edition of the *Guide to Physical Therapist Practice*. Achievement of this goal is necessary because current discussions of wellness are limited or flawed. It is noteworthy that the *Guide to Physical Therapist Practice* itself states that it is a "work in progress" (APTA, 2001b, p. 7) that will continue to evolve and be updated.

With that preface, my first recommendation is to provide a more appropriate definition of wellness. The *Guide to Physical Therapist Practice*'s current definition is, "Concepts that embrace positive health behaviors that promote a state of physical and mental balance and fitness" (APTA, 2001b, p. 691). The American Physical Therapy Association has since adopted the National Wellness Institute's definition; that is, "Wellness is an active process through which people become aware of, and make choices towards, a more successful existence" (National Wellness Institute, n.d., para. 3). However, this definition fails to recognize the WHO's (1947, 2009) triad of well-being.

My second recommendation is to include additional wellness-related terms in the Glossary, especially the terms that many physical therapists do not understand, such as *body composition* (Fair, 2007).

Thirdly, while a few of the Preferred Practice Patterns are related to fitness wellness (e.g., 6-B Impaired aerobic capacity/endurance associated with deconditioning), I propose that the third edition of the *Guide* add a chapter dedicated entirely to wellness. The reason is that an increasing number of physical therapists are expanding their practice into or indeed are specializing in wellness, particularly fitness wellness. These physical therapists deserve the same guidance that physical therapists who provide restorative care to patients are classified in what I affectionately refer to as the four powerhouses: the Musculuskeletal, Neuromuscular, Cardiovascular/Pulmonary, and Integumentary Preferred Practice Patterns.

The fourth wellness goal is to create and offer wellness seminars (perhaps with beginning, intermediate, and advanced levels) that culminate in written and practical examinations and a certificate. Although the association has considered reengineering the Fitness and Wellness Consultation course (Marilyn Phillips, Professional Development Director, APTA, personal communication, August 24, 2004; Janet Bezner, Senior Vice President of Education of the APTA, personal communication, June 24, 2006), as of the publication of this book, such a course has not been initiated.

The fifth goal is to establish a Fitness Wellness Section within the APTA. As of this publication, the APTA has 18 sections: Acute Care, Aquatic Physical Therapy, Cardiovascular and Pulmonary, Clinical Electrophysiology and Wound Management, Education, Federal Physical Therapy, Geriatrics, Hand Rehabilitation, Health Policy and Administration, Home Health, Neurology, Oncology, Orthopedic, Pediatrics, Private Practice, Research, Sports Physical Therapy, and Women's Health. The association touts that "APTA's sections give you the resources you need to stay current in your area of expertise and to continue your lifelong learning and professional development. With 18 special interest sections to choose from, you're sure to find something of interest to you!" (APTA, 2008b, para. 1). But what about fitness wellness specialists? Where do we fit in? Dr. Bezner, Senior Vice President of Education of the APTA, has suggested there should be a cross-sectional wellness special interest group (personal communication, June 24, 2006). While this would be a step in the right direction, even a cross-sectional special interest group (SIG) is unlikely to have the influence of a "full-fledged" section. Moreover, I suspect it would be cumbersome at best for the 18 current sections to be organized and managed to include a cross-sectional SIG that is wellness related. The founder and initial president of the Orthopedic Section, Stanley Paris, suggested that wellness should begin as a SIG within the Orthopedic Section and then mature into a section of its own (personal communication, 2006). However, such a course would be inappropriate because wellness is related to all physical therapy specialties, not just orthopedics.

Following the advent of a Fitness Wellness Section within our association, the sixth goal is to establish a Wellness Certified Specialist (WCS). The WCS would be on par with the specialists currently offered by the APTA, namely: Cardiovascular and Pulmonary Certified Specialist (CCS); Clinical Electrophysiologic Certified Specialist (ECS); Geriatric Certified Specialist (GCS); Neurologic Certified Specialist (NCS); Orthopedic Certified Specialist (OCS); Pediatric Certified Specialist (PCS); and Sports Certified Specialist (SCS). The WCS would either replace the previously discussed wellness certificate or the former could serve as part of the preparatory process to sit for the WCS examination. It is appropriate for a WCS to be made available because wellness requires a definitive proficiency and physical therapist members of our association are entitled to be recognized for their unique expertise. Furthermore, several disciplines are recognized already as possessing a significant amount of knowledge about one or more areas related to wellness. For example, exercise physiologists are educated in aspects related to fitness. If the appropriately qualified physical therapists are not soon credentialed, those who possess an expertise in fitness wellness may forever lose their ability to market themselves and be viewed by other medical professions and the public as the fitness wellness practitioners of choice.

A reasonable timetable for the APTA to adequately recognize fitness wellness as an expertise is as follows: Define the term *wellness* and develop a wellness model by the year 2010; make changes relating to wellness in the next edition of the *Guide to Physical Therapist Practice*; offer a Fitness Wellness course by 2011; establish a Fitness Wellness Section by 2012; and establish the curriculum and certification of Fitness Wellness Certification Specialist (WCS) by 2014. Of course, a more aggressive time frame might prompt more community members to seek out a physical therapist with an expertise in fitness wellness rather than turning to other practitioners or attempting to address the problem on their own.

Summary: Future Relationship Between Physical Therapy and (Fitness) Wellness

I suggest that the APTA establish a definition for and a model of wellness; the next edition of the *Guide to Physical Therapist Practice* incorporate advancements in their discussions of wellness; the APTA offer wellness seminars culminating in a certification after successfully completing an examination; and a Wellness Section be established within our association, one of whose initiates will be to sponsor a Fitness Wellness Certification Specialist (FWCS).

chapter four

Physical Wellness

Health is not valued till sickness comes.

■ ■ ■ ■ ■ ■ ■ ■ ■ ■ ■ ■ ■ ■ ■

Thomas Fuller, MD (1654–1734)

OBJECTIVES

Upon successful completion of this chapter, you should be able to:

1. Identify and briefly discuss each component of physical wellness.
2. Compare disease and physical wellness.
3. Discuss pharmaceutical and drug abuse and wellness.
4. List the reasons why physical therapists should possess an operational knowledge of physical wellness and its components.
5. Identify the relationships among persons who are classified in an APTA Preferred Practice Pattern, medical conditions, and medical wellness.
6. Determine the incidences of major medical conditions, smoking, and alcohol use.
7. Discuss the relationship between pharmaceutical and drug abuse and wellness, and the provision of physical therapy.
8. Determine the incidence of an inadequate nutritional and fitness wellness.

9. Identify why it is important for physical therapists to screen the nutritional, fitness, and body composition wellness of their patients/clients.
10. Describe ways in which physical wellness is linked to physical, mental, and social health.
11. Discuss how physical wellness can affect the ability to engage and progress in physical therapy.
12. Discuss the expansion of physical therapy in fitness wellness.
13. Discuss how physical therapists serve as wellness experts and role models.
14. Discuss the entry-level physical therapy accreditation requirements related to fitness/fitness wellness.

SECTION 1: PHYSICAL WELLNESS

Physical wellness consists of numerous components including, but not necessarily limited to, medical wellness, pharmaceutical and drug wellness, nutritional wellness, aerobic capacity wellness, muscular fitness wellness, flexibility wellness, and body composition wellness. If a patient/client strives to be and is knowledgeable about a component of physical wellness, is committed to a lifestyle that promotes it, and sufficiently participates in activities that promote it, then she or he possesses a satisfactory level of that component of physical wellness. In contrast, if a patient/client is not knowledgeable about a component of physical wellness, and/or is not committed to a lifestyle that promotes it, and/or does not engage in activities that promote it, then she or he has an unsatisfactory level of that component of physical wellness.

Diseases and Medical Wellness

Diseases and conditions that are primarily physical in nature, such as diabetes mellitus, obesity, Parkinson's disease, cancer, stroke, hypertension, viruses, bacterial infections, and fractures, are not static. For example, the signs and symptoms of type II diabetes mellitus can vary significantly from day to day. Because diseases and conditions are dynamic, they should be considered in terms of wellness rather than solely on health.

The medical wellness of a patient or client is determined by her or his knowledge about it, her or his commitment to it, and her or his related behaviors. Knowledge about medical wellness includes but is not necessarily limited to knowing risk factors for diseases, illnesses, and conditions and strategies (e.g., proper nutrition and exercise) to prevent or lessen the severity and/or duration of diseases, illnesses, and conditions. Behaviors related to medical wellness include preventative care, including periodic medical and dental examinations and periodic gynecological examinations for women and periodic prostrate exams for men, and medical self-care—that is, obtaining appropriate restorative and palliative care for diseases, illnesses, and conditions.

Medical wellness includes tertiary prevention. As discussed in Chapter 1, tertiary prevention can be defined as wellness for those with a chronic or irreversible condition. However, medical wellness is not related to whether a person has a disease. A person may be free of medical diseases, illnesses, and conditions but still be medically unwell. For example, a younger man who smokes cigarettes and ignores the risks of developing diseases linked to smoking, but who has not yet developed disease, is medically unwell. The reverse is also true: a person may have a chronic or irreversible disease and be medically well. For example, a woman who is a hemiplegic secondary to a stroke is well if she possesses and pursues medical knowledge, is committed to her medical wellness, and engages in behaviors that enhance her health (e.g., by getting regular exercise). Another example is a man with hypertension who advances his knowledge level about hypertension by researching it on the Internet, maintaining a commitment to leading a healthy lifestyle, and regularly exercising and engaging in stress reduction exercises.

Pharmaceuticals and Drugs and Drug Wellness

Pharmaceuticals are both prescription medications, such as clonazepam, temazepam, and oxycodone, and over-the-counter (OTC) medications, such as sleeping aids and ibuprofen. Drugs can be either illicit or street drugs (e.g., marijuana and cocaine) or legalized drugs. The primary legalized drugs are alcohol, tobacco, and caffeinated beverages. Alcohol includes beer, wine, and liquor. Tobacco includes smoking tobacco, such as cigarettes, cigars, and pipes, and nonsmoking tobacco, such as chewing tobacco and snuff. Caffeinated beverages include caffeinated coffee, tea, soda, and so on. Coffee is among the most commonly used legalized drugs in the world (Trunk, 2006).

Pharmaceutical abuse occurs when intake exceeds the prescribed or recommended dosage or if pharmaceuticals are used for nonmedical reasons, thus increasing the likelihood of dependence (National Institute on Drug Abuse, 2008b). Commonly abused classes of prescription drugs include opioids (often prescribed to treat pain), central nervous system depressants (often prescribed to treat anxiety and sleep disorders), and stimulants (prescribed to treat narcolepsy, attention deficit hyperactive disorder [ADHD], and obesity) (National Institute on Drug Abuse, 2008b). According to Craig P. Kurtz, Licensed Mental Health Counselor, Certified Addiction Professional (personal communication, February 12, 2009), a commonly abused OTC medication is Tylenol PM™.

Illicit drug abuse occurs whenever a street drug is used. The most commonly used street drug is marijuana (National Institute on Drug Abuse, 2008a). Alcohol abuse occurs when a person's intake exceeds recommended guidelines of an average of no more than one drink per day for women and no more than one to two drinks per day for men (with one drink equal to 12 ounces of beer, 5 ounces of wine, or 1½ ounces of spirits or hard liquor) (USDA, 2008c). Abuse also occurs in persons who drink alcohol who "cannot restrict their alcohol intake, women of childbearing age who may become pregnant, pregnant and lactating women, children and adolescents, individuals taking medications that can interact with alcohol, and those with specific medical conditions" (USDA, 2008c, para. 5). Some believe that consuming alcohol in any quantity negatively impacts wellness. Tobacco abuse occurs whenever a tobacco product is used. External tobacco abuse occurs when a person inflicts secondhand smoke on another. Caffeine abuse occurs when a person exceeds a moderate intake, generally regarded as 300 mg per day (International Food Information Council, 2007). An 8-ounce cup of drip-brewed coffee typically has 65 to 120 milligrams (mg) of caffeine; an 8⅓-ounce energy drink contains between 50 and 200 mg; an 8-ounce serving of brewed tea has 20 to 90 mg; caffeinated soft drinks have 30–60 mg per 12-ounce serving; and an ounce of milk chocolate has 1–15 mg (International Food Information Council, 2007).

Drug wellness is determined by a patient's/client's knowledge about it, commitment to it, and related behaviors. In terms of the behavioral component, satisfactory pharmaceutical and drug wellness includes abstinence from illicit drugs and tobacco products, not abusing prescription or OTC medications, and abstaining from or not abusing alcohol and caffeinated beverages.

Nutrition and Nutritional Wellness

Nutrition consists of the consumption status of calories, vitamins, and minerals such as sodium and iron, and substrates, including fats (e.g., healthy and unhealthy), carbohydrates (e.g., fiber and simple sugars), and protein. Nutrition also includes the consumption of alcohol and caffeine.

Nutritional wellness is determined by a patient's/client's knowledge about nutritional wellness, commitment to nutritional wellness, and nutrition-related behaviors. Nutrition and nutritional wellness are detailed in Chapter 5.

Aerobic Capacity and Aerobic Capacity Wellness

Aerobic capacity, also known as cardiovascular endurance, describes the functional status of the cardiopulmonary system. An individual's aerobic capacity is determined by her or his maximal oxygen consumption (VO_2max) or the "maximum volume of oxygen that the body can consume during intense, whole-body exercise, while breathing air at sea level" (Seiler, 2005, para. 2).

Aerobic capacity wellness is determined by a patient's/client's knowledge about it, commitment to it, and related behaviors. Aerobic capacity wellness is not necessarily related to aerobic capacity or VO_2max. For example, a man may be genetically predispositioned to possess a higher VO_2max, but he may not care about exercise and rarely exercise. Aerobic capacity and aerobic capacity wellness are detailed in Chapter 6.

Muscular Fitness and Muscular Fitness Wellness

Muscular fitness is one's level of strength, either generally to a muscle region or specifically to an individual muscle. There are several types of muscular fitness: muscular strength, muscular endurance, muscular power, and elastic strength. According to the *Guide to Physical Therapist Practice* (APTA, 2001b), muscular strength is "the muscle force exerted by a muscle or a group of muscles to overcome a resistance under a specific set of circumstances" (p. 688); muscular endurance is "the ability to sustain forces repeatedly or to generate forces over a period of time" (p. 688); and muscular power is "the work produced per unit of time or the product of strength and speed" (p. 688). Elastic strength is determined by the muscle's ability to exert forces quickly and to overcome resistance with a high speed of muscle action. A high level of elastic strength requires good coordination and a combination of speed and strength of muscle action. Elastic strength is important in explosive activities such as jumping and sprinting.

Muscular strength is determined by the ability to move a heavy weight a limited number of times (e.g., bench pressing 80 pounds eight times). Muscular endurance is determined by the ability to repeatedly move a lighter weight (e.g., performing 100 abdominal curls). Muscular power is determined by the ability to move the heaviest weight possible (e.g., bench pressing 120 pounds one time). Elastic strength is determined by the ability of the muscles to overcome a resistance with a fast contraction and thereby enable the patient/client to compete in a sport (e.g., a basketball game) without injuring the joints or muscles.

Muscular fitness wellness is determined by the patient's/client's knowledge about it, commitment to it, and related behaviors. Muscular fitness is not necessarily related to muscular fitness wellness. For example, a woman may be genetically predispositioned to be strong, but she may know little about muscular fitness and rarely if ever strength train. Muscular fitness and muscular fitness wellness are detailed in Chapter 6.

Flexibility and Flexibility Wellness

Flexibility is defined as the ability to move a joint or series of joints through their full range of motion, pain free and unrestricted. Flexibility is affected by the joint surfaces, capsule, ligaments, muscle length, and soft tissue (Prentice, 2006).

Flexibility wellness is determined by the patient's/client's knowledge about it, commitment to it, and related behaviors. Flexibility wellness is not necessarily related to flexibility. For example, a man may continually learn about flexibility and flexibility wellness, be committed to stretching, and regularly engage in stretching, but he may present with slightly impaired range of motion. Flexibility and flexibility wellness are detailed in Chapter 6.

Body Composition and Body Composition Wellness

Body composition can be defined as the percentage of body fat versus the percentage of lean body mass (McArdle, Katch, & Katch, 2006). Lean body mass is all tissue that is not fat—that is, skeletal muscle, smooth muscle, and the skeletal system.

Body composition wellness is determined by the patient's/client's knowledge about it, commitment to it, and related behaviors. Body composition wellness is not necessarily related to body composition or percentage of body fat. For example, a woman may know a lot about body composition and body composition wellness, be committed to living a lifestyle that promotes a healthy body composition, eat healthfully, and exercise regularly but still be overfat due to hypothyroidism. Body composition and body composition wellness are detailed in Chapter 7.

Summary: Physical Wellness

Physical wellness consists of numerous components, including but not necessarily limited to disease: medical wellness; pharmaceutical and drug wellness; nutritional wellness; aerobic capacity wellness; muscular fitness wellness; flexibility wellness; and body composition wellness. If a patient/client is knowledgeable about activities that promote a component of physical wellness, is committed to a lifestyle that promotes it, and participates in sufficient activities that promote it, she or he possesses a satisfactory level of that component of physical wellness.

Medical wellness is determined by medical self-care and includes tertiary prevention, but it is not related to whether a person has a disease or condition. Pharmaceutical and drug wellness includes abstaining from illicit drugs and tobacco products, not abusing prescription or OTC medications, and abstaining from or not abusing alcohol and/or caffeinated beverages. Maximal oxygen consumption determines a person's aerobic capacity. Muscular fitness is determined by a person's level of strength, either generally to a muscle region or specifically to an individual muscle, and includes muscular strength, endurance, power, and elasticity. Flexibility is defined as the ability to move a joint or series of joints through their full range of motion, pain free and unrestricted (Prentice, 2006). Body composition is determined by a person's percentage of body fat versus percentage of lean body mass. Aerobic capacity, muscular fitness, flexibility, and body composition wellness are not necessarily related to their corresponding aspects of health.

SECTION 2: WHY PHYSICAL THERAPISTS SHOULD POSSESS AN OPERATIONAL KNOWLEDGE OF PHYSICAL WELLNESS

Restorative Physical Therapy Patients Present with Impaired Physical Health

By definition, restorative physical therapy patients present with a medical diagnosis—for example, a disease, illness, or injury. All patients classified in an APTA Preferred Practice Pattern other than a preventative pattern necessarily present with impaired physical health. However, clients classified in only a preventative practice pattern (i.e., 4A: Primary prevention/risk reduction for skeletal demineralization, 5A: Primary prevention/risk reduction for loss of balance and falling, 6A: Primary prevention/risk reduction for cardiovascular/pulmonary disorders, and 7A: Primary prevention/risk reduction for integumentary disorders) may also present with an unrelated comorbidity. Common medical conditions include but are not limited to overweight and obesity, osteoarthritis, diabetes, and conditions related to the myocardium.

The prevalence of overweight, as defined by a body mass index (BMI) equal to or greater than 25, was 56% from 1988 to 1994, 64.5% from 1999 to 2000, 65.7% from 2001 to 2002, and 66.3% from 2003 to 2004 (National Center for Health Statistics [NCHS], 2008). Among European Americans, 57.6% of women and 71% of men are overweight; among African Americans, 79.6% of women and 67% of men are overweight (American Heart Association, 2008b).

The prevalence of obesity, as defined by a BMI of equal to or greater than 30, was 22.9% from 1988 to 1994, 30.5% from 1999 to 2000, 30.6% in 2001 and 2002, and 32.3% in 2003 and 2004 (NCHS, 2008). Among men, the prevalence of obesity was 31.1% from 2003 to 2004 and 33.3% from 2005 to 2006 (Ogden, Carroll, McDowell, & Flegal, 2007). Among women, the prevalence of obesity was 33.2% from 2003 to 2004 and 35.3% from 2005 to 2006 (Ogden et al., 2007). Among European Americans, 30.7% of women and 30.2% of men are obese; among African Americans, 51.1% of women and 30.8% of men are obese (American Heart Association, 2008b).

The prevalence of osteoarthritis among Americans is 7.4% (Corti & Rigon, 2003). The prevalence of hip osteoarthritis is slightly higher in women (8.0%) than in men (6.7%) (Quintana et al., 2008). In some people, evidence of osteoarthritic changes may exist by the second or third decade of life, but they are not usually accompanied by symptoms (Quintana et al., 2008). By age 40, almost everyone has some osteoarthritic changes in weight-bearing joints (e.g., hip and knee joints), and by age 75, virtually everyone has changes in at least one joint (Quintana et al., 2008).

According to the American Diabetes Association (ADA, n.d.), almost one-third of Americans are affected by diabetes, undiagnosed diabetes (using the ADA criteria of a fasting glucose of 126 mg/dL), or prediabetes (using the ADA criteria of a fasting glucose level of 100 to less than 126 mg/dL). About 6% have diagnosed diabetes, 2% have undiagnosed diabetes, and 20% have prediabetes. Prevalence by race/ethnicity and gender varies. Among Caucasian women, 6.8% have diagnosed diabetes, 1.7% have undiagnosed diabetes, and 21.6% have prediabetes. Among African American women, 13.2% have diagnosed diabetes, 2.3% have undiagnosed diabetes, and 13.2% have prediabetes. Among Caucasian men, 7.3% have diagnosed diabetes, 3.2% have undiagnosed diabetes, and 34.3% have prediabetes. Among African American men, 10.7% have diagnosed diabetes, 1.7% have undiagnosed diabetes, and 22.6% have prediabetes.

Coronary artery disease affects almost one out of every 10 American adults. Six percent of Caucasian women, 7.8% of African American women, 9.4% of Caucasian men, and 7.1% of African American men have coronary heart disease (American Heart Association, AHA, 2008a). Angina pectoris is diagnosed in 3.9% of Caucasian women, 4.3% of African American women, 4.8% of Caucasian men, and 3.4% of African American men (AHA, 2008a).

Significant numbers of American adults have hypercholesterolemia. Among Caucasian women, 49.7% have a total blood cholesterol level of 200 mg/dL or higher, and 33.8% have an LDL cholesterol of 130 mg/dL or higher. Among African American women, 42.1% have a total blood cholesterol level of 200 mg/dL or higher, and 29.8% have an LDL cholesterol of 130 mg/dL or higher. Among Caucasian men, 47.9% have a total blood cholesterol level of 200 mg/dL or higher, and 31.7% have an LDL cholesterol of 130 mg/dL or higher. Among African American men, 44.8% have a total blood cholesterol level of 200 mg/dL or higher, and 32.4% have an LDL cholesterol of 130 mg/dL or higher (AHA, 2008a).

Hypertension, defined as a systolic pressure of 140 mm Hg or higher or a diastolic pressure of 90 mm Hg or higher, is also prevalent. According to the AHA (2008a), 31.9% of Caucasian women, 46.6% of African American women, 32.5% of Caucasian men, and 42.2% of African American men have hypertension. Stroke occurs in 2.7% of Caucasian women, 2.4% of Caucasian men, and 4.1% of African Americans.

Because physical therapy patients/clients present with impaired physical health, they also present with impaired physical wellness. Physical therapists can and should help their patients/clients to enhance their physical health by educating them about physical wellness and, as indicated, directly addressing any physical wellness deficits.

Physical Therapy Patients/Clients Present with Impaired Drug Wellness

Many Americans have impaired drug wellness. About 18% of women and 24% of men smoke (AHA, 2009a). The percentages are even higher for certain groups. For example, the percentages are 29% for female Indian and Alaska natives and 36% for male Indian and Alaska natives (AHA, 2009a). About 48% of Americans consume three to four alcoholic drinks per occasion, and more than 20% consume more than five to seven alcoholic drinks per occasion (Johnson & Glassman, 1998). Consecutively, the typical female and male consume 2.2 and 3.2 alcoholic drinks per occasion, respectively (York, Welte, & Hirsch, 2003). At some time in their lives, more than 30% of Americans experience alcohol abuse or alcohol dependence (Johnson, 2007). In the year 2005, 11% of adults ages 26 to 35 and 4.5% of adults ages 35 or older reported that they used an illicit drug during the past month (CDC, 2007b). In the same year, 3.5% of adults ages 26 to 35 and 1.5% of adults ages 35 or older reported that they used a psychotherapeutic drug for a nonmedical purpose during the past month (CDC, 2007b). Rates of drug use are even higher in younger adults and minors. In 2005, 20% of adults ages 18 to 25 reported that they used an illicit drug during the past month, and 6.3% of them reported that they used a psychotherapeutic drug for a nonmedical purpose during the past month (CDC, 2007b). Younger individuals also use prescription pain medications for nonmedical purposes. In the year 2007, nearly 10% of high school seniors reported abusing Vicodin during the past month, and 5.2% reported abusing oxycontin during the past month (National Institute on Drug Abuse, 2008b).

Drug use can cause a person to require physical therapy. For instance, excessive alcohol consumption can cause a stroke or a fall (Horgan, Skwara, & Strickler, 2001). Physical therapists also provide care to those who have used illegal drugs and become infected with a disease, such as acquired immunodeficiency syndrome (AIDS). For instance, one of my patients had contracted the human immunodeficiency virus (HIV) secondary to heroin use and presented with an infected wound. I also provided physical therapy to a hospice patient who was so categorized because of his decreased life expectancy secondary to AIDS. While no one could reverse the disease state of these patients, I could and did enhance their wellness through their physical therapy sessions.

In some cases physical therapists provide direct intervention for drug use. A primary example is smoking cessation. Rea et al. (2004) found that a physical therapist's confidence in her or his ability to provide smoking cessation intervention is the largest factor in the provision of those services. To increase your confidence about providing smoking cessation, it is helpful to enhance your understanding of the addiction processes of smoking and smoking cessation. The provision of smoking cessation is an important portal into the physical wellness of Americans because of all the categories and types of drugs, tobacco has the greatest impact upon health. The effects of smoking are profound and are harmful to nearly every organ of the body (U.S. Department of Health and Human Services [DHHS], 2004). For example, smoking is linked to coronary heart disease, the leading cause of death in the United States (DHHS, 2004); cancers of the bladder, oral cavity, pharynx, larynx (voice box), esophagus, cervix, kidney, lung, pancreas, and stomach; acute myeloid leukemia (National Cancer Institute, 2004); and abdominal aortic aneurysm (Kurata et al., 1998). Smoking also doubles to quadruples the risk for coronary artery disease (AHA, 2009c), increases the risk of developing peripheral vascular disease more than tenfold (Fielding et al., 1998), and has a direct causal effect on stroke (Aldoori & Rahman, 1998). Compared with postmenopausal women who have never smoked, postmenopausal, chronically smoking women have lower bone density and an increased risk of hip fracture (American Lung Association, 2009).

Physical Therapy Patients Present with Impaired Nutritional, Fitness, and Body Composition Wellness

Many physical therapy patients/clients are deficient in nutritional and fitness wellness. The nutritional diet of about 90% of Americans is inadequate (Briefel & Johnson, 2004). For example, a typical American has an intake of fiber less than half of what is recommended (comparison of data from the Food and Nutrition Board, 2005, and Lanza, 1987) and consumes too much fat (comparison of data from Harvard School of Public Health, 2009c, and Briefel & Johnson, 2004). The most recent statistics from the National Center for Health Statistics (Barnes, 2007) indicate that 40% of adults spend most of their day sitting and engage in no leisure-time physical activity, and 70% do not engage in regular leisure-time physical activity.

Nutritional, fitness, and body composition wellness are linked to the prevalence of certain diseases. For example, good nutritional wellness decreases the risk of stroke in women (Manson, Willett, & Stampfer, 1994) and men (Gillman, Cupples, & Gagnon, 1995) and decreases the risk of hepatocellular cancer (Yu, Hsieh, & Pan, 1995), stomach cancer (Dorant, van den Brandt, & Goldbohm, 1996), and prostate cancer (Giovannucci, Ascherio, & Rimm, 1995).

Given the alarming number of Americans with impaired nutritional, fitness, and body composition wellness, I suggest physical therapists screen these components in the systems review of each patient/client. These screens should be problem focused and brief, similar to the screens detailed in the Systems Review sections of the APTA's *Guide to Physical Therapist Practice* (2001b). If the systems review suggests a wellness deficiency but the physical therapist does not possess the necessary expertise to further examine and treat it, then she or he should refer the patient/client to a physical therapist who does. If the physical therapist has the necessary expertise, then she or he should perform indicated nutritional, fitness, and body composition wellness examinations and the applicable evaluations; determine the condition(s); and describe the prognosis, preparing a plan of care and goals. Qualified physical therapists may provide the indicated interventions directly or supervise another healthcare practitioner to provide them. This choice should be made by considering the physical therapy practice legislation of the state in which the therapist is licensed, the knowledge and abilities of the ancillary practitioner, and if applicable, the patient's insurance coverage. Wellness therapy may be provided concurrently with or following restorative therapy.

Physical Wellness Affects Physical Health

Physical wellness is linked to physical health. A prime example is the relationship between fitness wellness and health. The National Center for Chronic Disease Prevention and Health Promotion (NCCDPHP, 1999) has stated that regular physical activity reduces blood pressure in people who already have hypertension; helps control body weight; helps build and maintain healthy bones, muscles, and joints; and decreases the risk of falls in the elderly.

Impaired body composition wellness has been shown to negatively impact the exercise capacity of both patients diagnosed with (type 2) diabetes (Ribisl et al., 2007) and patients diagnosed with osteoporosis (Zhao et al., 2007).

Physical wellness also impacts a person's risk for certain diseases. Aerobic capacity wellness decreases the risk of heart diseases (Megnien & Simon, 2008; Wilson, 2009), including hypertension, and the risk of dying of heart disease (NCCDPHP, 1999). It also reduces the risk of dying prematurely and of developing diabetes and colon cancer (NCCDPHP, 1999). In contrast, poor nutritional, fitness, and body composition wellness can increase the risk of diabetes, obesity, and certain types of cancer and cardiovascular diseases (e.g., "Exercise," 2008; McNaughton, Dunstan, Ball, Shaw, & Crawford, 2009; Norris et al., 2005; Weinstein, 2008).

Pharmaceutical and drug wellness is linked to health. For example, alcohol abuse can lead to liver cirrhosis, stroke, cancers, and heart disease (Schuckit, 2009).

Components of fitness wellness favorably affect their corresponding aspect of health and other aspects of fitness. In one study, those with modest aerobic capacity wellness (e.g., those who spent 3 hours per week jogging or doing aerobic dance) were able to perform more sit-ups and were more flexible (Ford, Pucket, Blessing, & Tucker, 1989). The study also found that those with modest muscular fitness wellness (via weight training) were more flexible.

Physical Wellness Is Linked to Mental and Social Health

Physical wellness is linked to mental and social health. Enhanced fitness wellness favorably affects body image (Ford et al., 1989; Reel et al., 2009; Tucker & Maxwell, 1992), depression and anxiety (De Matos, Calmeiro, & Da Fonseca, 2009; Juchmès-Férir et al., 1971; Landers, n.d.), self-esteem (Daley, Copeland, Wright, Roalfe, & Wales, 2006), quality of life (Martin, Church, Thompson, Earnest, & Blair, 2009), and mood (e.g., Folkins, 1976). Research also suggests that enhanced body composition wellness favorably affects body image, self-esteem, and quality of life (Foster et al., 2004). Improved nutritional wellness decreases depression and enhances quality of life (Grieger, Nowson, & Ackland, 2009). Alcohol abuse is associated with severe anxiety, insomnia, and depressive episodes (Donnelly, 2009; Schuckit, 2009), and there is a causal relationship between it and major depression (Fergusson, Bodden, & Horwood, 2009). Tobacco use is associated with anxiety and depression (Ziedonis et al., 2008).

Numerous studies indicate that fitness wellness improves the mental and social health of those with a chronic disease. A fitness wellness intervention improved mental health scales and self-efficacy for health behaviors in women with multiple sclerosis (Stuifbergen et al., 2003). Fitness wellness also counteracts depression and fatigue and may improve quality of life and produces an immunomodulatory effect in persons with multiple sclerosis (Waschbisch, Tallner, Pfeifer, & Mäurer, 2009). Pippenger and Scalzitti (2004) found that when children with cerebral palsy engage in strength training, their body image, level of satisfaction, and well-being improved, and they were more sociable and outgoing.

Physical Wellness Can Affect the Ability to Engage and Progress in Physical Therapy

Physical wellness affects a patient's/client's ability to engage in and progress in physical therapy. For instance, fitness wellness is linked to functional performance of elderly people living in a long-term care facility (Singh, Chin, Paw, Bosscher, & van Mechelen,

2006), and enhanced fitness and nutritional wellness can facilitate the progression from a transitional setting to participation in the community (Rimmer, 1999).

If a restorative patient's premorbid physical wellness is poor, then the patient may be able to tolerate only a conservative, if not initially a rather palliative, treatment plan. Patients/clients who are able to engage only in a conservative treatment plan may require an extended duration of rehabilitation and/or may not be able to achieve maximum benefit from the physical therapy. In contrast, if a patient's premorbid fitness and body composition wellness is good, then the patient may be able to tolerate a more aggressive treatment plan. I once provided physical therapy to an 80-year-old woman who had fallen and fractured her tibia and could bear only partial weight on her affected extremity. Prior to the accident, she had a high level of fitness wellness. Upon my examination of her, which was a few weeks after the fracture, she presented as a physically fit individual within her limitations secondary to her fractured tibia. While many individuals her age would have required a walker to ambulate secondary to her weight-bearing status, my patient was able to utilize crutches and engage in many of her activities of daily living (ADLs) independently and safely.

Physical Therapy Practice Is Expanding into the Fitness Wellness Arena

Historically, physical therapy has focused on restorative care (Moffat, 1996) rather than on wellness or even fitness wellness (Fair, 2005). One goal of the APTA (2006b) in its Vision 2020 plan is for physical therapists to be recognized as "exercise leaders." However, despite physical therapists' ability to play a larger role, they currently play a relatively small role in the fitness wellness arena. Figure 4-1 depicts the current status of physical therapists in the fitness wellness arena.

Fortunately, as in the classic Bob Dylan song, "The times they are a changin'" (1991, para. 1). Above and beyond the role as exercise leaders, I propose that physical therapists with an expertise in fitness wellness advance to providing all of the fitness wellness care for the U.S. population, just as the profession strives to provide all of other types of care (e.g., improving ambulation). Figure 4-2 depicts my proposal for the future status of the relationship between the practice of physical therapy and the arena of fitness wellness. Because an increasing number of physical therapists are achieving an operational knowledge of fitness wellness and specializing in fitness wellness, they are increasingly equipped to facilitate fitness wellness in the United States and, as a profession, should pursue this important initiative with vigor!

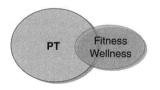

Figure 4-1 The Current Status of Physical Therapists in the Fitness Wellness Arena

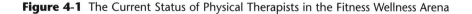

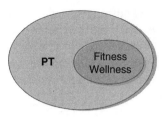

Figure 4-2 Fair's Proposal for the Future Status between the Practice of Physical Therapy and the Arena of Fitness Wellness

Physical Therapists Are Viewed as Wellness Experts and Role Models

Patients/clients ask physical therapists about wellness, particularly nutritional, fitness, and body composition wellness, because physical therapists are medical professionals and more and more often are also credentialed as doctors (Fair, 2004b). They are also viewed as fitness wellness role models (Fair, 2004b; Landry, 2004). Even when a physical therapist provides sound recommendations, a patient/client may mimic actions of the therapist that are contrary to the advice.

Physical therapists should possess a basic knowledge of nutritional, fitness, and body composition wellness and the ability and willingness to critically analyze the wellness information she or he has obtained to ensure that it is valid and reliable before applying it in the therapeutic realm or sharing it with patients. As with other types of physical therapy, wellness therapy should be evidence based, and advice must be based upon empirical research rather than only anecdotal data. The physical therapist should seek out additional information as necessary and then decide if she or he should answer the patient's/client's question or refer the patient to an appropriate specialist.

Case Scenarios:

Case 1. You are an outpatient physical therapist, and Betty is a patient under your care for restorative physical therapy secondary to tennis elbow. During one session, Betty confides that she'll be attending her 15th high school reunion in 2 weeks and she really wants to look good. She explains that her friend wore a plastic suit in a sauna, lost almost 5 pounds in just a few hours, and looked a lot thinner. Betty asks for your opinion. When you give Betty feedback, you would want to share with her that when a person sweats, she loses water weight. Sweating a lot does not cause fat loss, only dehydration. Excessive dehydration can cause weakness and lightheadedness and even more serious complications if fluid loss and electrolyte loss are excessive. You need to be sure that Betty understands that if she wears a plastic suit in a sauna she will lose weight, but it will be water weight rather than fat weight. The weight loss will be temporary and could be dangerous to her health. This scenario underscores why it so important that physical therapists have a basic knowledge of fitness wellness.

Case 2. You are a physical therapist in a private practice clinic, and one of your restorative patients, Sally, asks you about a diet that she has recently read about in *Shape* magazine. Your information about the diet might be based solely upon hearsay, or you may have read a peer-reviewed article about it. While it may be appropriate to supplement your evidence-based knowledge about the diet with your personal experience with other patients/clients, if you possess no evidence-based knowledge about the diet (or the mechanism of the diet), it would be imprudent to give her advice based upon anecdotal data. How you address Sally's inquiry about the diet is just as important as the traditional therapy you are providing to her, as both can have a significant impact upon her health. Above all, you must not cause Sally harm. For example, Sally may be a diabetic and the diet may be contraindicated. Not only do you not want to harm Sally, you also do not want to mislead her. For example, the magazine article might claim that the diet will cause those who follow it to lose 10 pounds in 2 weeks. What should your feedback be to Sally about this claim? Suppose you have a friend who tried the diet and did lose 10 pounds in 2 weeks—should you share your anecdotal information with Sally? How likely is it that Sally will lose 10 pounds in 2 weeks if she adheres to the diet? If she does, will most of the weight loss be in the form of fat, or will most of it be in the form of water-secondary-glycogen depletion and diuresis? Is the diet healthy? For example, does it supply an adequate amount of fiber, protein, vitamins, and so on? How much nutritional expertise do you possess? Should you refer Sally to a registered dietician (RD)? This scenario illustrates why it is important that physical therapists possess a basic knowledge of nutritional and body composition wellness, especially those dimensions that are likely to present themselves in physical therapy, and provide guidance only on issues about which they possess an expertise.

Case 3. You are an outpatient physical therapist, and one of your patients, Joe, is under your care for restorative physical therapy secondary to a sporting accident. Although you instruct Joe to hold each stretch you prescribe for 30 to 60 seconds, you hold your stretches for 6 seconds when you stretch in the clinic during your lunch break, and Joe happens to be present and notices you. Despite your request, Joe may mimic you, his doctor, and not hold his stretches for a significant duration.

Knowledge of Wellness and Physical Wellness Are Accreditation Requirements in Entry-Level Physical Therapy Curriculum

Given all of the previously discussed reasons for physical therapists to possess an operational knowledge of physical wellness, it should be no surprise that the accreditation body of entry-level physical therapy programs (i.e., the Commission on the Accreditation of Physical Therapist Education [CAPTE], 2004) requires an education in wellness (discussed in Chapter 2) and physical wellness (detailed in Chapters 5 through 7).

Summary: Why Physical Therapists Should Possess an Operational Knowledge of Physical Wellness

Physical therapists should possess an operational knowledge of physical wellness for numerous reasons: (1) physical therapy patients/clients present with physical diagnoses and comorbidities, and these conditions are linked to physical wellness; (2) physical therapy patients/clients present with impaired physical wellness, including drug wellness (e.g., American Heart Association, 2009a; CDC, 2007b; Johnson, 2007) and nutritional, fitness, and/or body composition wellness (e.g., Barnes, 2007; Briefel & Johnson, 2004); (3) components of physical wellness affect each other (Ford et al., 1989; Tucker & Maxwell, 1992); (4) enhanced nutritional and fitness wellness decreases the risk of certain diseases (e.g., Manson et al., 1994; Wilson, 2009), and decreased nutritional and fitness wellness increases the risk of certain diseases (e.g., McNaughton et al., 2009; Weinstein, 2008); (5) drug wellness is linked to health (e.g., Schuckit, 2009); (6) enhanced fitness wellness favorably affects mental health (e.g., De Matos et al., 2009; Martin, 2009); (7) enhanced nutritional wellness favorably affects mental health (e.g., Foster et al., 2004); (8) impaired drug wellness is associated with poor mental health (e.g., Schuckit, 2009; Ziedonis et al., 2008); (9) enhanced fitness wellness improves the mental and social health of those with a chronic disease (e.g., Stuifbergen et al., 2003; Waschbisch et al., 2009); (10) physical wellness can enhance, impede, or even contraindicate physical therapy; (11) physical therapy practice is expanding into the fitness wellness arena (APTA, 2006b); (12) physical therapists are viewed as wellness experts and models (Fair, 2004b; Landry, 2004); and (13) physical wellness is an accreditation requirement for all (U.S.) entry-level physical therapy programs (CAPTE, 2004).

chapter five

Physical Wellness and Nutrition

Tell me what you eat, and I will tell you what you are.

◾ ◾ ◾ ◾ ◾ ◾ ◾ ◾ ◾ ◾ ◾ ◾ ◾

Anthelme Brillat-Saravin

OBJECTIVES

Upon completion of this chapter, you should be able to:

1. Discuss the provision of nutritional wellness by physical therapists, including the concepts and expertise in nutritional wellness and scope of care.
2. Discuss concepts related to nutritional wellness, including caloric input, nutritional substrates, and food groups.
3. Explore the nutritional components of the history, systems review, and test measures.
4. Examine, apply, and critique templates of a Nutritional Wellness History, Nutritional Wellness Systems Review, and Nutritional Wellness Tests and Measures.
5. Explore the nutritional components of an evaluation.
6. Discuss nutritional wellness diagnoses and conditions.
7. Discuss concepts related to the nutritional wellness goals and a plan of care.
8. In terms of nutritional wellness, discuss prognosis, interventions, and outcomes.

SECTION 1: NUTRITIONAL WELLNESS AND SCOPE OF CARE OF PHYSICAL THERAPY PRACTICE

Addressing nutritional wellness is within the scope of physical therapy. While it is not expected that all physical therapists obtain an expertise in nutritional wellness, just as not all of them possess an expertise in such areas as neurology, home health, women's health, or aquatic therapy; all of them should possess a basic competence in this area (CAPTE, 2004). Each physical therapist should possess enough knowledge about nutritional wellness to examine basic aspects of nutrition during the Systems Review and analyze the results of the screens. If the results indicate there may be a nutritional wellness problem and the physical therapist possesses the expertise to address it, then she or he should examine nutritional wellness in the tests and measures. If the physical therapist does not possess the necessary expertise to address the potential nutritional problem, then she or he should refer the patient/client to a registered dietician. Nutritional concerns that are within the scope of appropriately educated physical therapists include but are not limited to the disease obesity (ICD-9-CM 278) and the conditions excessive caloric intake, deficient fiber intake, deficient intake of vegetables, and excessive intake of sugars and sweets. (Note: Nutritional conditions are discussed in Section 8.) Nutritional concerns that are outside the scope of physical therapy include but are not limited to diseases such as diabetes (ICD-9-CM 250), protein-calorie malnutrition (ICD-9-CM 262), and morbid obesity (ICD-9-CM 278.01).

Possessing at least a basic competence in nutritional wellness is indicated for many reasons. First, physical therapy patients/clients who are classified in an American Physical Therapy Practice Pattern (APTA, 2006b), including the preventative patterns, also may present with impaired nutritional wellness. For example, a restorative patient with the diagnosis of bilateral knee osteoarthritis (ICD-9-CM 715) and classified in the APTA's Preferred Practice Pattern 4D: Impaired joint mobility, motor function, muscle performance, and range of motion associated with connective tissue dysfunction may present also with the conditions overfat and excessive caloric intake.

Second, good nutritional wellness can prevent or delay chronic diseases, including diabetes mellitus, obesity, osteoporosis, stroke, and various types of cancer (Schlienger & Pradiqnac, 2009). For example, a diet lower in calories and saturated fat and higher in vegetables, whole grains, and fruits may reduce hyperinsulinic responses and thereby reduce the risk of developing diabetes (Schlienger & Pradiqnac, 2009). Joshipura et al. (2008) found that higher intakes of fiber, vegetables, and certain fruits decreases the risk of developing cardiovascular disease, including nonfatal and fatal myocardial infarction and ischemic stroke.

Third, nutritional wellness can enhance, impede, or even contraindicate physical therapy. For example, if a patient's/client's caloric intake is very low, it may be significantly difficult for her or him to engage in a vigorous exercise session. One study found that low carbohydrate dieting causes memory impairments during the times when available glycogen stores are at their lowest (D'Anci, Watts, Kanarek, & Taylor, 2009).

Fourth, physical therapists are sometimes viewed as nutritional experts and role models. Patients/clients ask physical therapists, perhaps especially those who are "doctors," questions related to nutritional wellness. For example, a restorative patient or wellness client might ask you what you think about the Atkins diet.

Finally, nutritional wellness is an accreditation requirement for all U.S. entry-level physical therapist programs (CAPTE, 2004). *A Normative Model of Physical Therapist Professional Education* (CAPTE, 2004) includes a nutrition section, which contends that physical therapists be able to compare diets for all populations for health, fitness, and wellness; and examine the diets (including any supplements) for all populations. It further states that examples of instructional objectives related to nutrition include but are not limited to:

- Describe the normal intake of carbohydrates, proteins, fats, vitamins, water and minerals in daily American diets.
- Compare the differences in diet in athletes of different sports.
- Describe effects of performing enhancing supplements and the side effects of usage of these supplements (p. 87).

Summary: Nutritional Wellness and Scope of Care

Nutritional wellness is within the scope of physical therapy. Possessing at least a basic competence in nutritional wellness is indicated for many reasons. All physical therapists should be able to screen nutritional wellness during a Systems Review.

SECTION 2: BASIC TERMINOLOGY AND CONCEPTS

Alcohol

Alcoholic beverages contain ethyl alcohol, carbohydrates, and calories. Ethyl alcohol, or ethanol, is an intoxicating ingredient found in wine, beer, and liquor (Centers for Disease Control and Prevention, 2008). A standard drink is equal to 0.6 ounces (13.7 grams) of pure alcohol: 12 ounces of beer, 8 ounces of malt liquor, 5 ounces of wine, or 1.5 ounces or a "shot" of 80-proof liquor (e.g., gin, rum, vodka, whiskey). Alcohol is not nutrient-dense. For example, 12 fluid ounces of regular beer is 146 calories, and contains 13 grams (g) carbohydrates, 0.7 g fiber, 1 g protein, no fat, 0.1 g iron, 18 milligrams (mg) calcium, 89 mg potassium, no vitamin A, 0.02 mg thiamin (vitamin B_1), 0.09 mg riboflavin (vitamin B_2), 1.6 mg niacin (vitamin B_3), and no ascorbic acid (vitamin C). Three and a half fluid ounces of red table wine is 74 calories and contains 2 g of carbohydrates, no fiber, a trace amount of protein, no fat, 0.4 g iron, 8 mg calcium, 115 mg potassium, no vitamin A, 0.01 mg thiamin, 0.03 mg riboflavin, 0.1 mg niacin, and no ascorbic acid (Gebhardt & Thomas, 2002).

Alcohol is produced by the fermentation of sugars, starches, and yeast (CDC, 2008). When alcohol is ingested, the body converts a small amount into fat and the liver converts the majority of alcohol into acetate (University of Rochester, 2008). Because the liver can only metabolize a small amount of alcohol at a time, the excess circulates in the bloodstream

(CDC, 2008) where it replaces fat as a source of fuel. Individual reactions to alcohol vary and are influenced by many factors, including but not limited to age, gender, ethnicity or race, physical condition, amount of food consumed before drinking, how quickly the alcohol was consumed, use of drugs or prescription medicines, and family history of alcohol problems (CDC, 2008).

The typical alcoholic beverage is high in calories and carbohydrates and devoid of protein, fat, and most micronutrients. For example, 12 fluid ounces of regular beer contains 146 calories; 13 g carbohydrate; 0.7 g fiber; no protein, fat, cholesterol, vitamin A, or ascorbic acid; 18 mg calcium, 0.1 mg iron, 89 mg potassium, 0.02 mg thiamin; 0.09 mg riboflavin; 1.6 mg niacin; and 18 mg sodium (Gebhardt & Thomas, 2002).

Athletes

In terms of nutrition, those who participate in a grueling exercise regimen should be considered an athlete. For example, an endurance-running athlete might run 2 to 3 hours each day, and a gymnast athlete might train for 5 hours per day, 6 days per week. Those who do not engage in a more moderate or heavy exercise regimen, rather than a grueling one, should not be considered an athlete for nutritional purposes. For example, those who engage in 30 minutes of moderate-intensity exercise on most days (i.e., those who meet the *Healthy People 2010* guidelines) and those who regularly engage in a moderate-strength training protocol should not be considered athletes insofar as their nutrition is concerned.

Beverages

Beverages include but are not limited to water, coffees, teas, milks, juice cocktails, sodas, and alcohol. Certain beverages are part of another food group. For example, 100% fruit juices are part of the fruit group and 100% vegetable juices are part of the vegetable group. Beverages vary in their caloric and nutrient content. For example, 1 cup of fruit punch contains 117 calories, 30 g carbohydrate, 0.2 g fiber, 0 g protein and fat, 0 g cholesterol, 20 mg calcium, 0.5 mg iron, 62 g potassium, 35 International Units (IU) of vitamin A, 0.5 g thiamin, 0.6 g riboflavin, 0.1 g niacin, 73 g ascorbic acid, and 55 mg sodium. In contrast, 6 fluid ounces of black brewed tea contains 2 calories; 1 g carbohydrate; no fiber, fat, protein, cholesterol, calcium, vitamin A, thiamin, niacin, or ascorbic acid; 66 mg potassium; and 5 mg sodium (Gebhardt & Thomas, 2002).

Calorie and Caloric Intake

A calorie is a unit of fuel. In this nutritional context, calories in food and beverages supply energy to the human body to sustain life. One calorie is defined as the amount of heat (energy) to raise 1 g of water 1°C (1.8°F). In the physical sciences, joules is used as the unit of measure, where 1 calorie = 4.184 joules. Most food packaging lists the nutritional content and ingredients in kilocalories, where 1 kilocalorie = 1000 calories. For example, 1 cup of popcorn is listed on the package as being 30 calories, meaning it is 30 kilocalories and 30,000 regular calories. Caloric intake refers to the number of calories consumed by an individual during a specific time frame, such as 1 day. Typically, caloric intake should be compared to caloric output, because it is the balance between input and output that impacts total body weight, fat weight, and muscle weight.

Carbohydrates

There are two major types of carbohydrates: simple and complex. Examples of simple carbohydrates include fructose, the sugar in fruit; glucose, the carbohydrate transported in the bloodstream for immediate energy needs; sucrose, common table sugar; and lactose, the sugar in milk. Examples of complex carbohydrates, called polysaccharides, include glycogen, which is stored in the liver and muscle cells and is used to resupply glucose as it is metabolized; starch, which is found in vegetables, grains, and, to a lesser extent, fruits; and dietary fibers, which are the parts of plants that cannot be digested and help move waste through the digestive organs for eventual elimination. Grains and vegetables contain a high percentage of complex carbohydrates. Meat products contain essentially no carbohydrates.

Carbohydrates have several essential roles in the chemical and chemical processes that maintain life in the human body.

1. Carbohydrates are an energy source particularly during anaerobic and high-intensity activities.
2. They help to preserve tissue protein.
3. They serve as the metabolic primer for fat catabolism, which is the process of breaking down complex molecules to obtain energy.
4. Carbohydrates are the primary fuel source in the central nervous system.

Coffee

"Coffee is reported to be among the most widely consumed beverages in the world" (Higdon & Frei, 2006, p. 101). Common foods and medications that contain caffeine include cold medicines, coffee beans, cocoa beans, soft drinks, tea leaves, cola nuts, and chocolate. According to Higdon and Frei:

> Coffee is a complex mixture of chemicals that provides significant amounts of chlorogenic acid and caffeine. Unfiltered coffee is a significant source of cafestol and kahweol, which are diterpenes that have been implicated in the cholesterol-raising effects of coffee. The results of epidemiological research suggest that coffee consumption may help prevent several chronic diseases, including type 2 diabetes mellitus, Parkinson's disease and liver disease (cirrhosis and hepatocellular carcinoma). Most prospective cohort studies have not found coffee consumption to be associated with significantly increased cardiovascular disease risk. However, coffee consumption is associated with increases in several cardiovascular disease risk factors, including blood pressure and plasma homocysteine. At present, there is little evidence that coffee consumption increases the risk of cancer. For adults consuming moderate amounts of coffee (3–4 cups/d providing 300–400 mg/d of caffeine), there is little evidence of health risks and some evidence of health benefits. However, some groups, including people with hypertension, children, adolescents, and the elderly, may be more vulnerable to the adverse effects of caffeine. In addition, currently available evidence

suggests that it may be prudent for pregnant women to limit coffee consumption to 3 cups/d providing no more than 300 mg/d of caffeine to exclude any increased probability of spontaneous abortion or impaired fetal growth. (p. 101)

Clinical implications of caffeine include: (1) Caffeine makes the heart work harder by raising blood pressure and heart rate; therefore, it is important to monitor your patients with heart conditions who may be under the influence of excessive amounts of caffeine (Higdon & Frei, 2006); (2) It may be wise for coronary artery patients to avoid caffeine consumption prior to exercising (Higdon & Frei, 2006); and (3) Caffeine consumption may increase blood lactate concentrations; therefore we, as therapists, should be able to understand why our patients may have acute muscle soreness during exercise (Shearer, 2007).

Dietary Reference Intake, Reference Daily Intake, and Recommended Daily Intake

In 1941, the Food and Nutrition Board of the National Academy of Sciences established the Recommended Dietary Allowances (RDAs) that were subsequently updated 10 times and were defined as "the levels of intake of essential nutrients that are judged to be adequate to meet the known needs of practically all healthy persons" (Penland, 2005, para. 1). In 1995, the Food and Nutrition Board deemed that a more comprehensive approach to establishing guidelines was required to promote health and prevent chronic diseases, and developed the *Dietary Reference Intakes (DRIs)*. The DRIs include the RDAs, which is the average daily dietary intake of a nutrient that is sufficient to meet the requirement of nearly all (97–98%) healthy persons, and *Adequate Intake (AI)*, a number based on observed intakes of the nutrient by a group of healthy persons and is only established when the RDA cannot be determined (USDA, 2004).

Dietician (Versus Nutritionist)

A dietician has graduated from a college or university with a degree in nutrition and has passed a licensure examination. A dietician has an expertise in food and nutrition. In contrast, there is no licensure requirement or minimal educational requirement to be a nutritionist. A nutritionist may have little or no education or practical experience in nutrition. Unlike dieticians, nutritionists are not regulated.

Fats

Most foods contain several different kinds of fats, including sterols and monounsaturated, polyunsaturated, saturated, and trans fats. Unsaturated fats are more healthy and saturated and trans fats are less healthy kinds.

Monounsaturated fats are found in oils such as olive oil (77% monounsaturated fatty acids), peanut oil, canola oil, and the oil in pecans, avocados, and almonds (Mayo Clinic, 2009a). Polyunsaturated fats are found in oils, such as sunflower, safflower, corn, and soybean. One type of polyunsaturated fat are Omega-3 fatty acids, which are found in fatty cold-water fish such as salmon, herring, and mackerel, flax oil, flaxseeds, and walnuts. Omega-3 fatty acids may help to reduce the blood pressure in those with hypertension, prevent arrhythmias, and reduce the risk of coronary artery disease (Mayo Clinic, 2009a).

Saturated fats are found in animal products such as butter (62% saturated fatty acids), beef (52% saturated fatty acids), chicken, lamb, pork, egg yolk, cheese, cream, and milk (Mayo Clinic, 2009a). Saturated fatty acids from the plant kingdom include vegetable shortening, hydrogenated margarine, coconut oil, and palm oil. Saturated fats are also plentiful in products such as cakes, cookies, and pies. A diet high in saturated fats is linked to increased low-density lipoprotein (LDL) blood levels and coronary artery disease (CAD) (Food and Nutrition Board, 2005).

Another lipid of importance are trans-fatty acids, which are found in partially hydrogenated vegetable oils, fried foods (such as doughnuts and French fries), shortening, and margarine, and products such as crackers, cookies, and cakes. Like saturated fats, trans-fatty acids are considered unhealthy. "As with saturated fatty acids, there is a positive linear trend between trans-fatty acid intake and LDL cholesterol concentration, and therefore increased risk of CHD" (Food and Nutrition Board, 2005, p. 1319).

Sterols are also fats. Dietary cholesterol is not technically a fat, but it is found in food derived from animal sources. Animal products include meat, poultry, seafood, eggs, dairy products, lard, and butter. Intake of dietary cholesterol increases blood cholesterol levels, but not as much as saturated and trans fats do (Mayo Clinic, 2009a).

Fats are essential to human function in several ways.

1. Fats are the primary energy source during rest and during all other aerobic activities.
2. Fat-soluble vitamins are transported and stored in fat.
3. Stored fat insulates the body and helps to regulate the body's temperature (thermodynamics).
4. Satiation from fats lasts longer than energy from carbohydrates and proteins, which is the reason for feeling full longer.

Fiber

Fiber is an important part of a healthy diet. Because humans do not have the enzymes to fully digest fiber, they do not yield a significant amount of energy to the body. There are two types of fiber: water soluble and water insoluble. Water soluble fiber is found primarily in oat bran, beans, brown rice, peas, carrots, and certain fruits. Water insoluble fiber is found primarily in wheat bran.

Fiber has many health-promoting benefits, especially when considering the prevention and treatment of colon cancer, cardiovascular diseases, obesity, gastrointestinal disorders, and diabetes (Marlett, McBurney, Slavin, & American Dietetic Association, 2002). Empirical research provides evidence that a high-fiber diet is helpful in the management of diabetes (Rodrigues, Dutra de Oliverira, de Souza, & Silva, 2005). A high intake of water soluble fiber also can help to reduce serum cholesterol (Brown, Rosner, Willett, & Sacks, 1999). One study found that each 10-gram daily increase of fiber produced a 14% decrease in coronary risk (Pereira, O'Reilly, Augustsson, Fraser, Goldbourt, et al., 2004). Water insoluble fiber may reduce constipation, adds bulk to feces, and aids in the prevention of gastrointestinal disorders (Bente, Hiza, & Fungwe, 2008). The typical U.S. low-fiber diet is considered to be the main cause of colonic diverticular disease (Korzenik, 2006). A low-fiber diet can contribute to reduced incidence to various types of cancer, such as prostate cancer (Walsh, 2003) and colon cancer (Jenab & Thompson, 1998; Schmitz & Folsch, 2000; Trock, Lanza, & Greenwalk, 1990). In contrast, a high-fiber diet is linked to a decreased body weight (i.e., less body fat) (Raben, Jensen, Marckmann, Sandstrom, & Astrup, 1995) and is recommended for those who are obese (Alfieri, Pomerleau, Grace, & Anderson, 1995).

Fruits

All fruits and 100% fruit juices are members of the fruit group. In general, 1 cup of fruit, 100% fruit juice, or one-half cup of dried fruit can be considered as one serving from the fruit group. Similar to vegetables, fruits may be raw or cooked; fresh, frozen, canned, or dried/dehydrated, and may be whole, cut up, or pureed. Examples of fruits are apple, apricot, avocado, banana, berries (cherries, raspberries, strawberries), grapefruit, grapes, Kiwi fruit, lemon, lime, mango, melons (cantaloupe, honeydew, watermelon), mixed fruits (fruit cocktail), nectarine, orange, papaya, peach, pear, pineapple, plum, prune, raisin, tangerine, and 100% fruit juice from any of the cited examples. The typical fruit is low calorie and nutrient-dense; and contains complex healthy carbohydrate (e.g., fructose), some fiber, some protein, minimal to no fat, and cholesterol. For example, 1 cup of sliced bananas is 138 calories and contains 35 g carbohydrate, 3.6 g fiber, 2 g protein, ½ g fat, 0 g cholesterol, 9 mg calcium, 0.5 mg iron, 594 mg potassium, 122 IU vitamin A, 0.07 mg thiamin, 0.15 mg riboflavin, 0.2 mg niacin, and 14 mg ascorbic acid (Gebhardt & Thomas, 2002).

Grains

Any food made from wheat, rice, oats, cornmeal, barley, or other cereal is a grain product. Examples of grains are bread, pasta, oatmeal, breakfast cereals, tortillas, and grits. In general, one serving or ounce of grain is equivalent to one slice of bread, 1 cup of ready-to-eat cereal, or ½ cup of cooked rice, cooked pasta, or cooked cereal. Grains are divided into two subgroups: whole grains and refined grains (USDA, 2008f).

Whole grains contain the entire grain kernel: the bran, germ, and endosperm. The typical whole grain is low-calorie and nutrient-dense, a good source of healthy carbohydrate, rich in fiber, contains some protein, and has little to no fat or cholesterol. Examples include whole wheat flour, bulgur (cracked wheat), oatmeal, whole cornmeal, and brown rice. The typical whole grain contains significant carbohydrate and fiber, some protein, minimal to no fat or cholesterol, and significant vitamins and minerals. For example, 1 cup of brown rice is 216 calories and contains 45 g carbohydrate, 3.5 g fiber, 5 g protein, 2 g fat, 0 g cholesterol, 20 mg calcium, 0.8 mg iron, 84 mg potassium, 0.19 mg thiamin, 0.05 mg riboflavin, and 3.0 mg niacin (Gebhardt & Thomas, 2002). Some whole-grain products contain significant amounts of bran, which is high fiber and important for health. However, products with added bran or bran alone (e.g., oat bran) are not necessarily whole-grain products.

Refined grains have been milled, a process that removes the bran and germ, two parts of the grain kernel. This is done to give grains a finer texture and improve their shelf lives, but it also removes dietary fiber, iron, and many B vitamins. The typical refined grain is low calorie but not nutrient-dense. It contains little fiber and a relatively small percentage of vitamins and minerals. For example, one piece (½) of a 9-inch yellow cake (made with water, egg whites, and no frosting) is 180 calories, and contains 37 g carbohydrate, 0.6 g fiber, 3 g protein, 2 g fat, 0 g of cholesterol, 69 mg calcium, 0.6 mg iron, 41 mg potassium, 6.0 IU of vitamin A, 0.06 mg thiamin, 0.12 mg riboflavin, 0.6 mg niacin, and 0 mg ascorbic acid (Gebhardt & Thomas, 2002).

When certain B vitamins (i.e., thiamin, riboflavin, niacin, folic acid) and iron are added back to a grain after processing, the grain is "enriched." Examples of enriched grains are white flour, degermed cornmeal, white bread, and white rice. The typical enriched grain is low calorie and nutrient-dense but contains significant carbohydrate, little fiber, some protein, and minimal to no fat or cholesterol. For example, 1 cup of enriched white rice is 205 calories and contains 45 g carbohydrate, 0.6 g fiber, 4 g protein, 0.5 g fat, 0 g cholesterol, 15 mg calcium, 1.9 mg iron, 55 mg potassium, 0.26 mg thiamin, 0.02 mg riboflavin, and 2.3 mg niacin (Gebhardt & Thomas, 2002). Comparatively, whole grains contain the greatest amount of vitamins and minerals and refined grains the least.

Milk and Dairy Products

All fluid milk products and many foods made from milk are considered part of the calcium-rich food group. Foods made from milk that retain their calcium content are part of the group, while foods made from milk that have little to no calcium—such as cream cheese, cream, and butter—are not. Some commonly consumed choices in the milk, yogurt, and cheese group are milk (fat-free/skim, low fat/1%, reduced fat/2%, whole milk), flavored milk (chocolate, strawberry), lactose-reduced and lactose-free milks, milk-based desserts (puddings made with milk, ice milk, frozen yogurt, ice cream), cheese (hard natural, e.g., cheddar, mozzarella, Swiss, parmesan; soft, e.g., ricotta, cottage, processed American); and yogurt (fat-free, low fat, reduced fat, whole milk). Milk and milk products contain carbohydrates (e.g., lactose), some protein, and often, fat. In general, 1 cup of milk or 2 cups of a milk product can be considered as one serving from the milk and dairy product group.

Food and drink items within this food group are high in carbohydrate and moderate in protein, contain no fiber, and vary in terms of fat, calories, and nutrient density. For example, 1 cup of whole milk is 150 calories and contains 11 g carbohydrate (primarily lactose), 8 g protein, 8 g fat, 291 mg calcium, 0.1 mg iron, 370 mg potassium, 307 IU of vitamin A, 0.09 mg thiamin, 0.40 mg riboflavin, 0.2 mg niacin, and 2 mg ascorbic acid; 1 cup of skim milk is 86 calories and contains 12 g carbohydrate (primarily lactose), 8 g protein, a trace amount of fat, 302 mg calcium, 0.1 mg iron, 370 mg potassium, 500 IU of vitamin A, 0.09 mg thiamin, 0.34 mg riboflavin, 0.2 mg niacin, and 2 mg ascorbic acid (Gebhardt & Thomas, 2002). While whole milk and skim milk are similar in terms of carbohydrate, protein, vitamins, and minerals, they are significantly different in terms of fat and calories. Because the amount of vitamins and minerals remains constant, the low-fat and low-calorie items are more nutrient-dense than the higher-fat and higher-calorie items.

Minerals

Dietary minerals other than the elements carbon, hydrogen, nitrogen, and oxygen (which are present in common organic molecules) are the chemical elements required by living organisms. At least seven minerals are required to support biochemical processes, many playing a role as electrolytes or in cell structure and function. Numerous minerals are required by humans in sufficient quantity (e.g., RDA $\geq$ 200 mg/d) and are referred to as *major minerals*: calcium (for muscle, heart, and digestive system health, builds bone, neutralizes acidity, and supports synthesis and function of blood cells), chloride (for production of hydrochloric acid in the stomach and in cellular pump functions), magnesium (to process adenosine 5'-triphosphate [ATP] and related reactions [health, builds bone, increases alkalinity]), phosphorus (a component of bones [see apatite], energy processing, and many other functions like bone mineralization), and potassium and sodium (each of which serve as a systemic electrolyte and is essential in coregulating ATP with sodium).

There are also numerous *trace minerals,* which are defined as RDAs less than 200 mg/d. Cobalt is required for biosynthesis of the vitamin B_{12} family of coenzymes and copper (which is a component of many redox enzymes, including cytochrome c oxidase). Fluorine helps to form tooth enamel, which contains fluoroapatite, iodine is required for the biosynthesis of thyroxine; iron is needed by many proteins and enzymes, notably hemoglobin; manganese is a cofactor in the function of antioxidant enzymes such as superoxide dismutase; molybdenum is required for xanthine oxidase and related oxidases; nickel is present in urease; selenium is required for peroxidase/antioxidant proteins; sulfur, an essential component of cysteine and methionine amino acids, participates as an enzyme cofactor; and zinc is required for several enzymes such as carboxypeptidase, liver alcohol dehydrogenase, and carbonic anhydrase. There is no evidence that other elements, such as chromium and vanadium, are important to maintaining human health.

Oils and Fats

All oils and fats are considered part of this group. In general, 1 tablespoon of oil, margarine, butter, or salad dressing is considered to be a single serving in this food group. Food items are high in fat and calories and contain no carbohydrate, fiber, vitamins, and minerals. Accordingly, items in this food group are nutrient-dense. While all items contain a significant amount of fat, they vary in the type of fat they contain. For example, while 1 tablespoon of safflower oil and 1 tablespoon of soybean oil each contain 120 calories, the safflower oil contains 0.8 g saturated fat, 10.2 g monounsaturated fat, and 2.0 g of polyunsaturated fat, while soybean oil contains 2.4 g saturated fat, 4.0 g monounsaturated fat, and 6.5 g polyunsaturated fat (Gebhardt & Thomas, 2002).

Protein

Dietary protein can be either complete or incomplete. Complete proteins, which are typically found only in the animal kingdom, contain each of the 10 essential *amino acids.* In contrast, incomplete proteins, which are typically found in the plant kingdom, are missing one or more of the essential amino acids. Although incomplete proteins lack one or more essential amino acids, an individual may consume two incomplete proteins during a meal (e.g., two different foods, such as beans and peas) and the human body recognizes what has been ingested as a complete protein. This is why vegans, who adhere to the strictest type of a vegetarian diet, can avoid animal products and yet still meet their daily protein intake requirement.

Protein serves essential functions in the human body, two of which are (1) amino acids help to build and maintain muscle; and (2) when carbohydrate intake is insufficient, proteins can be broken down. While a minimal amount of protein catabolism is normal and is balanced by protein anabolism, excessive protein catabolism is counterproductive and can be harmful or even fatal (Guyton & Hall, 2005).

Protein-Rich Foods

All foods made from fish, poultry, eggs, nuts, seeds, beans and peas, tofu, and meat are considered part of this group. Beans and peas are part of this group and the vegetable group. In general, 1 ounce of meat, poultry or fish, ¼ cup cooked dry beans, 1 egg, 1 tablespoon of peanut butter, or ½ ounce of nuts or seeds can be considered as one serving or ounce equivalent from this group.

Food items within this food group are moderate to high in protein; contain no carbohydrate or fiber (except beans and peas), and vary in terms of fat, calories, and nutrient density. For example, 3 ounces of an oven-cooked roast is 304 calories, and contains no carbohydrate or fiber, 19 g protein, 25 g fat (9.9 g saturated, 10.6 g monounsaturated, and 0.9 g polyunsaturated), 9 mg calcium, 2 mg iron, 256 mg potassium, no vitamin A, 0.06 mg thiamin, 0.14 mg riboflavin, 2.9 mg niacin, and no ascorbic acid. An equal amount of lean sirloin steak is 166 calories, and contains no carbohydrate or fiber, 26 g protein, 6 g fat (2.4 g saturated, 2.6 g monounsaturated, and 0.2 g polyunsaturated), 9 mg calcium, 0.25 mg riboflavin, 3.6 mg niacin, and no ascorbic acid (Gebhardt & Thomas, 2002). An example of an item within this food group that is moderate in protein is (brown and serve) sausage (i.e., 103 calories and 4 g protein in two links) (Gebhardt & Thomas, 2002).

Soda Beverages

The Food and Nutrition Board (2005) discourages the consumption of soda, such as Coca-Cola™, Diet Pepsi™, and hundreds of national and generic brands. Unless labeled "caffeine-free," soda drinks contain caffeine as well as many additives and chemicals. The implications of these chemicals are profound: Coke can be used to clean a toilet in an hour or remove stains from vitreous china. Coke and a ball of aluminum foil can be used to scrub rust from chrome, clean corrosion from car battery terminals, or loosen a rusted bolt. A can of Coke added to a load of greasy laundry will clean it of grease, and hazardous materials signs are required on trucks carrying Coke concentrate (TruthorFiction.com, 2009).

Soda beverages are typically high in carbohydrate and devoid of or low in other nutrients. For example, 12 fluid ounces of cola contains 152 calories, no fiber, protein, fat, vitamin A, thiamin, riboflavin, niacin, ascorbic acid, 11 mg calcium, 0.1 mg iron, 4 mg potassium, and 15 mg sodium.

Soups, Sauces, and Gravies

In general, 1 cup of soup, 1 tablespoon of sauce, or ¼ cup of gravy is considered as one serving in this food group. Foods within this food group vary in nutritional content. For example, 1 cup of New England clam chowder is 164 calories, and contains 17 g carbohydrate, 1.5 g fiber, 9 g protein, and 7 g fat (including 3 g saturated fat), while 1 cup of chicken noodle soup is 75 calories, and contains 9 g carbohydrate, 0.7 g fiber, 4 g protein, and 2 g fat (including 0.7 g saturated fat) (Gebhardt & Thomas, 2002).

Substrates and Substrate Intake

The nutritional substrates are carbohydrate, fat, protein, vitamins, and minerals. Vitamins and minerals are recognized as *micronutrients* because they should be consumed only in relatively small quantities. Carbohydrate, fat, and protein are *macronutrients* as they should be consumed in relatively large quantities. Respectively, a gram of fat, protein, and carbohydrate yield 9, 4, and 4 calories to the human body. Vitamins and minerals do not provide calories. As discussed previously, carbohydrates and fats can be directly metabolized for energy; protein is indirectly metabolized for energy. Each of the energy-yielding substrates also can be converted to fat and stored in adipose tissue, which is a special connective tissue that is the site for fat storage in the form of triglycerides (Guyton & Hall, 2005). (Note: Metabolism is explored in Chapter 7.)

Sugary Foods

All sugary foods, such as candy, chocolate, honey, jams, jellies, preserves, puddings, sugars, and syrups, are in this group. Examples of one serving in this food group are 1 bar of chocolate, ½₂ package of ready-to-eat frosting, 1 tablespoon of honey or syrup, ½ cup of pudding, and 1 teaspoon of sugar. Compared to their nutritive content, food items within this food group are very high in calories. For example, 1 tablespoon of pancake syrup is 57 calories and contains 15 g carbohydrate (primarily simple) but no protein or fiber, a trace amount of fat, and no trace amounts of various vitamins and minerals (Gebhardt & Thomas, 2002).

Vegetables

All vegetables and 100% vegetable juices are members of the vegetable group. In general, 1 cup of raw or cooked vegetables or vegetable juice or 2 cups of raw leafy greens are considered as one serving from the vegetable group. Vegetables may be raw or cooked; fresh, frozen, canned, or dehydrated; and may be whole, cut up, or mashed. Based upon their nutrient content, vegetables are organized into five subgroups: dark green vegetables, orange vegetables, dry beans and peas, starchy vegetables, and other vegetables (USDA, 2008g). Examples of dark green vegetables are broccoli, collard greens, dark green leafy lettuce, kale, romain lettuce, spinach, turnip greens, and watercress. Examples of orange vegetables are carrots, pumpkin, squash (acorn, butternut, and hubbard), and sweet potatoes. Examples of dry beans and peas are black beans, black-eyed peas, garbanzo beans (chickpeas), kidney beans, lentils, (mature) lima beans, navy beans, pinto beans, soy beans, split peas, and tofu. Examples of starchy vegetables are corn, green peas, lima beans, and potatoes. Examples of other vegetables are artichokes, asparagus, bean sprouts, beets, brussels sprouts, cabbage, cauliflower, celery, cucumbers, eggplant, green beans, green or red peppers, lettuce, mushrooms, okra, onions, parsnips, tomatoes, tomato juice, vegetable juice, turnips, wax beans, and zucchini.

The typical vegetable is very low calorie, very nutrient-dense, and contains significant healthy carbohydrate and fiber, some protein, and minimal to no fat or cholesterol. For example,

1 cup of spinach (from frozen) is 53 calories, and contains 10 g carbohydrate, 5.7 g fiber, 6 g protein, a trace amount of fat, 0 g cholesterol, 277 mg calcium, 2.9 mg iron, 566 mg potassium, 14,790 IU vitamin A, 0.11 mg thiamin, 0.32 mg riboflavin, 0.8 mg niacin, and 23 mg ascorbic acid (Gebhardt & Thomas, 2002).

Certain vegetables are quite high in protein. One cup of corn provides 5 g protein, 1 cup of broccoli has 5 g protein, 1 cup of spinach has 7 g protein, 1 cup of peas provides 9 g protein, and 1 cup of chickpeas provides 15 g protein (Gebhardt & Thomas, 2002). In addition to being part of the vegetable group, dry beans and peas are also part of the protein group. Protein from the plant kingdom is superior to the protein from the animal kingdom in two ways: (1) plant protein contains antioxidants and phytochemicals but animal protein does not; plant foods that are rich in protein are typically richest in phytochemicals and nutrients, and (2) while plant foods are low in saturated ("bad") fat (and fats in general), animal foods are typically high in saturated fat (American Heart Association, 2009c).

Vegetarians

Vegetarians emphasize relying upon foods from the plant kingdom as their dietary sustenance. The Vegetarian Society (n.d.) provides much information about vegetarianism. "A vegetarian is someone living on a diet of grains, pulses, nuts, seeds, vegetables and fruits with or without the use of dairy products and eggs. A vegetarian does not eat any meat, poultry, game, fish, shellfish or crustacea, or slaughter by-products" (para. 1). There are three categories of vegetarians: A lactovegetarian—the most common type of vegetarian—consumes only milk, milk products, and foods from the plant kingdom; an ovolactovegetarian consumes eggs, milk, milk products, and foods from the plant kingdom; and a vegan does not consume any animal products.

The American Dietetic Association (ADA) published a meta-analysis in 2003 summarizing important information about vegetarianism. A vegetarian, including vegan, diet can meet current recommendations for all nutrients, including protein, iron, zinc, calcium, vitamin D, riboflavin, vitamin B_{12}, vitamin A, n-3 fatty acids and iodine. In some cases, use of fortified foods or supplements can be helpful in meeting daily recommendations for individual nutrients. Well-planned vegan and other types of vegetarian diets are appropriate for all stages of the life cycle, including during pregnancy, lactation, infancy, childhood, and adolescence. Vegetarian diets offer a number of nutritional benefits, including lower levels of magnesium, potassium, folate, and antioxidants such as vitamins C and E and phytochemicals. Vegetarians have been reported to have lower body mass indices than nonvegetarians as well as lower rates of death from ischemic heart disease. They also show lower blood cholesterol levels, lower blood pressure, and lower rates of hypertension, type 2 diabetes, and prostate and colon cancers. Although a number of federally funded and institutional feeding programs can accommodate vegetarians, few have foods suitable for vegans at this time. Because of the variability of dietary practices among vegetarians, individual assessment of dietary intakes of vegetarians is required. Dietetic professionals have a responsibility to support and encourage those who express an interest in consuming a vegetarian diet. They can play key roles in educating vegetarian clients about food sources of specific nutrients, food purchase and preparation, and any dietary modifications that may be necessary to meet individual needs. Menu planning for vegetarians can be simplified by use of a food guide that specifies food groups and serving sizes. It is the position of the American Dietetic Association (2003) that appropriately planned vegetarian diets are healthful, nutritionally adequate, and provide health benefits in the prevention and treatment of certain diseases.

Vitamins

A vitamin is an organic compound required as a nutrient in tiny amounts by an organism (Lieberman & Bruning, 1990). A compound is called a vitamin when it cannot be synthesized in sufficient quantities by an organism and must be obtained from the diet. Vitamins are classified as either water soluble, meaning that they dissolve easily in water, or fat soluble, which are absorbed through the intestinal tract with the help of lipids (fats). In general, water-soluble vitamins are readily excreted from the body. Humans require 13 vitamins: four fat-soluble vitamins (A, D, E, and K) and nine water-soluble vitamins (eight B vitamins plus vitamin C).

Each vitamin is typically used in multiple reactions and therefore most have multiple functions (Dietary Reference Intakes, 2001). They function as hormones (vitamin D), antioxidants (vitamin E), mediators of cell signaling, and regulators of cell and tissue growth and differentiation (vitamin A). The largest number of vitamins, B complex vitamins, function as precursors for enzyme cofactor biomolecules (coenzymes) that help act as catalysts and substrates in metabolism.

Water

The human body contains 55% to 78% water depending on body size, body fat, and lean body weight (Guyton & Hall, 2005). About 20% of water intake comes from food with the remaining coming from drinking water and beverages. Water is excreted from the body in several forms: through urine and feces, sweating, and by exhalation of water vapor in the breath. Water has four primary functions in the human body: as a solvent, transportant, lubricant, and coolant (Guyton & Hall, 2005). Water does not contain calories unless an energy-yielding substance is added to it, such as flavoring with sugar.

Summary: Basic Terminology and Concepts

Basic terms and concepts related to nutritional wellness include alcohol; athletes; beverages; calorie and caloric intake; carbohydrate; coffee; Dietary Reference Intake (DRI), Reference Daily Intake (RDI), and Recommended Daily Intake (RDA); dietician (versus nutritionist); fat; fiber; milk and dairy foods; minerals; oils and fats; protein; protein-rich foods; soda beverages; soups, sauces, and gravies; substrates and substrate intake; sugary foods; vegetables and vegetable food group; vegetarians; vitamins; and water.

SECTION 3: NUTRITIONAL WELLNESS PYRAMIDS

The U.S. Department of Agriculture (USDA), in a chapter written by Davis and Saltos (2002), have detailed the history of their dietary recommendations. In 1894, before vitamins and minerals were even discovered, they published their first dietary recommendations.

In 1916, the first USDA's food guide was published. The guide was written by Caroline Hunt, a nutritionist, and divided food into five groups: milk and meat, cereals, vegetables and fruits, fats and fatty foods, and sugars and sugary foods.

Prompted by President Franklin Roosevelt, a National Nutrition Conference was called to action in 1941. For the first time, the USDA published Recommended Dietary Allowances (RDAs) that specified caloric intake and essential nutrients. In 1943, the USDA announced the Basic Seven, which was a special modification of the nutritional guidelines to help people deal with the shortage of food supplies during the war. Because of the complexity of the Basic Seven, the Basic Four were introduced. The Basic Four consisted of milk, meats, fruits and vegetables, and grain products.

In the late 1970s, in an effort to curtail the increasing prevalence of chronic diseases, the USDA revised the Basic Four to include the recommendation that fats, sweets, and alcoholic beverages be consumed in moderation. Although the USDA's food guide *A Pattern for Daily Food Choices* was being published annually since the 1980s, people were still not aware that it existed. Beginning in 1988, the USDA set out to create a graphic to represent the food groups. The Food Guide Pyramid was finally released in 1992. Both the graphics and text conveyed variety and proportionality by pictures of foods and the size of the food group.

The USDA changed the Food Pyramid to MyPyramid in 2005 in an effort to better educate the public about healthy nutrition. The MyPyramid is a rainbow of colored vertical stripes representing the food groups: Orange denotes grains; green denotes vegetables; red denotes fruits; yellow denotes fats and oils; blue denotes milk and dairy products; and purple denotes meat, beans, fish, and nuts. According to the USDA (2008c, para. 1), MyPyramid "offers personalized eating plans, interactive tools to help you plan and assess your food choices, and advise to help you: make smart choices from every food group; find your balance between food and physical activity; get the most nutrition out of your calories; stay within your daily calorie needs."

Harvard University asserts that the USDA's food pyramids are "based on out-of-date science and influenced by people with business interests in their messages" (2009c, para. 1). In response to the deficiencies in these pyramids, the faculty of the Department of Nutrition at Harvard School of Public Health created the Healthy Eating Pyramid in 2005 and updated it in 2008 (Figure 5-1). According to the developers, the Healthy Eating Pyramid is simple and trustworthy, is grounded in the most recent evidence, and is unaffected by organizations with a personal stake. Harvard School of Public Health critiques the USDA's food pyramids:

- The guidelines suggest that it is fine to consume half of our grains as refined starch. That's a shame, since refined starches, such as white bread and white rice, behave like sugar. They add empty calories, have adverse metabolic effects, and increase the risks of diabetes and heart disease (2009c, para. 15).
- In terms of protein, the guidelines continue to lump together red meat, poultry, fish, and beans (including soy products). They ask us to judge these protein

THE HEALTHY EATING PYRAMID

Department of Nutrition, Harvard School of Public Health

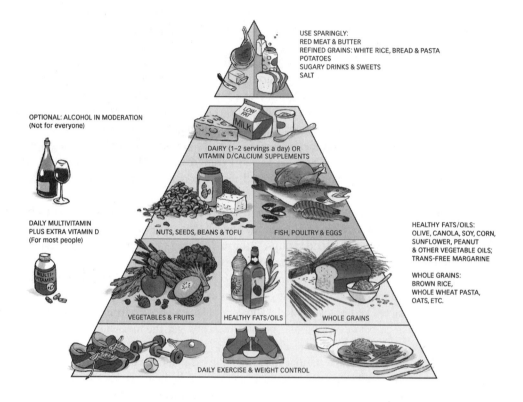

USE SPARINGLY:
RED MEAT & BUTTER
REFINED GRAINS: WHITE RICE, BREAD & PASTA
POTATOES
SUGARY DRINKS & SWEETS
SALT

OPTIONAL: ALCOHOL IN MODERATION
(Not for everyone)

DAIRY (1–2 servings a day) OR
VITAMIN D/CALCIUM SUPPLEMENTS

DAILY MULTIVITAMIN
PLUS EXTRA VITAMIN D
(For most people)

NUTS, SEEDS, BEANS & TOFU

FISH, POULTRY & EGGS

HEALTHY FATS/OILS:
OLIVE, CANOLA, SOY, CORN,
SUNFLOWER, PEANUT
& OTHER VEGETABLE OILS;
TRANS-FREE MARGARINE

WHOLE GRAINS:
BROWN RICE,
WHOLE WHEAT PASTA,
OATS, ETC.

VEGETABLES & FRUITS

HEALTHY FATS/OILS

WHOLE GRAINS

DAILY EXERCISE & WEIGHT CONTROL

For more information about the Healthy Eating Pyramid:

WWW.THE NUTRITION SOURCE.ORG

Eat, Drink, and Be Healthy
by Walter C. Willett, M.D. and Patrick J. Skerrett (2005)
Free Press/Simon & Schuster Inc.

Figure 5-1 The Healthy Eating Food Pyramid
Source: Copyright (c) 2008 Harvard University. For more information about The Healthy Eating Pyramid, please see The Nutrition Source, Department of Nutrition, Harvard School of Public Health, http://www.thenutritionsource.org, and *Eat, Drink, and Be Healthy*, by Walter C. Willett, MD and Patrick J. Skerrett (2005), Free Press/Simon & Schuster Inc.

sources by their total fat content, and "make choices that are lean, low-fat, or fat-free." This ignores the evidence that these foods have different types of fats. It also overlooks mounting evidence that replacing red meat with a combination of fish, poultry, beans, and nuts offers numerous health benefits (2009c, para. 16).

- The recommendation to drink three glasses of low-fat milk or eat three servings of other dairy products per day to prevent osteoporosis is another step in the wrong direction. Of all the recommendations, this one represents the most radical change from current dietary patterns. Three glasses of low-fat milk a day amounts to more than 300 extra calories a day. This is a real issue for the millions of Americans who are trying to control their weight. What's more, millions of Americans are lactose intolerant, and even small amounts of milk or dairy products give them stomachaches, gas, or other problems. This recommendation ignores the lack of evidence for a link between consumption of dairy products and prevention of osteoporosis. It also ignores the possible increases in risk of ovarian cancer and prostate cancer associated with dairy products (2009c, para. 17).

- MyPyramid contains no text. According to the USDA, it was "designed to be simple," and details are at MyPyramid.gov. Unless you've taken the time to become familiar with the Pyramid, though, you have no idea what it means (2009c, para. 20).

According to the Harvard School of Public Health, the Healthy Eating Pyramid is superior to the USDA's food pyramids because:

- [It] sits on a foundation of daily exercise and weight control (2009c, para. 24).
- The . . . guidelines emphasize the importance of controlling weight (2009c, para. 14).
- Exercise and weight control are . . . linked through the simple rule of energy balance: Weight change = calories in – calories out (2009c, para. 25).
- The recommendation on dietary fats makes a clear break from the past, when all fats were considered bad. The guidelines now emphasize that intake of trans fats should be as low as possible and that saturated fat should be limited. There is no longer an artificially low cap on fat intake. The latest advice recommends getting between 20 and 35 percent of daily calories from fats and recognizes the potential health benefits of monounsaturated and polyunsaturated fats (2009c, para. 15).
- Instead of emphasizing "complex carbohydrates," a term used in the past that has little biological meaning, the new guidelines urge Americans to limit sugar intake and they stress the benefits of whole grains (Harvard School of Public Health, 2009c, para. 16).

- [It emphasizes that a] diet rich in vegetables and fruits has bountiful benefits. Among them: It can decrease the chances of having a heart attack or stroke; possibly protect against some types of cancers; lower blood pressure; help you avoid the painful intestinal ailment called diverticulitis; guard against cataract and macular degeneration, the major causes of vision loss among people over age 65; and add variety to your diet and wake up your palate (2009c, para. 28)
- There's just one basic guideline to remember: A healthy diet includes more foods from the base of the pyramid than from the higher levels of the pyramid (2009c, para. 37).

Summary: Nutritional Wellness Pyramids

Over the years, the USDA has developed several nutritional wellness pyramids. Their most recent is MyPyramid (Harvard School of Public Health, 2009c). The School of Public Health of Harvard University has also developed nutritional wellness pyramids. Their most recent is the 2008 version of The Healthy Eating Pyramid (Harvard School of Public Health, 2009b). Unlike MyPyramid, the Healthy Eating Pyramid is simple to understand and apply, is grounded in the most recent evidence, and is unaffected by organizations with a personal stake (Harvard School of Public Health, 2009a).

SECTION 4: HISTORY OF NUTRITIONAL WELLNESS

History

The history component of a nutritional wellness examination is an aspect of the history section of the physical therapy examination. The physical therapist should complete a history of each client's alimentation detailing and summarizing a historical account of the client's nutritional habits and practices. The depth of the nutritional history should be based upon the client's chief complaints (initial presentation).

Historical data related to nutrition may be obtained through a patient/client self-report, family report, caregiver report, and/or the client's medical record. Patient/client self-reports should be obtained through a survey and/or interview using open and closed questions. It is unlikely that the patient's/client's nutritional medical record will be available unless it is obtained through an informed consent. The information from the external sources (e.g., family report, caregiver report) should be viewed as complementary rather than alternative. While the nutritional history can include data as early as childhood, often it is most important to include data from the past year.

Historical Nutrition Survey

Items that might be highlighted in the historical alimentation section include the patient's/client's ratings related to her or his history of healthy versus unhealthy eating and a historical summary of nutritional intake. My proposal for a historical nutrition survey is provided in Figure 5-2.

Nutritional Wellness History

(To be completed by the patient/client)

Surname: _____ First: _____ Date: ___/___/_____

Please answer each of the questions honestly. Your honesty will help us to better assist you meet any goals you may have related to your nutrition, body composition (i.e., fat weight versus muscle weight), and/or level of fitness.

1. During the *course of your life*, how healthy (or unhealthy) do you think your nutritional intake has been? (check only one)
   ❑ healthy ❑ somewhat healthy, somewhat unhealthy ❑ unhealthy ❑ I don't know

2. During the *past year*, how healthy (or unhealthy) do you think your nutritional intake has been? (check only one)
   ❑ healthy ❑ somewhat healthy, somewhat unhealthy ❑ unhealthy ❑ I don't know

3. Of the following, which describes your **low-calorie "dieting"**? (check all that apply)
   ❑ I've never been on a low-calorie diet
   ❑ I've been on a low-calorie diet once in my life and it lasted about _____ weeks / months / years
   ❑ I've been on a low-calorie diet about _____ times in my life, the average one lasted about _____ weeks / months / years, and the longest lasted about _____ weeks / months / years
   ❑ I've been on a low-calorie diet so many times in my life I can't count them

4. During the *course of your life*, has your diet been high, medium, or low in **dark green and orange vegetables**, such as broccoli, green beans, spinach, squash, and carrots?
   ❑ high ❑ medium ❑ low ❑ I don't know

5. During the *course of your life*, has your diet been high, medium, or low in **fruits**?
   ❑ high ❑ medium ❑ low ❑ I don't know

6. During the *course of your life*, has your diet been high, medium, or low in **whole grains** (e.g., whole-grain bread, pasta, rice)?
   ❑ high ❑ medium ❑ low ❑ I don't know

7. During the *course of your life*, has your diet been high, medium, or low in **healthy oils and fats**?
   ❑ high ❑ medium ❑ low ❑ I don't know

8. During the *course of your life*, has your diet been high, medium, or low in **nuts, seeds, beans, and tofu**?
   ❑ high ❑ medium ❑ low ❑ I don't know

9. During the *course of your life*, has your diet been high, medium, or low in **fish, poultry, and egg whites**?
   ❑ high ❑ medium ❑ low ❑ I don't know

10. During the *course of your life*, has your diet been high, medium, or low in **egg yolks**?
    ❑ high ❑ medium ❑ low ❑ I don't know

11. During the *course of your life*, has your diet been high, medium, or low in **red meat and butter**?
    ❑ high ❑ medium ❑ low ❑ I don't know

12. During the *course of your life*, has your diet been high, medium, or low in **refined grains** (e.g., white bread, white pasta, white rice)?
    ❑ high ❑ medium ❑ low ❑ I don't know

13. During the *course of your life*, has your diet been high, medium, or low in **sweets** (e.g., cookies, cake, candy) and **sugary drinks**?
    ❑ high ❑ medium ❑ low ❑ I don't know

14. During the *course of your life*, has your diet been high, medium, or low in **salt**?
    ❑ high ❑ medium ❑ low ❑ I don't know

15. During the *course of your life*, has your **alcohol** intake been high, medium, or low?
    ❑ high ❑ medium ❑ low ❑ I don't know

Figure 5-2 History of Nutritional Wellness

Analysis of History of Nutrition

For a broad overview of the patient's/client's alimentation history, examine her or his responses to items #1 and #2 in Figure 5-2. The optimal response for each is "healthy" and other responses are "unsatisfactory." Item #3 provides some information about the patient's/client's history of low-calorie dieting. This result will not only help to determine if nutritional wellness should be tested but also may help to determine if basal metabolic rate and/or body composition should be tested. Finally, examine the patient's/client's responses to items #4 through #15 to determine if she or he has likely been consuming healthy proportions of healthy and unhealthy foods. The satisfactory response for item #4 (dark green and orange vegetables) is high. The satisfactory response for item #5 (fruits) is medium or high. The satisfactory response for item #6 (whole grains) is high. The satisfactory response for item #7 (healthy oils and fats) is medium or high. To qualify for a satisfactory level of healthy protein-rich food, the response for #8 (nuts, seeds, beans and tofu) or the response for #9 (fish, poultry, and egg whites) must be high or the response to each item must be medium. The satisfactory response to item #10 (egg yolks) is medium or low. The satisfactory response to item #11 (red meat and butter) is low. The satisfactory response for item #12 (refined grains) is low. The satisfactory response to item #13 (sweets) is low. The satisfactory response to item #14 (salt) and #15 (alcohol) is low.

Summary: History of Nutritional Wellness

The physical therapist should complete an historical overview of the patient's/client's alimentation in the history section of the physical therapy examination. Items that might be highlighted in the nutrition history include the patient's/client's assessment of her or his general nutritional intake and questions to ascertain the patient's/client's nutrient intake over the course of her or his life. I recommend the use of the Nutritional Wellness History instrument (Figure 5-2).

SECTION 5: SYSTEMS REVIEW OF NUTRITIONAL WELLNESS

The Nutritional Wellness Examination—Systems Review should be a component of the systems review section of each physical therapy patient/client. It should be succinct, capturing a snapshot of the client's current nutritional habits and practices. Performing a nutritional wellness systems review on every patient/client enables the physical therapist to determine when a nutritional examination and/or a referral to a dietician is indicated.

The nutrition systems review should be problem-focused and brief. It should screen the patient's/client's compliance with the Healthy Eating Pyramid, which recommends significant intake of vegetables and fruits, whole grains, and healthy fats and oils; a moderate intake of fish, poultry, eggs, nuts, seeds, beans, and tofu; one to two servings of dairy products per day (or a calcium and vitamin D supplement); and a sparing intake of red meat, butter, refined grains, sugary foods, and beverages and salt; and when not contraindicated, a maximum of a moderate intake of alcohol.

To screen the client's nutritional status, you may utilize the nutrition systems review that I have proposed (Figure 5-3) or create one of your own. No matter what screening tool you choose, it is important to complete a nutritional wellness systems review and perform an analysis. My proposal for a nutritional wellness systems review is provided in Figure 5-3.

Nutritional Wellness Screen

(Note: To be completed by the patient/client)

Surname: _____ First: _____ Date: ___/___/_____

Please answer each of the questions honestly. Your honesty will help us to better assist you meet any goals you may have related to your nutrition, body composition (i.e., fat weight versus muscle weight), and/or level of fitness.

1. During the *past month*, how healthy (or unhealthy) do you think your nutritional intake has been? (check only one)
   ❏ healthy ❏ somewhat healthy, somewhat unhealthy ❏ unhealthy ❏ I don't know

2. During the *past week*, how healthy (or unhealthy) do think your nutritional intake has been? (check only one)
   ❏ healthy ❏ somewhat healthy, somewhat unhealthy ❏ unhealthy ❏ I don't know

3. Are you on a special diet (such as low-calorie or weight-loss diet or any type of diet prescribed by a physician or a dietician) at this time? ❏ yes ❏ no

4. Is your diet high, medium, or low in **dark green and orange vegetables**, such as broccoli, green beans, spinach, squash, and carrots?
   ❏ high ❏ medium ❏ low ❏ I don't know

5. Is your diet high, medium, or low in **fruits**?
   ❏ high ❏ medium ❏ low ❏ I don't know

6. Is your diet high, medium, or low in **whole grains** (e.g., whole-grain bread, pasta, rice)?
   ❏ high ❏ medium ❏ low ❏ I don't know

7. Is your diet high, medium, or low in **healthy oils and fats**?
   ❏ high ❏ medium ❏ low ❏ I don't know

8. Is your diet high, medium, or low in **nuts, seeds, beans, and tofu**?
   ❏ high ❏ medium ❏ low ❏ I don't know

9. Is your diet high, medium, or low in **fish, poultry, and egg whites**?
   ❏ high ❏ medium ❏ low ❏ I don't know

10. Is your diet high, medium, or low in **egg yolks**?
    ❏ high ❏ medium ❏ low ❏ I don't know

11. Is your diet high, medium, or low in **whole grains** (e.g., whole grain bread, pasta & rice)?
    ❏ high ❏ medium ❏ low ❏ I don't know

12. Is your diet high, medium, or low in **red meat and butter**?
    ❏ high ❏ medium ❏ low ❏ I don't know

13. Is your diet high, medium, or low in **refined grains** (e.g., white bread, white pasta, white rice)?
    ❏ high ❏ medium ❏ low ❏ I don't know

14. Is your diet high, medium, or low in **sweets** (e.g., cookies, cake, candy) and **sugary drinks**?
    ❏ high ❏ medium ❏ low ❏ I don't know

15. Is your diet high, medium, or low in **salt**?
    ❏ high ❏ medium ❏ low ❏ I don't know

16. Is your **alcohol** intake high, medium, or low?
    ❏ high ❏ medium ❏ low ❏ I don't know

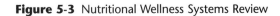

Figure 5-3 Nutritional Wellness Systems Review

Analysis of Nutritional Wellness Systems Review

For a broad overview of the patient's/client's current alimentation, examine her or his responses to items #1 and #2 in Figure 5-3. The optimal response for each is healthy and the other responses are unsatisfactory. Item #3 screens for a special diet. This result will not only help to determine if nutritional wellness should be tested, but may also help to determine if basal metabolic rate and/or body composition should be tested. Finally, examine the patient's/client's responses to items #4 through #15 to determine if she or he has likely been consuming healthy proportions of healthy and unhealthy foods. The satisfactory response for item #4 (dark green and orange vegetables) is high. The satisfactory response for item #5 (fruits) is medium or high. The satisfactory response for item #6 (whole grains) is high. The satisfactory response for item #7 (healthy oils and fats) is medium or high. To qualify for a satisfactory level of healthy protein-rich food, the response for #8 (nuts, seeds, beans, and tofu) or the response for #9 (fish, poultry, and egg whites) must be high or the response to each item must be medium. The satisfactory response to item #10 (egg yolks) is medium or low. The satisfactory response to item #11 (red meat and butter) is low. The satisfactory response to item #12 (refined grains), #13 (sweets and sugary drinks), #14 (salt), and #15 (alcohol) is low.

Summary: Systems Review of Nutritional Wellness

The physical therapist should complete a screen of each patient's/client's alimentation in the systems review section of the fitness wellness examination. This systems review should capture a brief overview of the patient's/client's nutritional current habits and practices. Specifically, it should screen her or his compliance with the Healthy Eating Pyramid of Harvard's School of Public Health (Figure 5-1). The systems review also may suggest whether the patient/client is a vegetarian and/or an athlete. I recommend the use of the Nutrition Wellness Screen (Figure 5-3).

SECTION 6: TESTS AND MEASURES OF NUTRITIONAL WELLNESS

If the nutritional wellness component of the systems review suggests that an aspect of the patient's/client's nutritional wellness is unsatisfactory, it is appropriate for the physical therapist to examine the patient's/client's nutritional wellness during the tests and measures section of the physical therapy examination. However, if the physical therapist does not possess the necessary expertise, she or he should refer the patient/client to a dietician.

Although the *Guide to Physical Therapist Practice* (APTA, 2001b) does not include a Preferred Practice Pattern related to nutritional wellness, nor do any of the Preferred Practice Patterns identify tests and measures that directly relate to nutritional wellness, they do state that the history may include a review of nutrition and hydration clinical tests (e.g., pp. 171, 439). Since physical therapy is expanding into the realm of nutritional wellness (as evidenced, for example, by CAPTE's inclusion of minimum competencies in nutrition in their *Normative Model of Physical Therapist Professional Education: Version 2004* and the APTA's inclusion of nutrition education in their 2001 Fitness and Wellness Consultation course), it is appropriate that physical therapists who possess the necessary expertise examine the nutritional wellness of patients/clients who may possess an unsatisfactory level of nutritional wellness.

As discussed in Chapter 3, it is appropriate to utilize a survey to test and measure an aspect of wellness. A survey to examine nutritional wellness should examine the patient's/client's (psychomotor) habits and practices related to nutrition, her or his cognitive knowledge of nutritional wellness, and her or his affective commitment to nutritional wellness.

Compared to the systems review, the tests and measures should more thoroughly examine the patient's/client's intake of various food groups including but not limited to vegetables, fruits, whole grains, refined grains, fish, poultry, eggs, nuts, seeds, beans and peas, tofu, red meat, milk and other dairy products, butter, healthy fats and oils, unhealthy fats, sugary foods and beverages, salt, and alcohol. I recommend the Nutritional Wellness Survey (Figure 5-4).

In some cases, such as when a patient/client is overfat, it is indicated to also test and measure caloric and substrate input. A food journal can be used to examine these aspects of nutritional wellness. I recommend the Food Journal (Figure 5-5). The instructions for the physical therapist and facility utilizing the Food Journal are provided in Figure 5-6.

Nutrition and Nutritional Wellness Survey
(Note: To be completed by the patient/client)

Surname: _____ First: _____ Date: ___/___/_____

Name of the Physical Therapist (PT): _____

Note to the PT: Dialog with the patient/client to complete these tests and measures. Utilize lay terminology unless there is direct evidence that more clinical terminology is indicated.

For the PT to state to the patient/client: I will be asking you numerous questions to obtain information about your nutritional habits. Please answer as honestly, accurately, and completely as possible. This will enable me to help you meet any goals you may have related to your nutrition, body composition (i.e., fat weight versus muscle weight), and/or level of fitness. At the end of this survey, you will have the opportunity to ask me questions. Are you ready to start?

Section A: Vegetarianism (Nutritional Status)
- Do you consider yourself to be a vegetarian? ❑ Yes ❑ No ❑ I don't know
- Do you consider yourself to be a vegan? ❑ Yes ❑ No ❑ I don't know
- Do you always avoid meat products? ❑ Yes ❑ No ❑ I don't know
- Do you always avoid eggs and egg products? ❑ Yes ❑ No ❑ I don't know
- Do you always avoid milk and milk products? ❑ Yes ❑ No ❑ I don't know

Section B: Athleticism
Note to the PT: There is no need to assess athleticism in both this exam and in the Tests and Measures related to fitness—just transfer the results.

1. During the past year, have you engaged in a "grueling" exercise program (i.e., at least 2 to 3 hours per day on at least 5 or 6 days per week)? ❑ Yes ❑ No ❑ I don't know

2. During the past month, have you engaged in a "grueling" exercise program (i.e., at least 2 to 3 hours per day on at least 5 or 6 days per week)? ❑ Yes ❑ No ❑ I don't know

3. In the foreseeable future, do you intend to engage in a "grueling" exercise program (i.e., at least 2 to 3 hours per day on at least 5 or 6 days per week)? ❑ Yes ❑ No ❑ I don't know

---

Figure 5-4 Nutritional Wellness Tests and Measures

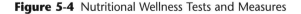

Section C: Cognitive Aspect of Nutritional Wellness

1. Tell me what you know about fiber:

_____

_____

_____

2. What do vegetables contain? For example, do they contain fat?

_____

_____

3. About how many cups of water should a person drink each day? _____

4. During the past week, how healthy (or unhealthy) do you think your nutritional intake has been?

_____

_____

_____

_____

Section D: Psychomotor (Behavioral) Aspect of Nutritional Wellness

1. Think about how many **refined grains** (e.g., white rice, white bread, white pasta, only the white part of a potato without the skin) you ate *during the past 3 days*. Did you eat:
   ❑ a lot almost every day or every day?
   ❑ some almost every day or every day?
   ❑ a lot on most days and none on other days?
   ❑ some on some days and none on other days?
   ❑ very little or none?

2. Think about how many **refined grains** you ate *during the past week*. Did you eat:
   ❑ a lot almost every day or every day?
   ❑ some almost every day or every day?
   ❑ a lot on most days and none on other days?
   ❑ some on some days and none on other days?
   ❑ very little or none?

3. Think about how many **whole grains** (e.g., whole grain bread, whole wheat pasta, brown rice, oats) you ate *during the past 3 days.* Did you eat:
   ❑ a lot almost every day or every day?
   ❑ some almost every day or every day?
   ❑ a lot on most days and none on other days?
   ❑ some on some days and none on other days?
   ❑ very little or none?

4. Think about how many **whole grains** you ate *during the past week.* Did you eat:
   ❑ a lot almost every day or every day?
   ❑ some almost every day or every day?
   ❑ a lot on most days and none on other days?
   ❑ some on some days and none on other days?
   ❑ very little or none?

Figure 5-4 Nutritional Wellness Tests and Measures (continued)

5. Think about how many **dark green and orange vegetables** (e.g., broccoli, green beans, spinach, carrots, squash, sweet potatoes) you ate *during the past 3 days*. Did you eat:
   - ❏ a lot almost every day or every day?
   - ❏ some almost every day or every day?
   - ❏ a lot on most days and none on other days?
   - ❏ some on some days and none on other days?
   - ❏ very little or none?

6. Think about how many **dark green and orange vegetables** you ate *during the past week*. Did you eat:
   - ❏ a lot almost every day or every day?
   - ❏ some almost every day or every day?
   - ❏ a lot on most days and none on other days?
   - ❏ some on some days and none on other days?
   - ❏ very little or none?

7. Think about how many **"starchy" vegetables** (e.g., corn, peas) you ate *during the past 3 days*. Did you eat:
   - ❏ a lot almost every day or every day?
   - ❏ some almost every day or every day?
   - ❏ a lot on most days and none on other days?
   - ❏ some on some days and none on other days?
   - ❏ very little or none?

8. Think about how many **"starchy" vegetables** you ate *during the past week*. Did you eat:
   - ❏ a lot almost every day or every day?
   - ❏ some almost every day or every day?
   - ❏ a lot on most days and none on other days?
   - ❏ some on some days and none on other days?
   - ❏ very little or none?

9. Think about how many dairy products you consumed *during the past 3 days*.
   - About how many cups of _____ skim, _____ 1%, _____ 2%, _____ whole milk did you drink each day?
   - About how many cups of other high-calcium foods did you eat per day? _____

10. Think about how many dairy products you consumed *during the past week*.
    - About how many cups of _____ skim, _____ 1%, _____ 2%, _____ whole milk did you drink each day?
    - About how many cups of other high-calcium foods did you eat per day? _____

11. Think about how much **red meat** you ate *during the past 3 days*. Did you eat:
    - ❏ a lot almost every day or every day?
    - ❏ some almost every day or every day?
    - ❏ a lot on most days and none on other days?
    - ❏ some on some days and none on other days?
    - ❏ very little or none?

12. Think about how much **red meat** you ate *during the past week*. Did you eat:
    - ❏ a lot almost every day or every day?
    - ❏ some almost every day or every day?
    - ❏ a lot on most days and none on other days?
    - ❏ some on some days and none on other days?
    - ❏ very little or none?

Figure 5-4 Nutritional Wellness Tests and Measures (continued)

13. Think about how many **nuts, seeds, beans, and tofu** fats you consumed *during the past 3 days.* Did you eat:
    ❑ a lot almost every day or every day?
    ❑ some almost every day or every day?
    ❑ a lot on most days and none on other days?
    ❑ some on some days and none on other days?
    ❑ very little or none?

14. Think about how many **nuts, seeds, beans, and tofu** fats you consumed *during the past week.* Did you eat:
    ❑ a lot almost every day or every day?
    ❑ some almost every day or every day?
    ❑ a lot on most days and none on other days?
    ❑ some on some days and none on other days?
    ❑ very little or none?

15. Think about how much **fish, poultry, and egg whites** you consumed *during the past 3 days.* Did you eat:
    ❑ a lot almost every day or every day?
    ❑ some almost every day or every day?
    ❑ a lot on most days and none on other days?
    ❑ some on some days and none on other days?
    ❑ very little or none?

16. Think about how much **fish, poultry, and egg whites** you consumed *during the past week.* Did you eat:
    ❑ a lot almost every day or every day?
    ❑ some almost every day or every day?
    ❑ a lot on most days and none on other days?
    ❑ some on some days and none on other days?
    ❑ very little or none?

17. Think about how many **egg yolks** you consumed *during the past week.* Did you eat:
    _____ 15 or more, _____ 8 to 14, _____ 5 to 7, _____ 1 to 4, or none?

18. Think about how much **healthy oils and fats** (e.g., olive, canola, soy, corn, sunflower, peanut, other vegetable oils) you ate *during the past 3 days.* Did you eat:
    ❑ a lot almost every day or every day?
    ❑ some almost every day or every day?
    ❑ a lot on most days and none on other days?
    ❑ some on some days and none on other days?
    ❑ very little or none?

19. Think about how much **healthy oils and fats** (e.g., olive, canola, soy, corn, sunflower, peanut, other vegetable oils) you ate *during the past week.* Did you eat:
    ❑ a lot almost every day or every day?
    ❑ some almost every day or every day?
    ❑ a lot on most days and none on other days?
    ❑ some on some days and none on other days?
    ❑ very little or none?

20. Think about how much **fried food** you ate *during the past 3 days.* Did you eat:
    ❑ a lot almost every day or every day?
    ❑ some almost every day or every day?

Figure 5-4 Nutritional Wellness Tests and Measures (continued)

❑ a lot on most days and none on other days?
❑ some on some days and none on other days?
❑ very little or none?

21. Think about how much **fried food** you ate *during the past week.* Did you eat:
❑ a lot almost every day or every day?
❑ some almost every day or every day?
❑ a lot on most days and none on other days?
❑ some on some days and none on other days?
❑ very little or none?

22. Think about how much **butter** you ate *during the past 3 days.* Did you eat:
❑ a lot almost every day or every day?
❑ some almost every day or every day?
❑ a lot on most days and none on other days?
❑ some on some days and none on other days?
❑ very little or none?

23. Think about how much **butter** you ate *during the past week.* Did you eat:
❑ a lot almost every day or every day?
❑ some almost every day or every day?
❑ a lot on most days and none on other days?
❑ some on some days and none on other days?
❑ very little or none?

24. Think about how many **sweets** (e.g., cookies, cake, candy) and sugary drinks you consumed *during the past 3 days.* Did you eat:
❑ a lot almost every day or every day?
❑ some almost every day or every day?
❑ a lot on most days and none on other days?
❑ some on some days and none on other days?
❑ very little or none?

25. Think about how many **sweets** (e.g., cookies, cake, candy) and sugary drinks you consumed *during the past week.* Did you eat:
❑ a lot almost every day or every day?
❑ some almost every day or every day?
❑ a lot on most days and none on other days?
❑ some on some days and none on other days?
❑ very little or none?

26. Think about how much **fruit** you ate *during the past 3 days.* Did you eat:
❑ a lot almost every day or every day?
❑ some almost every day or every day?
❑ a lot on most days and none on other days?
❑ some on some days and none on other days?
❑ very little or none?

27. Think about how much **fruit** you ate *during the past week.* Did you eat:
❑ a lot almost every day or every day?
❑ some almost every day or every day?
❑ a lot on most days and none on other days?
❑ some on some days and none on other days?
❑ very little or none?

Figure 5-4 Nutritional Wellness Tests and Measures (continued)

28. Think about how much **salt** you consumed *during the past 3 days*. Did you eat:
    ❏ a lot of foods high in salt?
    ❏ just a few salty foods?
    ❏ very few or no salty foods?

29. Think about how much **salt** you consumed *during the past week*. Did you eat:
    ❏ a lot of foods high in salt?
    ❏ just a few salty foods?
    ❏ very few or no salty foods?

30. Think about if you added **salt** to your food (at the table) *during the past week?* Did you:
    ❏ often or always add salt?
    ❏ sometimes add salt?
    ❏ never add salt?

31. Think about how much **alcohol** (e.g., beer, wine, liquor) you consumed *during the past 3 days.*
    About how many drinks did you drink each day? _____
    About how many total drinks did you drink total (during the past 3 days)? _____

32. Think about how much **alcohol** you consumed *during the past week.* About how many drinks
    did you drink each day? _____
    About how many drinks did you drink total (during the whole week)? _____

33. Think about how much **alcohol** you consumed *during the past month.*
    About how many drinks did you drink each day? _____

34. Do you regularly take a multivitamin? ❏ Yes ❏ No

35. Do you regularly take a supplement with calcium and vitamin D? (This may be as part of a multivitamin.) ❏ Yes ❏ No

36. If you are following any special diet (such as a low-calorie or weight-loss diet or any type of diet prescribed by a physician or dietician), please tell me about it:

    _____
    _____
    _____
    _____
    _____

37. Please tell me anything else that you believe is important about your current eating habits.

    _____
    _____
    _____
    _____
    _____

Section E: Affective Aspect of Nutritional Wellness
On a scale of 1 to 10, with 1 being no commitment and 10 being total commitment, how committed
are you to

1. Eating *some* dark green or orange vegetables (almost or) every day? _____

2. Eating *a lot* of dark green or orange vegetables (almost or) every day? _____

Figure 5-4 Nutritional Wellness Tests and Measures (continued)

3. Eating other kinds of vegetables (almost or) every day? _____

4. Eating some fruits (almost or) every day? _____

5. Choosing whole grains (e.g., whole grain bread, whole grain pasta, brown rice) rather than refined grains (e.g., white bread, white pasta, white rice) *some* of the time? _____

6. Choosing whole grains rather than refined grains *most or all* of the time? _____

7. Consuming some healthy oils (e.g., olive, canola, vegetable oils)? _____

8. Choosing fish, poultry, eggs, nuts, seeds, beans, and tofu rather than red meat *some* of the time? _____

9. Choosing fish, poultry, eggs, nuts, seeds, beans, and tofu rather than red meat *most or all* of the time? _____

10. Eating some fish, poultry, eggs, nuts, seeds, beans, or tofu? _____

11. Consuming two servings of milk or the equivalent of other high-calcium foods or taking a calcium/vitamin D supplement (almost or) every day? _____

12. Rarely or never eating red meat? _____

13. Rarely or never eating butter? _____

14. Rarely or never eating refined grains (e.g., white bread, pasta, rice)? _____

15. Rarely consuming sugary drinks (e.g., sodas)? _____

16. Rarely consuming sugary foods (e.g., cake, cookies)? _____

17. Limiting your salt intake? _____

18. If a man: Drinking less than one alcoholic drink per day? If a woman: Drinking less than one to two alcoholic drinks per day? _____

Section F: Food Preferences

1. What "healthy foods" do you like? Please be certain to list the kinds of vegetables you like.

_____
_____
_____
_____

2. What are your one or two favorite "unhealthy foods"?

_____
_____
_____

Section G: Nutritional Wellness Goal(s)

What is/are your goal(s) related to eating/nutrition?

_____
_____
_____
_____

Figure 5-4 Nutritional Wellness Tests and Measures (continued)

FOOD JOURNAL

** Please try to record information after each meal, or at the end of each day **

Date: ____/____/____ Day (circle one): Mon Tue Wed Thur Fri Sat Sun

Last Name: _____ First: _____

Time	Describe each food/drink you ate/drank	Where?	With Whom?	State of Mind?
Examples: 2 PM	*Examples:* McDonald's double cheeseburger, large fries, large diet Coke	*Examples:* driving in car, on way to pick up son	*Examples:* alone	*Examples:* hungry, in a hurry
9 PM	2 PBJ sandwiches (white bread, ~ 2 T peanut butter each, ~ 2 T jelly each), can diet Sprite	in bed	with husband	bored—watching tv show
9:45 PM	3 scoops chocolate ice cream	➡	➡	➡

Figure 5-5 Nutritional Wellness and Mental and Social Wellness Tests and Measures—Food Journal

Nutrition and Nutritional Wellness Tests and Measures Instructions

NOTE to the PT CLINIC:

When the patient/client calls the clinic to make the appointment for the first PT session, forward three blank Food Journals to her or him as an e-mail attachment, fax, or, as a last resort, through standard mail (if there are at least 1 to 3 days between the estimated day the patient/client will receive the Food Journal through the mail and the first PT session.)

NOTE to the PT:

- *If the patient/client has NOT completed at least 1 day of the Food Journal by the first PT session:* Provide the Food Journal to her or him and instruct her or him to record the items she or he has eaten so far that day and take the Journal home and complete the remainder of it at the end of the day. Also instruct the patient/client to complete the rest of the Food Journal over the next 2 days.

- *If the patient/client completed only 1 or 2 days of the Food Journal by the first PT session:* Collect what is completed and instruct her or him to complete the remainder.

- *If the patient/client completed 3 days of the Food Journal by the first PT session:* Collect it.

Figure 5-6 Nutritional Wellness Tests and Measures—Instructions

To test and measure a patient's/client's nutritional status, you may utilize the Nutritional Wellness Survey and the Food Journal that I have proposed or create your own tests and measures. Whether or not you utilize the instruments I have proposed, it is important to examine the nutritional wellness of a patient/client when it is indicated to do so.

SECTION 7: NUTRITIONAL WELLNESS EVALUATION

Evaluation

If the examination identifies issues related to nutritional wellness, the evaluation should include a section related to nutritional wellness. To evaluate a patient's/client's nutritional wellness and determine if it is satisfactory, analyze the nutritional wellness survey. To possess a satisfactory level of nutritional wellness, the patient/client must possess an adequate knowledge of nutrition and nutritional wellness, engage in healthy nutritional practices, and possess an acceptable level of commitment to healthy nutritional habits.

Evaluation of Vegetarianism

To determine if a patient/client is a vegetarian, assess her or his responses in Section A (Figure 5-4). If the patient/client indicates that she or he has avoided all meat, egg, and milk products and considers her- or himself a vegetarian and/or a vegan, then you may conclude that she or he is a vegan. If the patient/client indicates that she or he has avoided all meat, but consumes milk products and/or egg products and considers her- or himself a vegetarian, then you may conclude that she or he is a vegetarian.

Evaluation of Athleticism

To determine if a patient/client is an athlete, assess her or his responses to items #1 through #3 in Section B (Figure 5-4). If the patient/client indicates that she or he has regularly engaged in a grueling exercise program during the past month, if not year, and anticipates that she or he will continue to do so, then you may conclude that she or he is an athlete for nutritional purposes.

Evaluation of the Cognitive Aspect of Nutritional Wellness

To determine if a patient/client possesses an adequate knowledge of nutritional wellness, evaluate her or his responses to items #1 through #4 in Section C (Figure 5-4). A satisfactory response to items #1 through #3 could be an extremely abbreviated version of the elementary aspects (in lay terminology) of this chapter's discussions of nutritional wellness. Also determine if her or his response to item #4 ("During the past week, how healthy (or unhealthy) do you think your nutritional intake has been"?) matches her or his psychomotor nutritional behaviors (Section D, Figure 5-4). If they do, then you may conclude that her or his cognitive aspect of nutritional wellness is satisfactory.

Evaluation of the Psychomotor Aspect of Nutritional Wellness

To evaluate a patient's/client's psychomotor aspect of nutritional wellness as it relates to food groups, compare the responses to items #1 through #35 in Section D (Figure 5-4) to the Healthy Eating Pyramid of Harvard's School of Public Health (Figure 5-1). Patients/clients are asked to report on both the last 3 days and the last week because some of them will not be able to accurately recall the last week even though that is usually the more representative data.

The optimal level of nutritional wellness as it relates to food groups is a daily intake of very little or no refined grains; a lot of whole grains; a lot of dark green and orange vegetables and at least some intake of starchy vegetables; one to two servings of dairy products per day (or a calcium and vitamin D supplement); a lot of intake of nuts, seeds, beans, tofu, fish, poultry and/or egg whites; no more than 14 egg yolks; at least some fruit; very little to no red meat, fried foods, butter, sweets and sugary drinks, and salt; and no more than one alcohol drink per day if a woman and no more than two alcohol drinks per day if a man. The details of any special diet should be evaluated. If the diet is medically required but is outside of the expertise of the physical therapist, she or he should refer the patient/client to a registered dietician or medical doctor.

To evaluate a patient's/client's psychomotor aspect of nutritional wellness as it relates to substrate intake you will need to first analyze her or his food journal. To do this, you will need to access a nutritional software program, such as the NutriBase Junior Edition (available at http://www.dietsoftware.com/pricing.shtml). (Note: I do not endorse a particular nutrition software program, but provide the name of one as an example. There are many software programs available. You may obtain information about most of them by doing a Google search.) If you do not have access to a nutritional software program, you can manually analyze the data using *Nutritive Value of Foods* (available at http://www.nal.usda.gov/fnic/foodcomp/Data/HG72/hg72_2002.pdf). For example, one slice of wheat bread contains 65 calories, 12 g carbohydrate, 1.1 g fiber, 2 g protein, 1 g fat (0.2 g saturated fat, 0.4 g monounsaturated fat, and 0.2 g polyunsaturated fat), 26 mg calcium, 0.8 milligrams iron, 50 mg potassium, 133 mg sodium, 0 IU vitamin A, 0.10 mg thiamin, 0.07 mg riboflavin, 1.0 mg niacin, and 0 mg of ascorbic acid; and is equivalent to one serving in the grain group. For fiber and protein, you compute the total daily intake in grams and then calculate the average. For example, if the intake of fiber is 2 g, 5 g, and 11 g for days 1 through 3, the average is 9 g. For fat, you compute the daily total, calculate the averages, and then determine the percentage value of each. For example, if the intake of fat is 100 g and the total food intake is 2000 calories, the intake of fat is 45% of the total caloric intake (i.e., 100 g fat multiplied by 9 calories per gram equals 900 calories; 900 calories divided by 2000 calories is 45%).

The optimal level of nutritional wellness as it relates to fiber is a daily intake of at least 20 g for most women and at least 30 g a day for most men (Harvard School of Public Health, 2008). The Dietary Reference Intake (DRI) of fiber is 25 g for the reference woman and 38 g per day for the reference man (Food and Nutrition Board, 2005). For the reference individual; that is, not an athlete, the Dietary Reference Intake (DRI) of protein is 0.8 g protein per kilogram of body weight (Food and Nutrition Board, 2005). Fat intake should not exceed 25% to 30% of total caloric input (Harvard University, 2008). In addition, dietary cholesterol, trans fatty acids, and saturated fatty acids should be "as low as possible while consuming a nutritionally adequate diet" (Food and Nutrition Board, 2005, p. 1325).

The optimal level of nutritional wellness as it relates to caloric input is discussed in Chapter 7 because caloric intake is a critical component of body composition wellness.

The optimal level of nutritional wellness as it relates to the micronutrients is variable and Dietary Reference Intakes (DRIs) have been established for each of the vitamins and minerals. The DRIs sometimes vary according to gender and age and from the previous RDA values. The DRIs are vitamin A is 4000 IU for women and 5000 IU for men; vitamin D is 5 mg for those ages 19 to 50 and 10 mg for those older than 50; vitamin E is 8 mg for women and 10 mg for men; vitamin K is 60 mg for women over the age of 24, and 80 mg for men over the age of 24; vitamin B_1 is 1.0 mg for women 50 years of age and older, 1.1 mg for women up to 50 years of age, 1.2 mg for men 50 years of age and older, and 1.5 mg for men up to age 50; vitamin B_2 is 1.0 mg for women older than 50, 1.1 mg for women up to 50 years of age, 1.2 mg for men older than 50, and 1.5 mg for men up to 50 years of age; vitamin B_3 is 13 mg for women older than 50, 15 mg for women up to 50 years of age and men older than 50, and 19 mg for men up to 50 years of age; folate is 180 mg for women and 200 mg for men; vitamin B_6 is 1.6 mg for women and 2.0 mg for men; vitamin B_{12} is 2.0 mg; vitamin C is 60 mg; calcium is 1000 mg for men and women up to 50 years of age and 1200 mg for men and women older than 50; iron is 10 mg for all men and women older than 50 and 15 mg for women up to 50 years of age (Food and Nutrition Board, 2005).

The optimal level of nutritional wellness as it relates to the consumption of water is the daily intake of the equivalent of 11.5 cups for women and 15.5 cups for men (Harvard Health Publications, 2009). All the water in beverages and foods including fruits, vegetables, salads, and beverages count toward the daily intake of water.

Evaluation of the Affective Aspect of Nutritional Wellness

To determine if a patient/client possesses an adequate commitment to nutritional wellness, evaluate her or his responses to items #1 through #18 in Section E (Figure 5-4). If her or his commitment level is at least a 7 on the scale of 1 to 10 (with 1 being no commitment and 10 being total commitment), then you may conclude that the affective aspect of at least that nutritional component is satisfactory.

Evaluation of the Food Preferences

To evaluate the patient's/client's food preferences, examine her or his responses to items #1 and #2 in Section F (Figure 5-4).

Evaluation of the Patient's/Client's Goals

Evaluate the patient's/client's responses to Section G (Figure 5-4). Given the patient's/client's comprehensive status, determine which goals are realistic and which are not. Begin to consider the tentative time frame to achieve each reasonable goal. Also analyze each realistic goal in terms of its compatibility with other goals the patient/client has verbalized, including nutritional goals and non-nutritional goals.

The Typical Patient/Client

While each patient/client is unique, it is helpful to be familiar with the typical American's nutritional wellness because many physical therapy patients/clients will present with nutritional wellness deficits.

Caloric Intake

About 65% of Americans are overfat or obese (CDC, 2006a). Accordingly, it is likely that you will find that many physical therapy patients/clients present overfat or obese and have excessive caloric input. While similar patients/clients (by gender and age) can vary significantly in caloric intake, the average daily caloric intake (in 2000) of females was 2208 ages 20 to 39; 1828 ages 40 to 59; 1585 ages 60 to 74 (McArdle et al., 2006). In the same year, the average daily caloric intake of males was 2828 ages 20 to 39; 2590 ages 40 to 59; and 2123 ages 60 to 74 (McArdle et al., 2006). It is worthwhile to appreciate that these statistics indicate that the average man consumes more calories than the average woman and as an individual ages, she or he tends to consume fewer calories. The reduced caloric consumption associated with advancing age is despite the fact that the incidence of overweight and obesity increases with age.

Substrate Intake

As a percentage of total caloric input, the typical American consumption of fat, carbohydrate, and protein is 32%, 50%, and 18%, respectively (Briefel & Johnson, 2004). If the typical physical therapy patient/client mirrors these statistics, she or he will be consuming too much fat, too little carbohydrate, and perhaps too much protein. The excess in fat will likely be in the form of unhealthy fats, including saturated and trans fats; the deficit in carbohydrate will likely be a significant shortage of whole grains; and the excess in protein will likely be in the form of red meat. Because the typical American consumes 12 g of fiber per day (Lanza, 1987) many physical therapy patients/clients may also present with a deficient intake of fiber.

Quality of the Diet

Because only 10% of Americans consume a "good" diet, 74% need an improvement in their diet, and 16% consume a "poor" diet (Briefel & Johnson, 2004); it is likely you will find that many patients'/clients' intake of complex carbohydrate, fiber, vegetables, fruits, and/or milk products is deficient while their intake of saturated fats and/or sugars and sweets is excessive. Indeed, 70% of Americans do not consume enough milk and dairy products, 72% do not consume enough fruits, 83% do not consume enough vegetables, and 92% do not consume enough dark green, yellow, and orange vegetables (Briefel & Johnson, 2004). Accordingly, many, if not most, physical therapy patients/clients will present with an impaired intake of these food groups. In contrast, about 27% of the daily diet of the typical American consists of low-nutrient, energy-dense foods (excluding alcohol) (Briefel & Johnson, 2004). Almost two-thirds of the typical patient's/client's intake will be junk food.

Alcohol

More than 25% of Americans consume alcohol more than once per week, 48% have three to four alcoholic drinks per occasion, and more than 20% consume more than five to seven alcoholic drinks per occasion (Johnson & Glassman, 1998). So it is likely that any one of your patients/clients will imbibe. Moreover, because the typical woman drinks 2.2 alcoholic beverages per occasion and the typical man drinks 3.2 per occasion (York et al., 2003), those clients who do imbibe will surpass the recommended guidelines, which is no more than one drink per day for women and no more than two drinks per day for men (Harvard University, 2009a).

Categories of Reference Patients/Clients

Reference patients/clients can be categorized by differences in gender, age, and level of education. Compared to men, women tend to consume a healthier diet (Bailey & Lehigh, 1998; DeBate, Topping, & Sargent, 2001). The nutritional intake of women physical therapy students is healthier than that of their counterparts (Fair, 2005). Compared to younger individuals, older individuals tend to consume a healthier diet; enhanced nutritional intake is also associated with higher education levels (Briefel & Johnson, 2004).

Vegetarians

If the patient/client is a vegetarian, then her or his food intake will be significantly different from the reference patient/client. The caloric intake will likely be lower; the complex carbohydrate and fiber intake will be higher; the protein intake is likely to be adequate, but not excessive; the fat intake may be lower; the intake of the vegetable group will be higher; the intake of the fruit group may be higher; the intake of the milk and milk products will vary depending upon which type of vegetarian diet the patient/client follows; the intake of unhealthy fats will be lower; the intake of healthy fats may be higher; the intake of unhealthy sugars may be lower; the intake of certain vitamins and minerals may be higher; while the intake of certain other vitamins and minerals may be lower (e.g., calcium and iron).

Athletes

If your patient/client is an athlete, then the statistics are likely to be similar to the reference American in some aspects of nutritional wellness, but different in others. Like the reference patient/client, the athlete's diet is generally low in complex carbohydrates (Fielding & Parkington, 2002). The athlete also may present with a marginal intake of vitamins and minerals from the plant kingdom (Fielding & Parkington, 2002). In contrast to the reference patient/client, an athlete's intake of fat is generally not high but his or her intake of protein tends to be very high (Fielding & Parkington, 2002; Juhn, 2003). In fact, most consume more than 1.2 to 1.8 g of protein per kilogram of body weight (Juhn, 2003).

Summary: Nutritional Wellness Evaluation

If the examination identifies issues related to nutritional wellness, it should include a section related to nutritional wellness. The nutritional wellness evaluation is an analysis of the nutritional wellness information obtained in the examination, including the history, the systems review, and the tests and measures, particularly the information in the nutritional sections of the examination. If the Nutritional Wellness Survey is utilized as tests and measures, the evaluation should include an analysis of this instrument.

While each patient/client is unique, it is helpful to be familiar with the typical American's nutritional wellness because many physical therapy patients/clients will present with nutritional wellness deficits comparable to the reference individual. If the typical physical therapy patient/client mirrors the typical American, then she or he will present as overweight or obese; excessive in caloric input (hyperalimentation); excessive in unhealthy fat intake; high in protein intake; low in whole-grain and fiber intake; high in refined grains, sugar, and junk food intake; deficient in intakes of milk and dairy products, fruits, and vegetables; and have a high intake of alcohol. Statistically, only 10% of patients/clients will present with a good diet; 74% will need an improvement in their diet, and 16% will have a poor diet (Briefel & Johnson, 2004).

The nutritional wellness of a subgroup's reference individual may vary from the typical individual of another subgroup. For example, women, the elderly, and those with a higher education level tend to have a healthier nutrition intake. The typical patient/client will not be vegetarian or an athlete, but if a particular patient/client is one or both, it is likely that she or he will be at least somewhat dissimilar to the typical patient/client in terms of nutritional wellness.

SECTION 8: NUTRITIONAL WELLNESS CONDITIONS AND DIAGNOSES

Although it is outside their scope of care for physical therapists to assign a medical diagnosis, including those related to nutrition, we should be aware and versed in certain medical disorders related to nutrition. Nutrition-related diseases (i.e., diagnoses or V-codes) that are pertinent to physical therapy include but are not limited to dehydration (276.51);

abnormal weight gain (783.1); abnormal loss of weight and underweight (783.2); polyphagia or hyperalimentation NOS (783.6); obesity (278.00); morbid obesity (278.01); loss of weight (783.21); abnormal basal metabolic rate (794.7); V85.0 body mass index (BMI) < 19, adult; V85.1 BMI between 19 and 24, adult; V85.2 BMI between 25 and 29, adult; BMI between 30 and 39, adult; and V85.4 BMI ≥ 40, adult.

Like a diagnosis, a nutritional wellness condition is based upon information obtained in the examination, including the history, the systems review, and the tests and measures sections, particularly the information in the nutritional wellness section of the examination. A nutritional wellness condition, if any, is used to help guide the goals and plan of care and directly impacts the interventions and outcomes.

Conditions

Nutritional wellness conditions may be broad or specific. Generally, it is more appropriate to indicate a specific condition (or conditions), rather than rely upon a broad condition unless, of course, the patient's/client's condition is truly broad. An example of a broad condition is impaired alimentation. Examples of specific conditions include, but are not limited to, deficient protein intake; excessive vitamin or mineral intake; deficient vitamin or mineral intake, excessive intake of refined grains; deficient intake of whole wheat grain; deficient intake of milk and dairy products; deficient intake of vegetables; deficient intake of fruits; excessive intake of red meats; excessive intake of unhealthy fats; excessive intake of soups, sauces, and gravies; excessive intake of sugars and sweets; excessive intake of alcoholic beverages; and deficient intake of water beverages. These conditions are not diagnoses, but like diagnoses succinctly capture the nutritional findings in the examination, serve as a summation of the nutritional wellness evaluation, are used to guide the goals and plan of care, and impact the patient's/client's interventions and outcomes.

Vegetarianism

In the early 2000s, about 3% of adult Americans reported they followed a vegetarian diet (American Dietetic Association [ADA], 2003) and between 5% and 7% considered themselves "almost" vegetarians (McArdle et al., 2006). Interest in vegetarianism appears to be increasing (ADA, 2003). Vegetarian foods increasingly appear in supermarkets, restaurants, and college food services, and substantial growth in sales of foods attractive to vegetarians has occurred (ADA, 2003). Thus, although the typical physical therapy patient/client is not a vegetarian, some of them are. If a patient/client is a vegetarian, it is appropriate for the physical therapist to indicate this status. A vegetarian condition will not require a plan of care and interventions in and of itself, but if a related condition exists such as a deficient intake of the mineral iron, that condition will require a plan of care and intervention if not a referral to a dietician.

Athleticism

Although proportionately few individuals are genuine athletes, those who are have different nutritional requirements from the reference patient/client. Thus, it is appropriate for the physical therapist to indicate if a particular patient/client is an athlete. If the athlete's baseline nutritional wellness is deficient, she or he will require a nutritional wellness plan of care and interventions. For example, the athlete may need to increase her or his consumption of complex carbohydrates and fiber. If the physical therapist does not possess the necessary expertise to address the patient's/client's nutritional deficiencies, the patient/client should be referred to a dietician.

Summary: Nutritional Wellness Conditions and Diagnoses

A nutritional wellness condition is based upon information obtained in the examination, particularly the information in the nutritional sections of the examination. Although it is outside the scope of a physical therapist to assign medical diagnoses (either relating or not relating to nutrition), it is becoming increasingly acceptable for a physical therapist to assign a nutrition-related condition that is within her or his expertise in nutrition. Nutritional wellness conditions may be broad or specific. Conditions include vegetarianism and athleticism.

SECTION 9: PROGNOSIS, PLAN OF CARE, AND GOALS

Nutritional Wellness Prognosis

The nutritional wellness prognosis is a subset category within the physical therapy prognosis. The template wellness prognosis is for the patient/client to demonstrate optimal nutritional wellness and thereby enhance functioning in the home, leisure, occupation, and community environments. During the episode of care, the goals described in the plan of care will be achieved.

Nutritional Wellness Plan of Care

The nutritional wellness plan of care is a component within the broader physical therapy plan of care that you devise for your patient/client. It should be in alignment with her or his examination, evaluation, and condition/diagnosis.

Nutritional Wellness Goals

The nutritional wellness goals are a subset category within the physical therapy goals section. It may be indicated to develop one or more nutritional wellness goals. These goals should be guided by the patient's/client's evaluation (including the diagnosis and/or condition), nutritional guidelines, the patient's/client's personal goals, realistic expectations, and the physical therapist's clinical judgment. Factors that may influence these goals include a patient's/client's history, medical, and health status, personal goals, age, gender, her or his motivation, food preferences, and the physical therapist's expertise in nutritional wellness.

A nutritional wellness goal is related to the patient's/client's nutritional wellness; for example, the caloric intake and/or the intake of one or more of the food groups. Nutritional wellness goals may be general or specific. An example of general nutritional wellness goals is to reduce caloric intake. An example of a specific nutritional wellness goal is for the patient/client to achieve within 1 month a caloric intake of 1400 to 1500 calories per day. Typically, a nutritional wellness goal should be very specific because the patient/client should refer to it to guide her or him in her or his weekly nutritional regimen.

Each nutritional wellness goal should fully consider the stages of the wellness model: primordial, pre-contemplation, contemplation, assessment, action, maintenance, and permanent maintenance. Although as part of the examination you would have already assessed the patient's/client's nutritional wellness stage, she or he may in fact be in a lower wellness stage (e.g., primordial or pre-contemplation stage). If this is the case, then the immediate nutritional wellness goal(s) should be to achieve the contemplative stage in each area of nutritional wellness in which the patient/client has not achieved the contemplative stage. For example, if the physical therapist determines that the patient/client is in the contemplation stage for caloric intake but in the primordial stage for appropriate protein intake, an initial nutritional wellness goal should be to increase the patient's/client's awareness of appropriate protein intake to contemplation stage.

A physical therapist should always develop weekly short-term goals related to the wellness long-term goal(s) because these goals are actions the patient/client is supposed to be doing that build progress toward the final goals of treatment. Each weekly wellness goal should be able to be objectively measured with ease and precision.

It is critical that upon—if not before—discharge (or discontinuance), each long-term nutritional wellness goal is addressed. For example, if a goal was discharged/discontinued, then the incident should be documented. No goal should slip through the cracks.

Prognosis of Goals

The prognosis is a qualitative descriptor (i.e., excellent, above average, below average, or poor) of the likelihood that the patient/client will achieve a specific goal or a group of goals. It is helpful to determine the prognosis for each goal, including each nutritional wellness goal, rather than assign a global prognosis for all of the goals. For example, the prognosis to achieve the goal of improved nutritional intake might be excellent but the prognosis to achieve the goal of improved intake of whole-grain foods might be average. In addition to each specific prognosis, a more global prognosis may be identified.

Plan of Care and Goals Related to the Food Groups

As a general rule, individuals should emphasize a variety of healthy foods, including plenty of vegetables, grains, fruits, and water; and should consume a variety of foods both between and within the food groups (Food and Nutrition Board, 2005). To develop the plan of care of a patient/client who presents with food group deficits, I suggest you first compare the results of her or his Food Journal to the recommendations of MyPyramid (USDA, 2005b) as modified by The Healthy Eating Pyramid (Harvard University, 2009a) (Figure 5-1). I suggest that you integrate The Healthy Eating Pyramid because MyPyramid does not differentiate between healthy and unhealthy types of substrates. For example, while the USDA recommends that a 20-year-old woman who does not exercise eat 6 ounces of grains per day, it does not specify that the grains should be whole rather than refined. To compare the food group results of a patient's/client's Food Journal to MyPyramid, visit "My Pyramid Plan" at http://www.mypyramid.gov/mypyramid/index.aspx and input the patient's/client's age, gender, and activity level (i.e., less than 30 minutes, between 30 and 60 minutes, and greater than 60 minutes of moderate intensity physical activity per day) (USDA, 2005). Table 5-1 shows the recommended food group intake for 20-, 40-, and 60-year-olds.

Table 5-1 Recommended Food Group Intake for 20-, 40-, and 60-Year-Olds

	Daily Exercise	Grains	Vegetables	Fruits	Milk Group[a]	Protein Group[b]
Women						
20 y/o	< 30 min	6	2.5	2	3	5.5
	30–60 min	7	3	2	3	6
	> 60 min	8	3	2	3	6.5
40 y/o	< 30 min	6	2.5	1.5	3	5
	30–60 min	6	2.5	2	3	5.5
	> 60 min	7	3	2	3	6
60 y/o	< 30 min	5	2	1.5	3	5
	30–60 min	6	2.5	1.5	3	5
	> 60 min	7	3	2	3	6
Men						
20 y/o	< 30 min	9	3.5	2	3	6.5
	30–60 min	10	3.5	2.5	3	7
	> 60 min	10	4	2.5	3	7
40 y/o	< 30 min	8	3	2	3	6.5
	30–60 min	9	3.5	2	3	6.5
	> 60 min	10	3.5	2.5	3	7
60 y/o	< 30 min	7	3	2	3	6
	30–60 min	8	3	2	3	6.5
	> 60 min	9	3.5	2	3	6.5

[a] Milk and Dairy Group
[b] Meat, Poultry, Fish, Dry Beans, Eggs, and Nuts Group

Please visit "My Pyramid Plan" at http://www.mypyramid.gov/mypyramid/index.aspx to determine the amount of each food group you should consume. This activity will familiarize you with the MyPyramid.

Plan of Care and Goals Related to Caloric Input

The plan of care and goals related to caloric input is discussed in Chapter 7 because caloric input is a critical component of body composition, the focus of Chapter 7.

Plan of Care and Goals Related to the Nutritional Substrates

Certain medical diagnoses and conditions necessitate a diet that is significantly increased or decreased in carbohydrate, fat, protein, one or more vitamins, and/or one or more minerals. The guidelines discussed below do not apply to these individuals. The nutritional wellness of these individuals is outside the scope of physical therapists and these patients/clients should be referred to a dietician.

A goal related to carbohydrates should be established if the patient's/client's baseline carbohydrate intake is too low in whole grains, too high in refined grains, and/or too high in sugary foods and beverages. In many cases, it is indicated to decrease refined grain and simple sugar intake and simultaneously increase whole-grain intake. Added sugar should contribute no more than 25% of the total daily calories (Food and Nutrition Board,

2005). To positively affect carbohydrate intake, the patient/client should be instructed to choose whole grains over refined grains and nutrient-dense foods that taste sweet (e.g., fruits) over sugary foods (e.g., cookies).

A goal to increase fiber intake should be established if the patient's/client's baseline fiber intake is low; that is, less than 20 g/d if a woman or less than 30 g/d if a man. A reasonable goal is to increase fiber intake to at least 20 g/d if the patient/client is a woman and to increase it to at least 30 g/d if the patient/client is a man. To increase dietary fiber, the patient/client should be instructed to choose higher-fiber foods over lower-fiber foods. Higher-fiber foods include whole-grain products, vegetables, fruits, and legumes, which also provide vitamins, minerals, and water. Relatively small but consistent changes in the selection of food can significantly increase daily fiber intake. The best sources of fiber are fresh fruits and vegetables, nuts and legumes, and whole-grain foods (Harvard School of Public Health, 2009e). According to the Harvard School of Public Health (2009e, para. 17) ways to increase fiber intake are to eat whole fruits instead of drinking fruit juices; replace white rice, bread, and pasta with brown rice and whole-grain products; choose whole-grain cereals for breakfast; snack on raw vegetables instead of chips, crackers, or chocolate bars; and substitute legumes for meat two to three times per week in chili and soups. Table 5-2 compares the fiber content in typical food choices to the fiber content in healthier food choices.

A goal to decrease fat intake is indicated if the patient's/client's baseline fat intake is greater than 35% of total caloric input. A reasonable goal is to reduce fat intake to less than 30% of total caloric intake while maintaining an adequate intake of healthy fats. To increase the intake of healthy fats, a patient/client might be instructed to cook with and eat more monounsaturated and polyunsaturated oils, such as olive oil and safflower oil. To decrease the intake of unhealthy fats, a patient/client might be instructed to practice eating fewer fried foods.

A goal related to protein should be established if the patient's/client's baseline protein intake is too low or too high. When developing the plan of care related to protein intake, it is important to appreciate that the average requirement for protein is 0.6 g per kilogram of body weight and the RDA is set high, at 0.8 g protein/kg body weight, to cover the needs of essentially all Americans. This is equivalent to 0.367 g of protein per pound of body weight and meets 97.5% of the population's needs. For example, the RDA of protein for a 174-pound man is 63 g and for a 138-pound woman is 50 g. (Note: the protein requirement for athletes is subsequently explored.)

To increase the intake of healthful proteins, a patient/client might be instructed to consume more chicken or other lean protein-rich foods. To decrease the intake of protein, a patient/client might be instructed to consume less red meat.

A goal to increase (or more rarely decrease) one or more vitamins or minerals is indicated if that patient's/client's baseline intake is inadequate (or excessive).

To increase the intake of a particular vitamin or mineral, a patient/client might be instructed to add certain foods and beverages to his or her diet. For example, a patient/client who is deficient in iron intake might be instructed to select grain products that are fortified with iron, include 3 cups of green leafy vegetables in the daily diet, and consume 1 cup legumes on most days.

Table 5-2 Fiber Content of Selected Foods

Food Item	Calories	Fiber, grams
Bread		
White, 1 slice	70	0.5
Whole Wheat, 1 slice	70	3
Spaghetti		
Enriched, cooked	197	2.4
Whole Wheat, cooked	174	6.3
Donut—Dunkin' Donuts, Glazed	200	1
Cereal		
Captain Crunch, ¾ cup	110	1
Kellogg's Oat Bran, ¾ cup	110	4
Kellogg's 100% Bran, ¾ cup	130	4.5
Peach, canned in extra light syrup, ½ cup	50	0
Peach, fresh, 1	38	1.75
Snap Bean (cut)		
Yellow, from can	93	1.8
Yellow, raw or frozen	90	4.1
Green, from can	93	2.6
Green, raw or frozen	90	4.1
Sweet Potatoes		
Boiled, without skin	164	2.8
Baked, with skin	150	4.1

Source: Gebhardt, S.E. & Thomas, R.G. (2002). *Nutritive Value of Foods.* Beltsville, MD: United States Department of Agriculture (USDA). Available at: http://www.nal.uda.gov/fnic/foodcomp/Data/HG72/hg72_2002.pdf

To decrease the intake of a particular vitamin or mineral, a patient/client might be instructed to discontinue the supplement that provides an excessive amount of that macronutrient.

A goal to increase water consumption is indicated if that patient's/client's intake is inadequate. For example, if a patient/client typically drinks ½ cup of water per day, she or he might be instructed to gradually increase her or his consumption until she or he is drinking 6 to 8 cups of water per day. If drinking this much water is unreasonable for the patient/client, she or he might be instructed to drink 4 cups of water each day and significantly increase her or his consumption of foods and beverages that have a high water content such as watermelon and vitamin water.

Plan of Care and Goals Related to the Athlete

Secondary to the decreased carbohydrate intake of the athlete, glycogen synthesis may be inadequate. While athletes need more vitamins and minerals, these micronutrients are readily supplied by their increased food consumption that offsets an increased caloric output through exercise (Krasnopolsky-Levine & Olender-Russo, 1992). However, if the athlete consumes a hypo-caloric diet (e.g., suitable for a jockey, gymnast, or dancer), she or he may need to consume additional iron and calcium, particularly if the athlete is a woman (Fogelholm, 2003; Krasnopolsky-Levine & Olender-Russo, 1992).

The protein requirement of an athlete is typically higher than that of the average individual. While Krasnopolsky-Levine and Olender-Russo (1992) recommend 1.0 g protein/kg body weight, empirical evidence suggests that as much as 1.35 to 1.4 g protein/kg body weight may be required.

An investigation by Tarnopolsky, Atkinson, MacDougall, Phillips, and Schwarcz (1992) divided nonathletes and strength-training athletes into three groups of men. The first group consumed 0.86 g protein/kg body weight, the second consumed 1.4 g protein/kg body weight, and the third consumed 2.4 g protein/kg body weight. At the conclusion of the study, there was no difference in lean body mass in the three groups of nonathletes and those athletes ingesting 1.4 or 2.4 g protein/kg body weight, but the athletes who had consumed 0.86 g protein/kg body weight had a negative nitrogen balance. The results indicate that strength-training athletes require more than 0.86 g protein/kg body weight and 1.4 g protein/kg body weight to meet their protein needs.

A similar study by Lemon, Tarnopolsky, MacDougall, and Atkinson (1992) divided male bodybuilders into two groups; group 1 consumed 1.35 g protein/kg body weight and group 2 consumed 2.62 g protein/kg body weight. At the conclusion of the study, there was no difference between the groups in terms of total body mass, strength, or muscle mass (e.g., muscle density, creatinine excretion). The results indicate that there is no benefit of men bodybuilders consuming 2.62 g protein/kg body weight, rather than 1.35 g protein/kg body weight.

Despite the empirical evidence, Lemon (1998) recommended that male strength-training athletes *might* need to consume as much as 1.6 to 1.7 g protein/kg body weight and male endurance athletes *might* need to consume 1.2 to 1.4 g protein/kg body weight, "but future . . . studies are needed to confirm these recommendations" (p. 447). Despite that popular strength and conditioning textbook *Essentials of Strength Training and Conditioning* (Baechle & Earle, 2000) borrowed Lemon's conclusions, they subsequently have proven to be faulty. As healthcare professionals, we must critically analyze the literature and not propagate myths.

It is also important that as healthcare professionals we recognize the risks of an ultra-high protein diet. According to Williams (2001), these risks include a decreased intake of carbohydrate and fiber, an increased fat intake (since most animal protein is associated with a fat), and dehydration (secondary to excess nitrogen excretion). An ultra-high protein diet stresses renal function and is contraindicated if kidney function is impaired (Brenner, Meter, & Hosteler, 1982).

As a summation, the "nutritional needs of athletes are not much different from those of typically healthy adults" (Krasnopolsky-Levine & Olender-Russo, 1992, p. 321). In fact, the "basic nutritional prescription for athletes is simple—a normal diet, regular meals, ample fluids, a variety of foods and caloric intake sufficient to meet the demands of energy expenditure for a particular sport" (Manjarrez & Birrer, 1983).

Summary: Prognosis, Plan of Care, and Goals

The nutritional wellness goals, plan of care, prognosis, interventions, and outcomes are subsets within the physical therapy goals, plan of care, prognosis, interventions, and outcomes, respectively. A nutritional wellness goal may be broad or specific. Short-term goals should be linked to the long-term goals. Each goal may be assigned a prognosis. Nutritional wellness plan of care, goals, prognosis, and interventions can focus on the nutritional substrates, or nutritional considerations for the athlete.

SECTION 10: NUTRITIONAL WELLNESS INTERVENTIONS AND GLOBAL OUTCOMES

Interventions

The nutritional wellness interventions are identified in the same section as the other physical therapy interventions.

The predominant interventions related to nutritional wellness are patient/client education and a home program. The educational intervention includes teaching the patient/client about aspects of nutritional wellness. A nutritional wellness home program is also an educational intervention but includes the added component of instructing the patient/client to practice the nutritional program (e.g., cooking with olive oil or adherence to a lower-calorie diet). Both the educational intervention and the home intervention can include cognitive education in nutritional wellness, instruction in the psychomotor aspect of nutritional wellness, and/or an affective component, such as motivation.

A referral is also an intervention. In some cases, the physical therapist informs that patient/client that a referral may be appropriate and the physician is being notified. In this case, it is the physician who will decide whether a referral (order) is indicated. An example is a referral to a dietician. In other cases, a recommendation is made directly to the patient/client. An example is a referral to a class about healthy cooking at the local community college.

Global Outcomes

Nutritional wellness global outcomes are the cumulative effects that physical therapy has upon the nutritional wellness of the patient/client. As a goal is achieved, an outcome is realized. Upon discharge from physical therapy, each goal that has been met contributes to the nutritional wellness outcome of the patient/client.

Summary: Nutritional Wellness Interventions and Global Outcomes

The nutritional wellness interventions is a subset of the physical therapy interventions. The predominant interventions related to nutritional wellness are patient/client education and a home program. An intervention also can be a referral. Nutritional wellness outcomes are the cumulative effects that physical therapy has upon the nutritional wellness of the patient/client.

chapter six

Physical Wellness and Fitness

Walking is [woman's and] man's best friend.

■ ■ ■ ■ ■ ■

Hippocrates

OBJECTIVES

Upon completion of this chapter, you should be able to:

1. Discuss the provision of fitness and fitness wellness by physical therapists, including the concepts of an expertise in fitness and fitness wellness and scope of care.
2. Define and discuss terms and concepts related to fitness and fitness wellness.
3. Explore the fitness and fitness wellness components of a history, systems review, and tests and measures of a physical therapy patient/client.
4. Examine, apply, and critique the fitness wellness template.
5. Explore the fitness and fitness wellness components of an evaluation of a physical therapy patient/client.
6. Discuss fitness and fitness wellness diagnoses and conditions.
7. Explore fitness and fitness wellness goals and plans of care.
8. Discuss the variables that may affect a prognosis related to a fitness and/or fitness wellness problem of a physical therapy patient/client.
9. Discuss fitness and fitness wellness interventions and outcomes.

SECTION 1: SCOPE OF PHYSICAL THERAPY PRACTICE

As detailed in the previous chapters, *fitness* consists of aerobic capacity, muscular fitness, and flexibility. *Fitness wellness* refers to the habits and practices related to aerobic capacity, muscular fitness, and flexibility.

Addressing fitness and fitness wellness is within the scope of physical therapy. However, to provide fitness and fitness wellness to patients/clients, the physical therapist should possess at least some expertise in these areas. This degree of expertise is similar to that which a physical therapist should possess to provide manual physical therapy to an orthopedic patient, neurological physical therapy to a brain-injured patient, home health to a geriatric home-bound patient, women's physical therapy to a female patient with incontinence, or aquatic physical therapy. Thus, while a goal of the American Physical Therapy Association (APTA; 2006a) is for physical therapists to be "exercise leaders," not all will obtain an expertise in fitness and fitness wellness, just as not all physical therapist will obtain an expertise in manual therapy, neurology, home health, women's therapy, or aquatic therapy.

Restorative physical therapy patients who are classified in an American Physical Therapy Practice Pattern (APTA, 2001b) also may present with impaired fitness and/or fitness wellness. For this reason alone, all physical therapists should possess at least a minimum understanding of fitness and fitness wellness, just as they should possess at least a minimum understanding of each of the specialties of physical therapy. This basic understanding can vary from a minimum competence in the respective subdiscipline (e.g., manual therapy), which would enable the physical therapist to provide basic treatments (e.g., stretching), to an awareness of the subdiscipline (e.g., women's therapy), which would enable the physical therapist to screen and refer the patient. Possessing at least an awareness of fitness and fitness wellness is necessary to each physical therapist because a patient's/client's fitness and fitness wellness affects her or his health (The National Center for Chronic Disease Prevention and Health Promotion [NCCDPHP], 1999) and ability to engage and/or progress in physical therapy (Rimmer, 1999; Singh et al., 2006). Fitness wellness enhances the health status of those with chronic conditions (e.g., Pippenger & Scalzitti, 2004; Ribisl et al., 2007; Zhao et al., 2007). One component of fitness wellness impacts other components of fitness wellness and may impact mental wellness, too (Ford et al., 1989; Tucker & Maxwell, 1992). Patients/clients ask their physical therapists, especially those considered as their "doctors," questions about their fitness/fitness wellness (Fair, 2004b). Physical therapists serve as fitness wellness role models (Fair, 2004b; Landry, 2004). Finally, fitness and fitness wellness is an accreditation requirement for all U.S. entry-level physical therapist programs.

Summary: Scope of Physical Therapy Practice

Fitness and fitness wellness is well within the scope of physical therapy. All physical therapists should possess an adequate amount of knowledge about fitness and fitness wellness to examine and analyze the results of the systems review. If the results indicate there is a fitness wellness problem, then the physical therapist should address the problem if she or he possesses the necessary expertise to do so or refer the patient/client to a physical therapist who has the necessary expertise.

SECTION 2: BASIC TERMS AND CONCEPTS

There are many concepts that are pertinent to fitness wellness, including anabolic steroids, the athlete, caloric output, dehydration and hydration, maximal oxygen consumption, substrate supplementation, types strength training (isometric, isotonic, isokinetic), and warm-up and cool-down. Each physical therapist must possess a basic understanding of such terms and concepts to at least conduct a systems review of the fitness/fitness wellness of patients/clients and refer them or, if sufficiently trained, be able to examine and evaluate the patients/clients and devise their diagnosis, prognosis, and plan of care.

Anabolic Steroids

Anabolic steroids have been available since the 1930s and are now used therapeutically to stimulate bone growth and reduce wasting in patients with acquired immune deficiency syndrome (AIDS), kidney disease, some types of cancers, and other diseases (BBC News, 1999). Anabolic steroids help increase muscle mass and physical strength and consequently are used by some athletes, including bodybuilders. Bodybuilders and other athletes are more likely to use anabolic steroids for nonmedical purposes than the general population (Sjöqvist, Garle, & Rane, 2008). It is also more common for males than females to use anabolic steroids for nonmedical purposes (Sjöqvist et al., 2008). Risks of anabolic steroid abuse include multi-organ abnormal functioning and damage, which can be fatal in some cases (Samaha et al., 2008). Specific dysfunctions include nausea, diarrhea, vomiting, headaches, muscle cramps, aching joints, blood clots, stroke, hypertension, hypercholesterolemia, kidney failure (America Academy of Pediatrics, 2008), liver disease, liver cancer, and heart disease (Volkow, 2009). Steroid abuse can also affect mental health by causing "roid rage" (that is, severe aggressive behavior that may result in violence), mania, and delusions (Volkow, 2009). The use of anabolic steroids is banned by all major sporting bodies, including the International Olympic Committee.

Athletes

In terms of fitness wellness, those who participate in a "grueling" exercise regimen should be considered an athlete (Glick & Horsfall, 2005). For example, an athlete who is an endurance runner might run for 2 to 3 hours each day and a gymnast might train for 5 hours per day, 6 days per week. Those who engage in a more moderate or heavy exercise regimen rather than a grueling one should not be considered an athlete. For example, those who engage in 30 minutes of moderate intensity exercise on most days (i.e., those who meet the *Healthy People 2010* guideline) and/or regularly engage in a moderate strength-training protocol should not be considered athletes.

Caloric Output

The components of caloric output are basal metabolic rate (BMR), dietary thermogenesis, and physical activity above the baseline rate. Each of these components of caloric output are discussed in Chapter 7.

Dehydration and Hydration

Dehydration is characterized by a prolonged time without consuming an adequate amount of fluid (water), especially when engaging in physical activity and/or in a hot and humid environment. Dry air can exacerbate dehydration (Sawka, Francesconi, Pimental, & Pandolf, 1984). *Hydration* is the replenishment of water through the consumption of water or water-based beverages. It is advisable to drink water (or a water-based beverage) before and during an exercise session, especially in hot and humid weather (Gisolfi, 1983) and hot and dry weather (Sawka et al., 1984).

Examination of Fitness Wellness

While it is appropriate and feasible to directly examine fitness wellness (e.g., via a step test to estimate maximal oxygen consumption), it is not efficient or practical to directly assess fitness wellness because by definition it is the habits and practices related to fitness. To directly examine fitness wellness, the physical therapist would have to monitor the patient/client throughout her or his daily activities and record the observed data over a proscribed period of time. An appropriate alternative to the prohibitively time-intensive and costly task of directly monitoring a patient's/client's fitness-related activities over the course of days, weeks, or longer is the survey method. Chapter 3 details this issue.

Isometrics, Isotonics, and Isokinetics

In an isometric exercise, the skeletal muscle is contracted, but there is no significant amount of movement in the muscle or the affected joint(s). Isometrics are done with the patient/client in static positions. To complete an isometric exercise, the individual holds a maximum contraction for 1 second or holds ⅔ of the maximum contraction for 6 seconds (McArdle et al., 2006). Examples of isometric exercises include gluteal sets and quadriceps sets. Advantages of isometric are (1) they are less likely than other types of strength training to cause injury, (2) they are time efficient, (3) they can be done anywhere, (4) they do not require equipment, and (5) they help a patient/client to develop the static strength needed to push, pull, or hold up a heavy object. The only significant disadvantage of isometric exercises is that the muscle gains strength only at the angle at which the patient/client exercises.

In an isotonic exercise, the skeletal muscle is contracted and the muscle's length is lengthened or shortened. Examples of isotonic contractions include walking and lifting a weight. Isotonic strength training involves concentric and eccentric contractions. In a concentric contraction, the muscle tension exceeds the resistance and the muscle shortens. In an eccentric contraction, the muscle lengthens due to force greater than that which the muscle can produce. Although muscle strengthening may be greatest using exercises that involve eccentric contractions, muscle injury and soreness are selectively associated with eccentric contraction (Frident & Lieber, 1992). While isotonic strength-training exercises can be performed without the use of weights (e.g., calisthenics), weights such as free weights are often utilized. The primary advantage of isotonic exercises is that they strengthen the affected muscles throughout their range of motions. The primary disadvantage of isotonic exercises is that they may cause muscle soreness secondary to the eccentric contraction phase.

Plyometrics is a type of isotonic strength training that targets and enhances elastic strength; it involves a forcible and rapid stretch in the eccentric phase immediately before the concentric phase (National Strength and Conditioning Association [NSCA], 2009). An example of a plyometric exercise is rebound jumping up and down. A primary goal of plyometric strength training is to enhance athletic performance (NCSA, 2009). Examples of athletes who may benefit from this type of training include those who play sports such as volleyball, basketball, and gymnastics.

In *isokinetic* strength training, there is muscle overload at constant speed throughout the full range of motion (McArdle et al., 2006). In theory, isokinetic strength training activates the largest number of motor units. It requires a specialized apparatus to provide variable resistance to a movement, so that no matter how much is exerted, the movement takes place at a constant speed. Isokinetic exercises are typically used in restorative physical therapy rather than fitness wellness. Advantages of isokinetic exercises are that the affected muscles gain strength evenly throughout the range of motion and muscle strength is gained relatively rapidly. The primary disadvantage of isokinetic exercises is that the required equipment is cost prohibitive to most individuals, health clubs, and even many physical therapy clinics.

In restorative physical therapy, isometrics are "level one" exercises, isotonics and isokinetics are "level two" exercises, and plyometrics are "level three" exercises. Typically, it is not necessary or appropriate to advance a patient/client to plyometric exercises because they are more likely to cause orthopedic injury and their unique purpose is to enhance elastic strength, which is critical in sport performance but not in fitness wellness.

Substrate Supplementation

Substrate supplementation includes the addition of extra carbohydrates and/or protein in the diet to enhance athletic performance. The original glycogen-loading protocol was created by Dr. Per-Olof Astrand and was popularized in the late 1960s. Astrand's (as cited by Manjarrez & Birrer, 1983) protocol was: One week before event, deplete glycogen by exercising to exhaustion specific muscle and consuming a high-protein, high-fat, low-carbohydrates (100 grams) diet. Then, during the 3 days prior to the event, consume a moderate protein, low-fat, high-carbohydrate (70% to 80% of total calories from carbohydrates or to 525 grams of carbohydrates) diet and refrain from exercise.

Warm-Up and Cool-Down

The *warm-up* precedes the exercise session and may last 5 to 10 minutes (Correa, Conde, & Santini, 1989). The warm-up period prepares the body for exercise and prevents injury (Howard, Blyth, & Thornton, 1966; Start, 1963; Start & Hines, 1963). The warm-up accomplishes these goals by dilating local vascular beds, which increases blood flow through active tissues, increases local muscle temperature and metabolism, and increases the release of oxygen from hemoglobin. The warm-up also enhances motor recruitment and sport performance (Grodjinovsky & Magel, 1970; Richards, 1968). An example of a warm-up is performing the exercise mode at a lower intensity. For example, the warm-up for a jogging session might be a moderately paced walk.

The cool-down period follows the exercise session and may last 5 to 10 minutes (Correa et al., 1989). The primary purposes of the cool-down are to safely return the body to a post-exercise state and prevent injury (Perryman, 1980). The cool-down assists in dissipation of lactic acid and other waster products, decreases adrenaline in the blood, decreases venous blood pooling in the distal extremities that decreases the risk of dizziness and fainting, and reduces the risk of delayed-onset muscle soreness (DOMS) (McArdle et al., 2006). The cool-down may be the same type of exercise as the warm-up; for example, a moderately paced walk. To enhance flexibility, it is helpful to stretch following the cool-down as it helps to cool down the body.

Summary: Basic Terms and Concepts

Many concepts are pertinent to fitness wellness, including anabolic steroids, athlete, caloric output, dehydration and hydration, an examination of fitness wellness, maximal oxygen consumption, substrate supplementation, types strength training (isometric, isotonic, isokinetic), and warm-up and cool-down. The physical therapist must possess a basic understanding of such terms and concepts to be able to conduct an effective systems review of the fitness and fitness wellness of patients/clients and refer them if necessary, or evaluate and devise her or his diagnosis, prognosis, and plan of care.

SECTION 3: EXAMINATION: HISTORY

During the completion of the history of a patient/client, the physical therapist should examine the history of fitness and fitness wellness. This historical information may be obtained through self-report, family report, and/or the medical record. A patient's/client's self-report can be obtained through the use of open and closed types of questions. The information from the family should be viewed as complementary rather than alternative. It is unlikely that the medical record, if available, will include fitness-related data. Relatively few patients/clients will be able to provide detailed information about, for example, their fitness level or their maximum oxygen consumption. In contrast to the history of a patient's/client's fitness, a physical therapist can obtain a rather thorough history of her or his fitness wellness. The depth of the fitness wellness history should be based upon the patient's/client's chief complaints and stated goals.

The *Guide to Physical Therapist Practice* (APTA, 2001b) includes two Preferred Practice Patterns related to aerobic capacity ("6A, primary prevention/risk reduction for cardiovascular/pulmonary disorders" and "6B, impaired aerobic capacity/endurance associated with deconditioning"), one related to muscular fitness ("4C, impaired muscle performance"), and eight related to muscular fitness and flexibility ("4D, impaired joint mobility, motor function, muscle performance, and range of motion associated with connective tissue," "4E, impaired joint mobility, motor function, muscle performance, and range of motion associated with localized inflammation," "4F, impaired joint mobility, motor function, muscle performance, and range of motion associated with spinal disorders,"

"4G, impaired joint mobility, motor function, muscle performance, and range of motion associated with fracture," "4H, impaired joint mobility, motor function, muscle performance, and range of motion associated with joint arthroplasty," "4I, impaired joint mobility, motor function, muscle performance, and range of motion associated with bony or soft tissue surgery," and "4J, impaired motor function, muscle performance, and range of motion, gait, locomotion associated with amputation"). It is noteworthy that each of these Preferred Practice Patterns, with the exception of 6A, are geared to restorative patients; that is, those who will require traditional physical therapy rather than wellness patients/clients. (Chapter 2, Section 2 discusses restorative and traditional physical therapy). Each of these Preferred Practice Patterns state that the patient/client history could include general demographics, social history, employment/work/school/play, growth and development, living environment, general health status, social/health habits (past and current), family history, medical/surgical history, current condition(s)/chief complaint(s), functional status and activity level, medications, and other clinical tests.

While the recommendations of the *Guide to Physical Therapist Practice* for the history are certainly helpful when conducting the history of a patient/client who presents with impaired fitness and fitness wellness, a fitness and fitness wellness history also should include—and indeed emphasize—the patient's/client's perception of her or his fitness status and fitness wellness during the course of her or his life and during the past year. My proposal for a survey to examine a patient's/client's fitness and fitness wellness history is provided in **Figure 6-1**. Whether you utilize this proposed instrument, it is important to complete a fitness and fitness wellness history and perform an analysis of that examination.

Analysis of the History of Fitness and Fitness Wellness Survey

If you utilized the History of Fitness Wellness form (Figure 6-1) to examine a patient's/client's fitness and fitness wellness history, then you can use the information in this section to analyze the results. The answers to questions #1 through #4 and #5 through #8 will provide a glimpse of the patient's/client's fitness history during her or his life and during the past year, respectively. For example, if the patient/client describes her- or himself as a "couch potato" during the course of her or his life as well as during the past year, it may be more difficult to enact a change at this time without enhanced compliance strategies. If the patient/client engaged in little to no exercise in the last year, it is important to appreciate this fact throughout the rest of the physical therapy episode of care. For example, you probably would select a test that is not physically as challenging as some other tests. Also you might need to progress the patient's/client's physical activity more gradually, at least initially. The last item on this form assesses whether the patient/client has the results from a maximal oxygen consumption exam. If so, then the test results will be helpful to integrate into the information you have gathered about the patient's/client's current aerobic capacity.

Summary: History

During the history portion of a physical therapist's examination of a patient/client, the therapist should complete a history of her or his fitness and fitness wellness. This history is

Fitness Wellness History
(To be completed by the patient/client)

Surname: _____ First: _____ Date: __/__/____

1. If you consider yourself throughout the **course of your life**, how would you best describe yourself?
   ❑ a "couch potato"   ❑ an occasional exerciser   ❑ a regular exerciser   ❑ an "athlete"

2. Over the **course of your life**, how often have you done physical activities (such as jogging or carrying boxes at least 12 minutes) that increase your **endurance**?
   ❑ regularly   ❑ occasionally   ❑ rarely   ❑ never   ❑ I don't know

3. Over the **course of your life**, how often have you done physical activities (such as weight lifting or strengthening calisthenics) that increase your **strength**?
   ❑ regularly   ❑ occasionally   ❑ rarely   ❑ never   ❑ I don't know

4. Over the **course of your life**, how often have you done activities (such as stretching or yoga) that increase your **flexibility**?
   ❑ regularly   ❑ occasionally   ❑ rarely   ❑ never   ❑ I don't know

5. If you consider yourself throughout the course of the **past year**, how would you best describe yourself?
   ❑ a "couch potato"   ❑ an occasional exerciser   ❑ a regular exerciser   ❑ an "athlete"

6. During the **past year**, how often have you done physical activities (such as jogging or carrying boxes at least 12 minutes) that increase your **endurance**?
   ❑ regularly   ❑ occasionally   ❑ rarely   ❑ never   ❑ I don't know

7. During the **past year**, how often have you done physical activities (such as weight lifting or strengthening calisthenics) that increase your **strength**?
   ❑ regularly   ❑ occasionally   ❑ rarely   ❑ never   ❑ I don't know

8. During the **past year**, how often have you done activities (such as stretching or yoga) that increase your **flexibility**?
   ❑ regularly   ❑ occasionally   ❑ rarely   ❑ never   ❑ I don't know

9. Tests to measure endurance (or, technically, maximal oxygen consumption) include walking on a treadmill, walking and then jogging on a treadmill, riding a stationary bike, and walking or jogging on a track. Have you ever had any of these tests?
   ❑ yes   ❑ no

If you have had an endurance test (i.e., to measure maximal oxygen consumption), provide as much information about the test as you can:

- Approximate date and year of the test: _____
- The result of the test: ❑ excellent   ❑ good   ❑ okay   ❑ poor
- Your maximum oxygen consumption: _____ mL/kg·min
- Did you wear an air mask?   ❑ yes   ❑ no

Figure 6-1 History of Fitness Wellness

often largely obtained through a self-report. Among other items discussed in the History sections of various Preferred Practice Patterns included in the *Guide to Physical Therapist Practice* (APTA, 2001b), the patient's/client's fitness and fitness wellness history should detail her or his past fitness status (e.g., during the past year as well as her or his entire life), how often she or he has exercised in the past (especially during the last year), and the results of a past test assessing maximal oxygen consumption (if any). To assess the history of a patient's/client's fitness and fitness wellness, you can utilize the form in Figure 6-1.

SECTION 4: EXAMINATION: SYSTEMS REVIEW

As discussed in the previous section, the *Guide to Physical Therapist Practice* (APTA, 2001b) includes one Preferred Practice Pattern related to the primary prevention of aerobic capacity disorders and numerous Preferred Practice Patterns related to restorative physical therapy that focus on aerobic capacity, muscular fitness, and/or flexibility. Each of these Preferred Practice Patterns stated that the systems review may include the anatomical and physiological status of the cardiovascular/pulmonary, integumentary, musculoskeletal, and neuromuscular system as well as communication, affect, cognition, language, and learning style. While the recommendations of the *Guide to Physical Therapist Practice* for the systems review are certainly helpful when conducting the systems review of a patient/client who presents with impaired fitness and fitness wellness, a fitness and fitness wellness systems review also should emphasize screening results related to fitness and fitness wellness. This typically includes the patient's/client's perception of her or his current fitness level, a "snapshot" of her or his current exercise, a screen of her or his commitment to fitness, and a screen of her or his involvement in and/or commitment to issues related to exercise, such as warming-up and cooling-down, hydration, and the use of anabolic steroids. To complete a systems review of a patient's/client's fitness and fitness wellness, you can utilize my Fitness Wellness Screen form (**Figure 6-2**). Using this screen or another, it is important to complete a fitness and fitness wellness systems review.

Analysis of the Fitness Wellness Systems Review

If you utilized the Fitness Wellness Screen (Figure 6-2) during a patient's/client's systems review, the information in this section can be used to analyze the results. For a broad overview of the patient's/client's current fitness wellness, examine her or his responses to items #1 and #2 in Figure 6-2. A satisfactory response for each is a regular exerciser or an athlete. Items #3 through #5 screen aerobic capacity wellness. A satisfactory response for items #3 and #4 is regularly. A satisfactory response for item #5 is at least 3 to 3.5 hours. Items #6 through #7 screen muscular fitness wellness and a satisfactory response for each is regularly. Items #8 and #9 screen muscular fitness wellness and flexibility wellness, respectively, and a satisfactory response for each is regularly.

The patient's/client's response to item #10 is a screen for anabolic steroid use. If the patient/client responds affirmatively, then you can ask detailed questions about her or his usage in the tests and measures section. Even if the patient/client denies steroid use in the systems review, she or he may not be disclosing the truth. Questions about anabolic

Fitness Wellness Screen

(To be completed by the patient/client)

Surname: _____   First: _____   Date: ___/___/_____

Please answer each of the questions honestly. Your honesty will help us to better assist you meet any goals you may have related to your fitness and/or body composition (e.g., fat weight versus muscle weight).

1. If you consider yourself throughout the **past month**, how would you best describe yourself?
   ❑ a "couch potato"   ❑ an occasional exerciser   ❑ a regular exerciser   ❑ an "athlete"

2. If you consider yourself throughout the **past week**, how would you best describe yourself?
   ❑ a "couch potato"   ❑ an occasional exerciser   ❑ a regular exerciser   ❑ an "athlete"

3. Over the **past month**, how often have you done physical activities (such as jogging or carrying boxes at least 12 minutes) that increase your **endurance**?
   ❑ regularly   ❑ occasionally   ❑ rarely   ❑ never   ❑ I don't know

4. Over the **past week**, how often have you done physical activities (such as jogging or carrying boxes for at least 12 minutes) that increase your **endurance**?
   ❑ regularly   ❑ occasionally   ❑ rarely   ❑ never   ❑ I don't know

5. Over the **past week**, for about how many hours did you do physical activities that increase your endurance?
   _____ hours

6. Over the **past month**, how often have you done physical activities (such as weight lifting or strengthening calisthenics) that increase your **strength**?
   ❑ regularly   ❑ occasionally   ❑ rarely   ❑ never   ❑ I don't know

7. Over the **past week**, how often have you done physical activities (such as weight lifting or strengthening calisthenics) that increase your **strength**?
   ❑ regularly   ❑ occasionally   ❑ rarely   ❑ never   ❑ I don't know

8. Over the **past month**, how often have you done activities (such as stretching or yoga) that increase your **flexibility**?
   ❑ regularly   ❑ occasionally   ❑ rarely   ❑ never   ❑ I don't know

9. During the **past week**, how often have you done activities (such as stretching or yoga) that increase your **flexibility**?
   ❑ regularly   ❑ occasionally   ❑ rarely   ❑ never   ❑ I don't know

10. Do you ever use anabolic steroids?   ❑ yes   ❑ no

Figure 6-2 Fitness and Fitness Wellness Systems Review

steroids in the tests and measures section will provide more insight into her or his behavior with anabolic steroids.

Summary: Systems Review

Among other items discussed in the systems review sections of various Preferred Practice Patterns included in the *Guide to Physical Therapist Practice* (APTA, 2001b), the fitness and fitness wellness aspect should screen the patient's/client's perception of her or his current fitness wellness and use of anabolic steroids. To complete a systems review of the client's fitness wellness, you can utilize the Fitness Wellness Screen found in Figure 6-2. It is important to complete a fitness wellness systems review using this or another screen.

SECTION 5: EXAMINATION: TESTS AND MEASURES

A physical therapist should examine her or his patient's/client's fitness wellness during the tests and measures section of the physical therapy examination. Unless otherwise medically contraindicated (e.g., by a diagnosis/condition of the patient/client at presentation), the physical therapist also should examine the patient's/client's level of fitness. It may be helpful to assess additional areas associated to the patient's/client's fitness and fitness wellness including but not limited to her or his knowledge and practices related to warming-up and cooling-down, dehydration and hydration (linked to exercise), and possible anabolic steroid use.

Fitness Wellness Tests and Measures

As discussed in Chapter 1, it is appropriate to utilize a survey to test and measure wellness, including fitness wellness; that is, aerobic capacity fitness wellness, muscular fitness wellness, and flexibility wellness. The survey should examine the patient's/client's habits and practices related to fitness wellness, cognitive knowledge of fitness wellness, and affective commitment to fitness wellness.

My proposal for a fitness wellness survey is provided in **Figure 6-3**. (Note: A discussion of the analysis of the fitness wellness survey is provided in Section 6.) Although several instruments measure aspects of physical wellness, such as the TestWell Wellness Inventory (National Wellness Institute [NWI], 2009), the Perceived Wellness Inventory (Adams et al., 1997), the Paffenbarger Physical Activity Questionnaire (Paffenbarger, Wing, & Hyde, 1978), and the Baecke Questionnaire (Baecke, Burema, & Frijters, 1982), none adequately examines the practices and habits that promote physical fitness. The survey in Figure 6-3 incorporates the strengths from earlier instruments and adds questions specific to fitness wellness.

Of the 100 items in the TestWell Wellness Inventory (NWI, 2009), only five relate to fitness. More importantly, the validity of three of the five fitness items is poor. For example, the first item on it stipulates that for an activity to qualify as an aerobic activity, it must cause the participant to sweat. Another fitness item asks the respondent to signify if "stretching is a routine part of my exercise program" is almost always, very often, often, occasionally, or almost never true (NWI, 2009, item #2). While responses to the questions

Fitness and Fitness Wellness Survey

(PT to examine patient/client and fill in this survey)

Surname: _____ First: _____ Date: ___/___/_____

Name of the Physical Therapist (PT): _____

Note to the PT: Dialog with the patient/client to complete these tests and measures. Utilize lay terminology unless there is direct evidence that more clinical terminology is indicated.

For the PT to state to the patient/client: I will be asking you numerous questions to obtain information about your exercise and fitness habits. Please answer as honestly, accurately, and completely as possible. This will enable me to help you meet any goals you may have related to your fitness and/or body composition (e.g., fat weight versus muscle weight). At the end of this survey, you will have the opportunity to ask me questions. Are you ready to start?

Section A: Cognitive Aspects of Fitness Wellness

1. Please rate the amount of cardiovascular/endurance/aerobic capacity exercise in which you've engaged during the past month:
   ❑ much too little   ❑ too little   ❑ just right   ❑ too much   ❑ I don't know

2. Please rate the amount of strength training/muscular fitness exercise in which you've engaged during the past month:
   ❑ much too little   ❑ too little   ❑ just right   ❑ too much   ❑ I don't know

3. Please rate the amount of stretching/flexibility exercise in which you've engaged during the past month:
   ❑ much too little   ❑ too little   ❑ just right   ❑ too much   ❑ I don't know

4. Tell me what you know about what a person should do in terms of cardiovascular/endurance/aerobic capacity exercise:

   _____

   _____

5. Tell me what you know about what a person should do in terms of strength training/muscular fitness exercise:

   _____

   _____

6. Tell me what you know about what a person should do in terms of stretching/flexibility exercises:

   _____

   _____

7. Under what circumstances can leisure activities (such as cleaning the house, playing basketball, and shoveling snow) "count" as cardiovascular/endurance/aerobic capacity exercise?

   _____

   _____

Figure 6-3 Fitness Wellness Tests and Measures

8. Under what circumstances can leisure activities (such as cleaning the house, playing basketball, and shoveling snow) "count" as strengthening/muscular fitness exercise?

_____

_____

9. What is the purpose of a warm-up?

_____

_____

10. What is the purpose of a cool-down?

_____

_____

11. Tell me what you know about exercise and dehydration:

_____

_____

12. Tell me what you know about anabolic steroids:

_____

_____

13. Do you believe it can be safe to use anabolic steroids?   ❑ yes   ❑ no   ❑ I don't know
14. Tell me what you know about the **risks** of anabolic steroids:

_____

_____

Section B-1: Psychomotor Aspects of Aerobic Capacity Wellness

1. Have you engaged in cardiovascular (aerobic capacity) exercise during the past week?

   ❑ yes   ❑ no

If yes: Please describe your cardiovascular (aerobic capacity) routine during the past week by telling me what type of exercise you did and on what day.

If no, but usually does: Complete this section and indicate when this aerobic capacity program was last performed. *If no, and does not usually:* Skip to the next section (Muscular Fitness Wellness).

DESCRIPTION OF EXERCISE	Monday	Tuesday	Wednesday	Thursday	Friday	Saturday	Sunday
Duration (in minutes)	_____	_____	_____	_____	_____	_____	_____
Mode of exercise (e.g., bike, swim, aerobic dance)	_____	_____	_____	_____	_____	_____	_____
Intensity of exercise utilizing the Perceived Activity Scale or terms *light, moderate,* or *heavy*	_____	_____	_____	_____	_____	_____	_____

Figure 6-3 Fitness Wellness Tests and Measures (continued)

2. If what you've just told me about your cardiovascular program is not typical behavior, tell me what you usually do and why it was different last week. (*Note to PT*: Specify what is typically performed in previous table and provide additional data below.)

_____

_____

Section B-2: Psychomotor Aspects of Muscular Fitness Wellness

1. Have you engaged in strengthening exercises during the past week?

    ❑ yes   ❑ no

If yes: Please describe your strengthening routine during the past week by telling me what type of exercise you did and on what day.

If no, but usually does: Complete this section and indicate when this strengthening program was last performed. *If no, and does not usually:* Skip to the next section (Flexibility Wellness).

Muscle–Strengthened	# of days	# of repetitions	# of sets	Mode (e.g., calisthenics, free)
Back of arms	_____	_____	_____	_____
Front of arms	_____	_____	_____	_____
Shoulder	_____	_____	_____	_____
Chest	_____	_____	_____	_____
Upper Back	_____	_____	_____	_____
Lower Back	_____	_____	_____	_____
Abdomen	_____	_____	_____	_____
Front of thighs	_____	_____	_____	_____
Back of thighs	_____	_____	_____	_____
Outer thighs	_____	_____	_____	_____
Inner thighs	_____	_____	_____	_____
Calves	_____	_____	_____	_____

2. If what you've just told me about your strength training program is not typical behavior, tell me what you usually do and why it was different last week. (*Note to PT*: Specify what is typically performed in previous table and provide additional data below.)

_____

_____

_____

Figure 6-3 Fitness Wellness Tests and Measures (continued)

Section B-3: Psychomotor Aspects of Flexibility Wellness

1. Have you engaged in a flexibility program during the past week, such as stretching, yoga, or tai chi?

   ❑ yes ❑ no

If yes: Please describe your stretching routine during the past week by telling me what type of exercise you did and on what day.

If no, but usually does: Complete this section and indicate when this flexibility program was last performed. *If no, and does not usually:* Skip to the next section (Leisure Wellness).

Muscle Group	# of days	Duration (in seconds)	Intensity (*no, mild,* or *severe* discomfort)	Mode (e.g., stretch on own, yoga position)
Chest	_____	_____	_____	_____
Shoulders	_____	_____	_____	_____
Back of upper arms	_____	_____	_____	_____
Back	_____	_____	_____	_____
Hips	_____	_____	_____	_____
Front of thighs	_____	_____	_____	_____
Back of thighs	_____	_____	_____	_____
Calves	_____	_____	_____	_____
Other:	_____	_____	_____	_____

2. If what you've just told me about your stretching (flexibility) program is not typical behavior, tell me what you usually do and why it was different last week. (*Note to PT*: Specify what is typically performed in previous table and provide additional data below.)

_____

_____

_____

Section B-4: Psychomotor Aspects of Leisure Wellness

Note to the PT: Based upon what the patient/client reports, select the most appropriate section of this survey in which to record each activity. Do **not** record an item in this section as well as in either of the Exercise sections. For example, if a patient/client plays 1 hour of basketball per day, do not include it in this section *and* in the Aerobic Capacity Wellness section.

1. During the past week, what was the average number of hours per day during which you engaged in a **sedentary activity** (e.g., sleeping, reading, being on the Internet/computer, watching TV/playing video games)? *Note*: Because the total includes sleep, the minimum hours recorded should typically be 7 or 8.

   _____ hours

Figure 6-3 Fitness Wellness Tests and Measures (continued)

2. During the past week, what was the average number of hours per day during which you engaged in an **activity of light intensity** (e.g., cleaning windows, raking leaves, weeding, painting, lawn mowing with a power mower, slowly waxing floor, playing doubles tennis)?

   _____ hours

3. During the past week, what was the average number of hours per day during which you engaged in an activity of **moderate intensity** (e.g., easy digging in a garden, pushing a lawn mower, light backpacking, house cleaning, skating, moderate-intensity basketball)?

   _____ hours

4. During the past week, what was the average number of hours per day during which you engaged in an activity of **heavy intensity** (e.g., sawing wood, heavy shoveling, carrying a heavy weight, digging a ditch, canoeing without rests, mountain climbing, high-intensity basketball)?

   _____ hours

5. During the past week, what was the average number of hours per day during which you engaged in an activity of **very heavy intensity** (e.g., carrying a very heavy weight or a load up steps, shoveling heavy snow, or playing paddleball, touch football, handball, or vigorous basketball)?

   _____ hours

6. If what you have just told me about your household activities is not typical behavior, tell me what you usually do and why it was different last week:

   _____

   _____

   _____

Section B-5: Other Dimensions of Fitness Wellness

1. Do you warm-up before you exercise?   ❑ yes   ❑ no

   If yes, what do you do?

   _____

2. Do you cool-down after you exercise?   ❑ yes   ❑ no

   If yes, what do you do?

   _____

3. If you warm-up before you exercise, about how often do you do it (e.g., 100% of the time, once per week)?

   _____

4. If you cool-down after you exercise, about how often do you do it (e.g., 100% of the time, once per week)?

   _____

   _____

Figure 6-3 Fitness Wellness Tests and Measures (continued)

5. Do you drink water or another beverage before, during, or after you exercise? ❑ yes ❑ no
If yes, what, when, and how much do you drink?

_____

_____

6. Have you used a tobacco product within the past month? ❑ yes ❑ no
If yes, tell me about your usage.

_____

_____

Specific directions to the physical therapist for items 7 and 8: If the patient/client talks positively and openly about anabolic steroids, it is important the physical therapist not speak to him or her in a judgmental tone. In an open atmosphere, the patient/client may more readily admit that she or he uses steroids.

7. Have you ever used anabolic steroids? ❑ yes ❑ no
If yes, tell me about it.

_____

_____

8. Do you currently use anabolic steroids? ❑ yes ❑ no
If yes, tell me about it.

_____

_____

Section C: Affective Aspects of Fitness Wellness

On a scale of 1 to 10, with 1 being no commitment and 10 being total commitment,

1. How committed are you to engaging in cardiovascular (aerobic capacity) exercise?
2 times/wk? _____; 3 times/wk? _____; 4 times/wk? _____; 5 times/wk? _____;
6 times/wk? _____; every day? _____

2. How committed are you to engaging in strengthening exercises 2 times/wk? _____;
3 times/wk? _____

3. How committed are you to engaging in flexibility exercises 2 times/wk? _____,
3 times/wk? _____

4. How committed are you to performing leisure activities that promote cardiovascular (aerobic capacity), e.g., tennis and other sports, laser tag, sand or snow art/play, gardening? _____

5. How committed are you to performing leisure activities that promote strength (muscular fitness), e.g., heavy yard work or house cleaning, carrying items that are heavy for you? _____

6. What kinds (modes) of exercise do you like and what kinds (modes) of exercise do you not like? (For example, one person might really like to swim, "kind of" like to strength train, and hate to use the treadmill.)

_____

_____

_____

Figure 6-3 Fitness Wellness Tests and Measures (continued)

Section D: Athleticism

Note to the PT: If you are examining both nutritional and fitness wellness, examine athleticism in one section only.

1. Over the past year, have you engaged in a "grueling" exercise program (i.e., at least 2 to 3 hours per day on at least 5 or 6 days per week)?

   ❑ yes   ❑ no   ❑ I don't know

2. Over the past month, have you engaged in a "grueling" exercise program (i.e., at least 2 to 3 hours per day on at least 5 or 6 days per week)?

   ❑ yes   ❑ no   ❑ I don't know

3. In the foreseeable future, do you intend to engage in a "grueling" exercise program, (i.e., at least 2 to 3 hours per day on at least 5 or 6 days per week)?

   ❑ yes   ❑ no   ❑ I don't know

Section E: Fitness Wellness Goal(s)

What is/are your fitness goal(s)?

_____

_____

_____

Figure 6-3 Fitness Wellness Tests and Measures (continued)

provide some information about the frequency of the stretching routine, they provide no information about the specific muscles being stretched or the quality of the stretches, including the duration of the stretches. Finally, item #4 on the TestWell Wellness Inventory is vague and overly subjective in that it invites the participant to indicate how often she or he engaged in an "adequate amount" of aerobic, strengthening, and flexibility exercise. The final two items related to fitness wellness also are weak. For example, item #3 asks the respondent to indicate if she or he increases her or his "physical activity by walking or biking for transportation whenever possible" almost always, very often, often, occasionally, or almost never (NWI, 2009, item #3). This item is a screen rather than a test and measure.

The other instruments designed to measure aspects of physical wellness also are deficient in their assessment of fitness wellness. While some of the items in the Perceived Wellness Survey (Adams et al., 1997) relate to the individual's beliefs and attitudes about his or her physical health, none relate to her or his behaviors. For example, one item is, "My physical health is excellent" and another is, "My body seems to resist physical illness very well" (Adams et al., 1997, p. 218). In fact, the creators of the Perceived Wellness Inventory declared that the survey emphasized the affective constructs of wellness (Adams et al., 1997). Finally, the Paffebarger Physical Activity Questionnaire (Paffenbarger et al., 1978) and the Baecke Questionnaire (Baecke et al., 1982) were designed to assess activity level at work, in sports, and or during leisure time; neither separately assesses muscular fitness wellness, aerobic capacity wellness, or flexibility wellness.

Fitness and Fitness Wellness Survey

The fitness wellness survey, which is a modification of the survey developed as part of my Philosophy Doctorate coursework, is provided in Figure 6-3. The purpose of the survey is to test and measure the fitness wellness of physical therapy patients/clients. In contrast to my surveys related to the fitness wellness history and systems review, the fitness wellness survey is designed to be completed by the physical therapist as she or he asks the patient/client a series of questions. As necessary, the examining physical therapist should facilitate the understanding of any questions that are unclear to the patient/client. Whether or not you utilize Figure 6-3 as your survey, it is important to complete one and be able to analyze it.

Fitness Tests and Measures

Aerobic Capacity: Preferred Practice Patterns

The *Guide to Physical Therapist Practice* (APTA, 2001) includes two Preferred Practice Patterns related to aerobic capacity: "6A, primary prevention/risk reduction for cardiovascular/pulmonary disorders" and "6B, impaired aerobic capacity/endurance associated with deconditioning." Both of these Preferred Practice Patterns state that the tests and measures may examine aerobic capacity and endurance, anthropometric characteristics, arousal, attention, and cognition; circulation; ergonomics and body mechanics; muscle performance (including endurance, strength, and power); posture, self-care and home management (including activities of daily living and instrumental activities of daily living), ventilation and respiration; and work (work/play/school), leisure, and community integration or reintegration. In addition, the "impaired aerobic capacity" of the tests and measures may also include assistive and adaptive devices; environmental, home, and work barriers; gait, balance, and locomotion; motor function (motor learning and motor control); range of motion (including muscle length); and sensory integration.

Test of Aerobic Capacity

Broadly speaking, there are two methods to assess aerobic capacity: (1) a direct assessment of the maximal oxygen consumption ($\dot{V}O_{2max}$), and (2) an indirect assessment of $\dot{V}O_{2max}$ through a submaximal test.

The direct assessment of $\dot{V}O_{2max}$ requires sophisticated equipment and procedures that may include oxygen and carbon dioxide analyzers, an ergometer on which workload may be modified, or collection of expired air volume measured via Douglas bags or a Tissot tank, or measured by a pnuemotach or turbine ventilometer. The direct assessment is costly, maximally strenuous to the participant, and may require the supervision of a physician. During a direct assessment, a participate is considered to have reached her/his $\dot{V}O_{2max}$ if there is a plateau (or *peaking over*) in oxygen uptake, a respiratory exchange ratio of 1.0 to 1.15 or greater attained, or the participant reaches volitional exhaustion.

In contrast to the rigors of the direct assessment of maximal oxygen consumption $\dot{V}O_{2max}$, indirect and submaximal tests are a popular alternative. A common type of indirect measurement relies upon the measurement of heart rate (HR) in response to a given workload. Maximal oxygen consumption may be predicted from the measurement of HR in response to a given exercise load because $\dot{V}O_{2max}$ and maximum heart rate (MHR) are correlated.

Indirect exams to predict $\dot{V}O_{2max}$ may over or underestimate an individual's true maximal oxygen consumption for several reasons. First, the MHR of an individual is estimated using the formula, 220 minus age. For example, if a female client is 40 years old, we could estimate that her MHR is 180 beats per minute (BPM), but her actual rate might be higher (185 BPM) or lower (175 BPM). (Note: Even if we directly measure our client's $\dot{V}O_{2max}$, we may not be able to assess her MHR because she may stop the test before reaching her maximum workload.) Second, during indirect examinations, a standard mechanical efficiency is assumed (McArdle et al., 2006). It is assumed that the individual utilizes a certain oxygen consumption at a given work rate, but the actual oxygen consumption at a given work rate may be somewhat higher or somewhat lower. Third, during indirect examinations to assess maximal oxygen consumption, it is assumed that the individual reaches a steady-state HR during each workload, but this may not be the case. Finally, it is also assumed that there is a linear relationship between heart rate and work rate during a submaximal examination, but, again, this may not be the case either. Secondary to these factors as well as human error, the predication of maximal oxygen consumption through submaximal tests is not 100% valid and the result should be critically analyzed (by comparing them to other factors including but not limited to the patient's/client's self-report of her or his exercise habits and the patient's/client's resting heart rate (if the patient/client is not taking a medication that affects her/his resting heart rate, of course).

There are numerous indirect examinations to estimate $\dot{V}O_{2max}$, including walk tests, jog tests, bicycle tests, and step tests. The following indirect examinations to estimate $\dot{V}O_{2max}$ are not all-inclusive.

Walk Test: Rockport The Rockport Walk Test is an appropriate examination to use if you suspect that the patient/client is less physically fit or has an orthopedic condition that precludes running. Benefits of this and similar walk tests are that they require only minimal equipment and resources and are not expensive. Moreover, you can assess multiple patients/clients at one time. While the Rockport Walk Test, like other walk tests, are less rigorous than those that require jogging, nonetheless they can require maximal exertion from a poorly conditioned individual. The Rockport Walk Test was validated ($r = 0.93$) by Kline, Porcari, Hintermeister, and colleagues in 1987. The test is also valid for women over the age of 65 (Fenstermaker, Plowman, & Looney, 1992). It is valid for college students (Dolgener, Hensey, Marsh, & Fjelstul, 1994), and a modified version is specifically designed for college-age men and women (George, Fellington, & Fisher, 1998).

To conduct the Rockport Walk Test, you will require a flat, nonslippery surface of a reasonable length (preferably a quarter-mile track) and a stopwatch. Instruct the patient/client to walk 1 mile (four laps around a quarter-mile track) as fast as possible. During the (estimated) final minute of the walk, the patient/client measures her or his heart rate. At the conclusion of the mile, record the length of time (in minutes and seconds expressed in decimal form) it took the patient/client to complete the mile. To calculate the patient's/client's $\dot{V}O_{2max}$, utilize the formula developed by Kline et al. (1987): $\dot{V}O_{2max}$ mL/kg·min = 132.853 − 0.1692 (weight in kilograms) − 0.3877 (age in years) + 6.315

(gender: 0 for female, 1 for male) − 3.2649 (time in minutes) − 0.1565 (heart rate at end of walk). A web site where this can be calculated is http://www.exrx.net/Calculators/Rockport.html.

Without a walking protocol, such as this test, estimating maximal oxygen consumption cannot be estimated reliably by measuring the heart rate during walking (Harrison, Bruce, Brown, & Cochrane, 1980).

Run Test: 1.5 Mile The 1.5-Mile Run Test is an appropriate examination to use if you suspect that the patient/client is physically fit. Benefits of this and similar run tests are that they require only minimal equipment and resources, and are not expensive. Moreover, multiple patients/clients can be assessed at one time. The 1.5-Mile Run Test and other run tests are more rigorous than walking tests, and the participant can cause it to be a maximal test if she or he sprints rather than maintains a steady pace. As early as 1980, run tests were found to be as valid and reliable in the measurement of $\dot{V}O_{2max}$ as treadmill tests (Harrison et al., 1980). The 1.5-Mile Run Test was validated by Kline et al. in 1987 and its validity has not been subsequently refuted.

To conduct the 1.5-Mile Run Test, you will require a flat, nonslippery surface of a reasonable length, preferably a quarter-mile track, and a stopwatch. Instruct the patient/client to run 1.5 miles (e.g., six laps around a quarter-mile track) at a steady rate but as fast as possible. At the conclusion of the run, record the length of time (in minutes and seconds expressed in decimal form) it took the patient/client to complete the mile. To calculate $\dot{V}O_{2max}$, utilize the formula: $\dot{V}O_{2max}$ mL/kg·min = 3.5 plus (483 divided by the time in minutes) (American College of Sport Medicine [ACSM], 2000, p. 307).

Run Test: 12 Minute The 12-Minute Run Test, devised by Kenneth H. Cooper, M.D., was developed in the late 1960s to assess servicemen in the U.S. Air Force (Cooper, 2008). The 12-Minute Run Test is an appropriate examination to use if you suspect that the patient/client is physically fit. Benefits of the 12-Minute Run Test, like the tests discussed above, are that it requires only minimal equipment and resources, is inexpensive, and multiple patients/clients can be assessed at one time. The 12-Minute Run Test is more rigorous than walking tests, and the participant can cause it to be a maximal test if she or he sprints rather than maintains a steady pace. As early as 1980, run tests were found to be as valid and reliable in the measurement of maximal oxygen consumption as treadmill tests (Harrison et al., 1980). The 12-Minute Run Test was validated by Cooper in 1968 and its validity has not been subsequently refuted.

To conduct the 12-Minute Run Test you will require a flat, nonslippery surface of a reasonable length, preferably a quarter-mile track, and a stopwatch. To conduct the test, instruct the patient/client to run for 12 minutes at a steady rate, but as fast as possible. At the conclusion of the run, record the distance (in meters) that the patient/client covered during the 12-minute period.

To calculate the patient's/client's $\dot{V}O_{2max}$, utilize the formula: $\dot{V}O_{2max}$ mL/kg·min = (distance covered in meters minus 504.9) divided by 44.73 (Cooper, 1968). Two web sites that can perform the calculations are http://www.brianmac.demon.co.uk/gentest.htm and http://revelsports.com/Articles/VO2_Max.htm.

Recognize that there are numerous field tests to estimate maximal oxygen consumption. For example, Léger and Lambert (1982) developed the Multi-Stage Fitness Test, which is a maximal multistage 20-meter shuttle run test. To review a modified version of the Multi-Stage Fitness Test, you may visit http://www.brianmac.demon.co.uk/beep.htm.

Treadmill Tests The treadmill is an appropriate mode to assess the $\dot{V}O_{2max}$ of most any patient/client because the machine can be programmed for walking, jogging, or running speeds. The advantage of testing a patient/client maximally is that you can obtain his or her MHR without relying upon his or her age-predicted MHR when prescribing his or her training HR range. The primary disadvantage of a treadmill test is the cost. Unlike a track, which can be freely and readily accessed at a local public school or other facility, the cost of a good treadmill is at least $3,000, if not significantly more. There are numerous treadmill protocols, including but not limited to the Bruce protocol, modified Bruce protocol, Balke protocol, Ellestad protocol, and continuous multistage running protocol. Research indicates that there are significant differences between tests to determine MHRs and $\dot{V}O_{2max}$ except between the Balke and the running protocols (39 vs 41 mL/kg·min) (Pollock et al., 1976).

To conduct a treadmill test, you will need a treadmill machine, with adjustments in slope and speed, a stopwatch, and an assistant. To conduct the test, instruct the patient/client to keep pace with the treadmill until she or he can no longer continue or experiences a contraindication (e.g., dizziness or angina).

The Bruce protocol was established in 1963 by Robert A. Bruce, M.D. It was independently validated in 1972 and continues to be utilized as the "gold standard" (Speer, 2005). The Bruce protocol consists of progressive stages that are 3 minutes each in length. The speed and incline for each stage are 1.7 mph and 10%, 2.5 mph and 12%, 3.4 mph and 14%, 4.2 mph and 16%, 5.0 mph and 18%, 5.5 mph and 20%, 6.0 mph and 22%, 6.5 mph and 24%, 7.0 mph and 26%, and 7.5 mph and 28%, respectively (Bruce, Blackmon, Jones, & Strait, 1963). The generic conversion to maximal consumption is $\dot{V}O_{2max}$ (mL/kg·min) = $14.76 - (1.379 \times T) + (0.451 \times T^2) - (0.012 \times T^3)$ (ACSM, 2007). To calculate a female patient's/client's $\dot{V}O_{2max}$, utilize the formula described by Pollock and colleagues (1982): $\dot{V}O_{2max}$ mL/kg·min = $4.38 \times T - 3.9$, where T is the total time of the test expressed in minutes and fractions of a minute (e.g., 13 minutes 15 seconds = 13.25 minutes). To calculate a male patient's/client's $\dot{V}O_{2max}$, utilize the formula described by Foster (1984): $\dot{V}O_{2max}$ mL/kg·min = $14.8 - (1.379 \times T) + (0.451 \times T^2) - (0.012 \times T^3)$, where T is the total time of the test expressed in minutes and fractions of a minute. A web site that can perform the calculations is http://www.exrx.net/Calculators/Treadmill.html.

The Balke protocol was established in the 1970s by Bruno Balke, M.D. For men the treadmill speed is set at 3.3 mph with the gradient starting at 0%. After 1 minute it is raised to 2%, and then 1% each minute thereafter. For women the treadmill speed is set at 3.0 mph with the gradient starting at 0% and increased by 2.5% every 3 minutes.

Other researchers used a constant walking speed at 3k/h with an increase in grade by 2.5% every 2 minutes (Froelicher, Thompson, Davis, Stewart, & Triebwasser, 1975). To calculate a woman's $\dot{V}O_{2max}$, utilize mL/kg·min = 1.38 (T) + 5.22; a man's $\dot{V}O_{2max}$ is mL/kg·min = 1.444 (T) + 14.99 where T is the total time of the test expressed in minutes and fractions of a minute (Pollock et al., 1982, as cited in Hanson, 1984).

Step Test: Queens College The Queens College Step Test is an appropriate examination to use if you need to test the patient/client indoors. It requires minimal equipment, is inexpensive, and you can assess multiple patients/clients at one time. In fact, the Queens College Step Test was specifically designed to test a large number of people by utilizing the bleachers commonly found in high school and university gymnasiums. This as well as many other step tests are biased against individuals of shorter stature, a factor that should be considered when interpreting the results. Similarly, step tests may overestimate the $\dot{V}O_{2max}$ of individuals who have extremely long legs. The Queens College Step Test was validated by McArdle, Katch, and Katch in 1972 (as cited by McArdle et al., 2006) and its validity has not been subsequently refuted. As early as 1980, step tests were found to be as valid and reliable in the measurement of maximal oxygen consumption as treadmill tests (Harrison et al., 1980).

To conduct the Queens College Step Test you will need access to a gymnasium bleacher or a step of the same height (16.25 inches), a stopwatch, and a metronome. To conduct the test, the metronome is set at a cadence of 88 BPM for women and 96 BPM for men. The duration of the test is 3 minutes. Instruct the patient/client to step up and then down from the bleacher (e.g., up right foot, up left foot, down right foot, down left foot). At the conclusion of the 3 minutes, ask the patient/client to sit on the bleacher and locate her or his pulse. After a 5-second period (during which time the patient/client locates her or his pulse), have the patient/client count the number of beats for a 15-second period (i.e., second 5 through second 20 of recovery). Multiply the result by four to obtain the recovery heart rate.

To calculate a woman's $\dot{V}O_{2max}$, utilize the formula: $\dot{V}O_{2max}$ mL/kg·min = 65.81 − (0.1847 × recovery heart rate) (McArdle et al., 2006). For men the formula is $\dot{V}O_{2max}$ mL/kg·min = 111.33 − (0.42 × recovery heart rate) (McArdle et al., 2006).

There are numerous step tests to estimate $\dot{V}O_{2max}$. For example, there is the Harvard Step Test. Visit http://www.topendsports.com/testing/tests/step.htm for details.

Bicycle Test The bicycle is an appropriate mode to assess $\dot{V}O_{2max}$ if the patient/client is uncomfortable using a treadmill or she or he regularly bicycles and it can be used if an outdoor mode of testing is not available. Compared to the field tests, the primary disadvantage of a bicycle test is the cost. Unlike a track, which can be freely and readily accessed at a local public school or other facility, the cost of an appropriate stationary bicycle is approximately $1,000. While there are numerous bicycle protocols, one of the most well-known is the Astrand–Ryhming (A-R), which was initially developed in 1954 (Legge & Banister, 1986). While the Astrand protocol was validated (r = .83) in 1981 by Cink and Thomas, there was a consistent tendency of the test to underestimate $\dot{V}O_{2max}$ with the original protocol.

A revised nomogram was developed and validated (r = .98) in 1986 by Legge and Banister for trained, moderately trained, and untrained males.

Test of Muscular Fitness

While muscular fitness can be assessed through traditional manual muscle tests, manual muscle testing will not be discussed in this book because it is extensively explored in numerous other textbooks, such as *Musculoskeletal Assessment: Joint Range of Motion and Manual Muscle Test and Muscles* by Clarkson and Gilewich (1999) and *Muscle Testing and Function with Posture and Pain (5th edition)* by Kendall, McCreary, and Provance (2005). In the "wellness" arena of muscular fitness, however, it is sometimes more appropriate to use other tests, such as calisthenics and weight equipment, because these modes of exercise are often included in a fitness wellness plan of care. To assess a patient's/client's muscular fitness using calisthenics and weight equipment, select exercises that will examine a variety of muscle groups, such as crunches, lumbar extensions, push-ups and/or pec deck, tricep extension, bicep curl, lat pull-down, seated knee extension, and hamstring curl. In cases involving weights, typically it is not appropriate to assess the one-repetition maximum as such a test can cause injury. A more reasonable option is the 5-repetition maximum test or even the 10-repetition maximum test if the patient/client has been previously sedentary. In calisthenic muscular fitness tests, it is often appropriate to have the patient/client perform as many repetitions as possible. However, if a patient/client has been previously sedentary, it may be better to have her or him complete as many repetitions as is felt as moderate, rather than easy or exhausting. In some cases there is a time limit and/or a cadence is required. Examples of calisthenic muscular fitness tests are in **Figures 6-4** and **6-5**.

Test of Flexibility

Flexibility can be assessed through traditional range of motion and/or muscle length tests. These tests are not discussed in this book as they are extensively explored in numerous other textbooks, such as *Musculoskeletal Assessment: Joint Range of Motion and Manual Muscle Test and Muscles* by Clarkson and Gilewich (1999) and *Muscle Testing and Function with Posture and Pain* by Kendall, McCreary, and Provance (2005).

Summary: Tests and Measures

The tests and measures section of a physical therapy examination assesses a patient's/client's fitness wellness and fitness. While it is appropriate to directly assess fitness, the same is not true for fitness wellness. Instead, the fitness wellness section of the tests and measures should utilize a written survey, such as my Fitness Wellness Survey, which fully examines a patient's/client's habits and practices related to fitness wellness.

Tests and measures for aerobic capacity include the walking tests (e.g., Rockport Walk Test), run tests (e.g., the 1.5-Mile Run Test and the 12-Minute Run Test), treadmill tests (e.g., Bruce protocol), step tests (e.g., Queens College Step Test), and bicycle tests (e.g., Astrand protocol). Tests and measures for muscular fitness include manual muscle

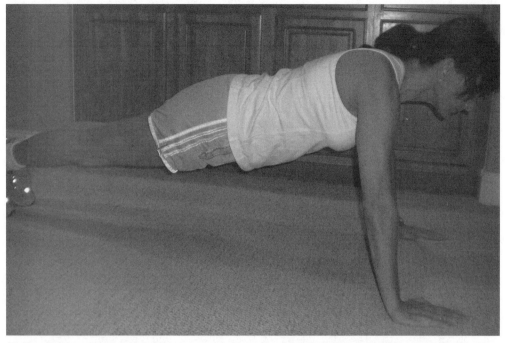

(A) Phase 1: Start position. The body is prone with elbows extended, back flat, and feet together.

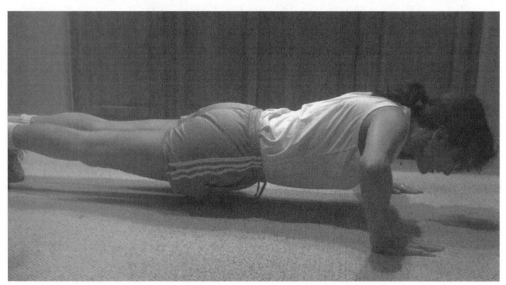

(B) Phase 2: Lower the entire length of the body, keeping the back flat and bending the elbows until the upper arms are parallel to the floor. Phase 3: Slowly push the arms against the floor, bringing the body up in a controlled fashion and finishing at the starting position.

Figure 6-4 Push-up test. The maximum number of push-ups performed consecutively without rest is counted as the score. The duration of the test is limited to 3 minutes. The maximum score is 75 repetitions.

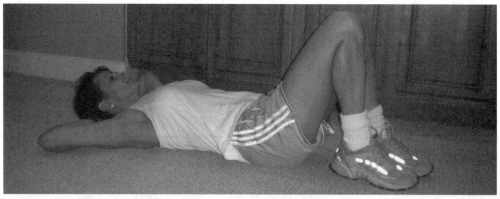

(A) Phase 1: Start position. Lay supine with the back in a posterior pelvic tilt (flat), knees bent, feet flat on the floor, and hands placed behind the head.

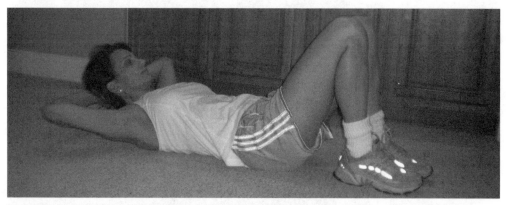

(B) Phase 2: While keeping the back in a posterior pelvic tilt, engage the abdominal muscles and curl upwards. Initiate the movement by gently flexing the cervical spine and dropping the chin slightly.

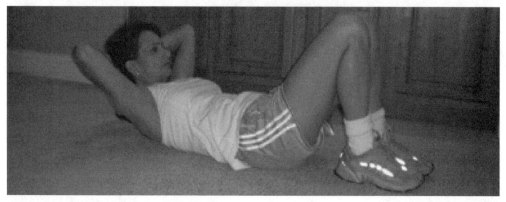

(C) Phase 3: Activate the abdominal muscles by raising the shoulders and upper back off of the floor toward the pelvis, and contract the abdominal muscles at the top of the movement. Phase 4: Return to the starting position while maintaining the posterior pelvic tilt.

Figure 6-5 Abdominal curl test. The maximal number of abdominal curls performed to a cadence of 25 repetitions per minute (the metronome is set at 50 beats per minute) consecutively without rest is counted as the score. The duration of the test is limited to 3 minutes and the maximum score is 75 repetitions. (*Source:* Modification of a test described by Sparling, Millard-Stafford, & Snow, 1997.)

tests, calisthenic tests, and weight equipment tests. Flexibility tests include range of motion tests and muscle length tests.

SECTION 6: EVALUATION OF FITNESS AND FITNESS WELLNESS

If the examination includes tests and measures related to fitness and fitness wellness, the evaluation must include a section related to fitness and fitness wellness. The fitness and fitness wellness evaluation is an analysis of the fitness and fitness wellness information obtained in the complete examination, including the history, the systems review, and the tests and measures. This evaluation may be influenced by other information obtained in the physical therapy examination, such as the patient's/client's mental status and motivation. In terms of components of fitness wellness, it is important that the psychomotor, cognitive, and affective dimensions are evaluated.

Evaluation of the Fitness Wellness Survey

If you utilized the Fitness Wellness Survey in Figure 6-3 to examine a patient's/client's fitness wellness, you may use the information in this subsection to evaluate her/his fitness wellness.

Aerobic Capacity Wellness

To determine if a patient's/client's aerobic capacity wellness is satisfactory, assess the applicable items in the fitness and fitness wellness survey. To possess a satisfactory level of aerobic capacity wellness, the patient/client must possess an adequate knowledge of aerobic capacity wellness, engage in a sufficient amount of aerobic capacity activities, and possess an acceptable level of commitment to aerobic capacity wellness.

Cognitive Aspect To determine if a patient/client possesses an adequate knowledge of aerobic capacity wellness, evaluate her/his response to items #4 and #7 in Section A (Figure 6-3). A satisfactory response to item #4 could be an extremely abbreviated version of the elementary aspects (in lay terminology) of this chapter's discussions of aerobic capacity wellness. Also determine if her/his response to item #1 in Section A matches her/his responses to Section B-1 and items #2 through #4 in Section B-4. If the patient/client accurately answers items #4 and #7 in Section A and her/his response to item #1 in Section A matches her/his responses in Section B-1 and items #2 through #4 in Section B-4, then you may conclude that her/his cognitive aspect of aerobic capacity wellness is satisfactory.

Psychomotor Aspect To determine if a patient/client engages in a sufficient amount of aerobic capacity activity, evaluate her or his responses in Section B-1 (Figure 6-3) in conjunction with her or his responses to items #2 through #4 in Section B-4 to the aerobic capacity wellness guidelines. Because the APTA (2001b) discusses aerobic capacity, but does not provide prescriptive guidelines, I suggest that physical therapists consider the guidelines of the *Healthy People 2010* (U.S. DHHS, 2000) and the ACSM (2006). Both resources recommend that individuals engage in at least 30 minutes of aerobic capacity exercise 5 or most days per week. Of course, one may exercise more than the minimum. For example, it is typically perfectly well to exercise for 4 hours per week. However, one may exercise too much. If a client/patient reports that she or he engages in aerobic capacity exercise more than 2 hours every day, then the physical therapist should examine the patient/client for an overuse injury as well as examine her or his mental wellness more thoroughly and screen for such disorders as bulimia nervosa. (Note: Bulimia nervosa and other mental disorders are discussed in Chapter 8.) If a patient/client engages in an appropriate amount of aerobic capacity exercise, then you can conclude that the psychomotor aspect of her/his aerobic capacity wellness is satisfactory.

Affective Aspect To determine if a patient/client possesses an adequate commitment to aerobic capacity wellness, evaluate her/his response to item #1 in Section C (Figure 6-3). If her or his commitment level to exercising 5 times per week is at least a 7 on the scale of 1 to 10 (with 1 being no commitment and 10 being total commitment), then you can conclude that the affective aspect of her/his aerobic capacity wellness is satisfactory.

Muscular Fitness Wellness

To determine a patient's/client's muscular fitness wellness, assess the applicable items in the Fitness and Fitness Wellness Survey. To possess a satisfactory level of muscular fitness wellness, the patient/client must possess an adequate knowledge of muscular fitness wellness, engage in a sufficient amount of muscular fitness activities, and possess an acceptable level of commitment to muscular fitness wellness.

Cognitive Aspect To determine if a patient/client possesses an adequate knowledge of muscular fitness wellness, evaluate her/his response to items #5 and #8 in Section A (Figure 6-3). A satisfactory response to item #5 could be an extremely abbreviated version of the elementary aspects (in lay terminology) of this chapter's discussions of muscular fitness wellness. Also determine if her/his response to item #2 in Section A matches her/his responses in Section B-2 and item #5 in Section B-4. If the patient/client accurately answers items #5 and #8 in Section A and her/his response to item #2 in Section A matches the responses in Section B-2 and item #5 in Section B-4, then you can conclude that her or his cognitive aspect of muscular fitness wellness is satisfactory.

Psychomotor Aspect To determine if a patient/client engages in a sufficient amount of muscular fitness activity, evaluate her/his responses in Section B-2 (Figure 6-3) in conjunction with her/his responses to item #5 in Section B-4 and muscular fitness wellness guidelines. Because the APTA (2001b) discusses muscular fitness wellness but does not provide prescriptive guidelines, I suggest that physical therapists consider the guidelines of the ACSM.

Perform a minimum of 8 to 10 separate exercises that train the major muscle groups . . . perform a minimum of one set of 8 to 12 repetitions . . . for individuals approximately 50 to 60 years of age or a more frail person, 10 to 15 repetitions may be more appropriate . . . perform these exercises 2 to 3 [days per week] (ACSM, 2006, p. 159).

Of course, one may exercise more than the minimum. For example, it is often perfectly fine to engage in strength training 3 or more days per week. However, one may exercise too much. For example, if strength training is performed on consecutive days, it is not advisable to (maximally or near maximally) strength train a particular muscle group on consecutive days (e.g., bicep muscles on both Mondays and Tuesdays). Instead, one should alternate muscles and days; for example, biceps on day 1, triceps on day 2, biceps again on day 3, and triceps again on day 4. However, if the physical therapist uncovers that a patient/client is strength training in a grueling fashion 6 or 7 days per week, the patient/client should be examined for an overuse injury as well as mental wellness to screen for such disorders as body dysmorphic disorder. (Note: This and other mental disorders are discussed in Chapter 8.) If a patient/client engages in an appropriate amount of aerobic capacity exercise, then you can conclude that the psychomotor aspect of her/his muscular fitness wellness is satisfactory.

Affective Aspect To determine if a patient/client possesses an adequate commitment to muscular fitness wellness, evaluate her or his response to item #2 in Section C (Figure 6-3). If her/his commitment level is at least a 7 on the scale of 1 to 10, then you may conclude that the affective aspect of her or his muscular fitness wellness is satisfactory.

Flexibility Wellness

To determine if a patient's/client's flexibility wellness is satisfactory, assess the applicable items in the fitness and fitness wellness survey. To possess a satisfactory level of flexibility wellness, the patient/client must possess an adequate knowledge of flexibility wellness, engage in a sufficient amount of flexibility activities, and possess an acceptable level of commitment to flexibility wellness.

Cognitive Aspect To determine if a patient/client possesses an adequate knowledge of flexibility wellness, evaluate her/his response to item #6 in Section A (Figure 6-3). A satisfactory response could be an extremely abbreviated version of the elementary aspects (in lay terminology) of this chapter's discussions of aerobic capacity wellness. Also determine if her/his response to item #3 in Section A matches the responses in Section B-3. If the patient/client accurately answers item #6 in Section A and item #3 in Section A matches her/his responses in Section B-3, then you can conclude that her/his cognitive aspect of flexibility wellness is satisfactory.

Psychomotor Aspect To determine if a patient/client engages in a sufficient amount of flexibility activity, evaluate her/his responses in Section B-3 (Figure 6-3) to flexibility wellness guidelines. Because the APTA (2001b) discusses flexibility but does not provide prescriptive guidelines, I suggest that physical therapists consider information contained in publications related to the American Physical Therapy Association as well as other reputable sources, such as *ACSM's Guidelines for Exercise Testing and Prescription* (2006).

Similar to their muscular fitness guidelines, the ACSM (2006) recommend that each major muscle and/or tendon group be stretched during the 30-minute exercise session a minimum of 2 to 3 days per week. Of course, it is perfectly fine to engage in flexibility activities more frequently, including up to every day. In terms of the duration of a stretch, empirical evidence in articles published in journals affiliated with the APTA, recommend 30 seconds or more (Felend, 2001; Manzari, Ruddy, Woycik, & Pfalzer, 2001). The intensity of a stretch, whether it be a traditional stretch on one's own or a yoga pose in a group exercise class at a health club, should be to the point of mild discomfort (ACSM, 2006), rather than without discomfort or to the point of severe discomfort. There is an array of acceptable modes of flexibility exercises, including but not limited to, static stretching, yoga poses, and the stretching that occurs with proprioceptive neuromuscular facilitation.

Affective Aspect To determine if a patient/client possesses an adequate commitment to flexibility wellness, evaluate her/his response to item #3 in Section C (Figure 6-3). If her/his commitment level is at least a 7 on the scale of 1 to 10, then you can conclude that the affective aspect of her/his flexibility wellness is satisfactory.

Leisure Activity

To determine if a patient's/client's leisure activity wellness is satisfactory, assess the applicable items in the fitness and fitness wellness survey. To possess a satisfactory level of leisure activity wellness, the patient/client must possess an adequate knowledge of leisure activity wellness, engage in adequate amount of non-sedentary leisure activities, and possess an acceptable level of commitment to leisure activities that promote aerobic capacity wellness and muscular fitness wellness.

Cognitive Aspect To determine if a patient/client possesses an adequate knowledge of aerobic capacity wellness, evaluate her/his response to items #7 and #8 in Section A (Figure 6-3). A satisfactory response could be an extremely abbreviated version of the elementary aspects (in lay terminology) of this chapter's discussions of aerobic capacity wellness. Also determine if the responses to items #1 and #2 in Section A match the responses to Section B-4. If the patient/client accurately answers items #1 and #2 in Section A and these match her/his responses in Section B-4, then you can conclude that her/his cognitive aspect of leisure activity wellness is satisfactory.

Psychomotor Aspect To determine if a patient/client engages in a sufficient amount of leisure activity, evaluate her/his responses in Section B-4 (Figure 6-3). When evaluating the psychomotor aspect of leisure activity of wellness, it is appropriate to consider the typical day as a whole rather than each section separately (i.e., evaluating the sedentary section by itself, and then evaluating the light-intensity section by itself, etc.). For example, if a patient/client engages in more hours per week of very heavy-intensity or heavy-intensity activity, it still would be satisfactory if she or he engaged in little or no moderate-intensity activity. In contrast, if a patient/client engages in no very heavy- or heavy-intensity activity, it is expected that she or he would engage in a significant amount of moderate-intensity and light-intensity activities.

Affective the Aspect To determine if a patient/client possesses an adequate commitment to leisure activity wellness, evaluate her/his response to items #4 and #5 in Section C (Figure 6-3). If her/his commitment level to each of the two items is at least a 7 on the scale of 1 to 10, then you can conclude that the affective aspect of her/his leisure activity wellness is satisfactory.

Additional Aspects of Fitness Wellness

Warm-Up and Cool-Down To determine if a patient/client is satisfactory in terms of warming-up and cooling-down, evaluate her/his response to items #9 and #10 in Section A (Figure 6-3) and items #1 through #4 in Section B-5. A satisfactory response to these items can be determined by several means, one of which is to compare the response to the information provided in the "Warm-Up and Cool-Down" subsection in Section 1 of this chapter. For example, a brisk walk or slow jog is an appropriate warm-up for a faster jog, whereas only stretching the hamstrings is not.

Dehydration and Hydration To determine if a patient/client is satisfactory in terms of dehydration and hydration (as they relate to exercise), evaluate her/his response to item #11 in Section A and item #5 in Section B-5. A satisfactory response to these items can be determined by several means, one of which is to compare the response to the information provided in the "Dehydration and Hydration" subsection in Section 1 of this chapter. For example, the patient/client might report that she or he drinks about ½ cup of water before her or his exercise session, about 1 cup of water during her or his 30-minute bicycle ride, and 1 cup of water following her or his exercise session.

Anabolic Steroids To determine if the patient/client is (or possibly is) using anabolic steroids, assess her/his responses to items related to anabolic steroids in the Fitness Wellness Survey (Figure 6-3). If the patient/client shares a significant amount of information about anabolic steroids (items #12, Section A) and/or insists that is safe to use them (item #13, Section A), and/or insists that there are no risks to using them (item #14, Section A), and also is a bodybuilder or an athlete and is also a man, then she or he may be using them even having previously denied taking them (e.g., in the systems review). Also assess the patient's/client's responses to items #7 and #8 in Section B-5.

Athleticism

To determine if a patient/client is an athlete, assess her or his responses in Section D. If the patient/client responds that she or he has been engaging in a grueling exercise program (i.e., she or he exercises at least 2 to 3 hours per day on at least 5 or 6 days per week) and these data are at least somewhat corroborated from the aerobic capacity and muscular fitness tests and measures, then you can conclude that the client is an athlete. (Keep in mind that a patient/client may engage in a grueling exercise program but not be genetically predisposed to a high maximal oxygen consumption or a high level of muscular strength.)

Patient/Client Goals

Evaluate the patient's/client's response to Section E (Figure 6-3). Given the patient's/client's comprehensive status, determine which goals are realistic and which are not. Begin to consider the tentative time frame to achieve each reasonable goal. Also analyze each realistic goal in terms of its compatibility with other goals the patient/client has verbalized, including fitness and non-fitness goals.

The Typical Patient's/Client's Fitness Wellness

While each person is unique, it is helpful to be familiar with the typical American's fitness wellness because many physical therapy patients/clients will present with similar fitness wellness deficits. In 2005, the prevalence of those engaging in regular physical activity was 47% among women and 50% among men (Kruger, 2007). These statistics represent an increase from 2001, when 43% of women and 48% of men regularly engaged in physical activity. Fitness wellness varies among racial/ethnic groups. In 2005, 49.6% of non-Hispanic white women, 52.3% of non-Hispanic white men, 31.5% of non-Hispanic black women, 40.5% of non-Hispanic black men, 36.5% of Hispanic women, and 40.3% of Hispanic men regularly engaged in physical activity.

Aerobic Capacity

Gender and Age While some women possess a higher $\dot{V}O_{2max}$ than some men, the typical man has a higher maximal oxygen consumption than the typical woman. Wood (2006a) identified the average $\dot{V}O_{2max}$ of a 30-year-old man as 40 to 42 mL/kg·min while the average for a same aged woman was 31 to 33 mL/kg·min. Generally speaking, younger adults possess a higher maximal oxygen consumption than older adults. That same study found that the average $\dot{V}O_{2max}$ of a 60-year-old man is 30 to 31 mL/kg·min and an age-matched woman was 25 to 27 mL/kg·min. Although advancing age negatively impacts maximum oxygen consumption, consistent training throughout life will lessen the effects of aging on maximal oxygen consumption (Hawley, Myburgh, & Noakes, 1999).

Maximal Oxygen Consumption and Occupation Aerobic capacity appears to be occupation-dependent (McArdle et al., 2006). If gender and age are accounted for, a more active job is positively correlated to a higher $\dot{V}O_{2max}$. Pafnote, Vaida, and Luchian (1979) found that the maximal oxygen consumption of foresters ranged from 39 to 57 mL/kg·min, miners ranged from 35 to 49 mL/kg·min, and toolmakers and panel operators ranged from 32 to 45 mL/kg·min. These investigators also reported that the highest $\dot{V}O_{2max}$ values were found in the foresters, with miners, toolmakers, and panel operators in descending order. In 20- to 29-year-olds, values of 50 mL/kg·min or above were found in 88% of the foresters, 54% of the miners, 37% of the toolmakers, and 27% of the panel operators.

Maximal Oxygen Consumption and Athletes The $\dot{V}O_{2max}$ of certain athletes, particularly endurance athletes, is significantly higher than that of even those individuals who engage in aerobic exercise on a regular basis. For example, a professional male athlete may have a $\dot{V}O_{2max}$ rated as excellent at 80 to 83 mL/kg·min and a female professional athlete may rate as 60 to 65 mL/kg·min (McArdle et al., 2006). Perhaps the highest $\dot{V}O_{2max}$ in a man was 96 mL/kg·min, which was measured in the winner of 29 Olympic and World Championship medals for cross-country skiing, Bjørn Daehlie Verdens Gang ([VG], 2001). A U.S. study measured 94 mL/kg·min in another Olympic champion (Montana State University, 1998). Perhaps the highest maximal oxygen consumption for a woman was 75 mL/kg·min, which was reported for a professional skier (*Physiology and Psychology*, 1998).

It is important to note that maximal oxygen consumption is determined not only by training, but also by a genetic predisposition. Independently from how intensely an individuals trains, if that individual does not have a genetic predisposition for an exceptionally high maximal oxygen consumption, she or he will never achieve an exceptional level. Athletes, as groups, differ in their maximal oxygen consumption. In one study, the $\dot{V}O_{2max}$ of distance runners was 54.4 mL/kg·min while for sprinters was 47.2 mL/kg·min. (Barnard, Grimditch, & Wilmore, 1979).

Maximal Oxygen Consumption Normative Values

Pollock, Schmidt, and Jackson's (1980) $\dot{V}O_{2max}$ normative values for women and men are provided in **Table 6-1** and **Table 6-2**, respectively.

Evaluation of Aerobic Capacity

To evaluate a patient's/client's aerobic capacity, the physical therapist should compare the patient's/client's $\dot{V}O_{2max}$ to the normative guidelines and assign a value of excellent, above average, average, below average, or poor. If an examination of $\dot{V}O_{2max}$ was not possible or appropriate, the physical therapist should estimate the client's level of aerobic capacity by

Table 6-1 Maximal Oxygen Consumption Normative Values for Women $\dot{V}O_{2max}$ (mL/kg·min)

Age (yrs)	Poor	Below Average	Average	Above Average	Excellent
Women					
20–29	< 24	24–30	31–37	38–48	49+
30–39	< 20	20–27	28–33	34–44	45+
40–49	< 17	17–23	24–30	31–34	42+
50–59	< 15	15–20	21–27	28–37	38+
60–69	< 13	13–17	18–23	24–34	35+

Table 6-2 Maximal Oxygen Consumption Normative Values for Men

Age (yrs)	Poor	Below Average	Average	Above Average	Excellent
Men					
20–29	< 25	25–33	34–42	45–52	53+
30–39	< 23	23–30	31–38	39–48	49+
40–49	< 20	20–26	27–35	36–44	45+
50–59	< 18	18–24	25–33	34–42	43+
60–69	< 16	16–22	23–30	31–40	41+

Source: Pollock ML, Schmidt DH, Jackson AS. (1980) Measurement of cardio-respiratory fitness and body composition in the clinical setting. *Comprehensive Therapy, 6(9),* 12–27 (p. 16).

considering her or his medical status, functional status, and self-reported habits and practices related to aerobic capacity (e.g., frequency, intensity, and duration of activities that promote aerobic capacity). For example, if the patient's/client's history includes a diagnosis of coronary artery disease, she or he reports having a sedentary job, and sedentary leisure activities (e.g., watches television and plays cards), and does not exercise, it is reasonable to presume that her/his aerobic capacity is below average to poor.

Evaluation of Muscular Fitness

If muscular fitness was examined with traditional manual muscle tests, the physical therapist need not assign a value of excellent, above average, average, below average, or poor. However, if muscular fitness was examined with calisthenics and/or weight equipment, it is indicated to assign a category value. In such cases, standardized values can be used. **Tables 6-3** and **6-4** show the values for push-up and abdominal curl tests respectively by age and gender.

Flexibility

If flexibility was examined with traditional range of motion and/or muscle length tests, the physical therapist may assign a value. However, instead of using the categories excellent to poor, the categories of within normal limits, within functional limits, minimally impaired, moderately impaired, and maximally impaired may be utilized. For example, a shoulder flexion of zero to 180 degrees can be assigned the value of within normal limits,

Table 6-3 Muscular Fitness: Standard Push-Up Test

% Score	Age 20–29	Age 30–39	Age 40–49	Age 50–59
Women				
Excellent	16	15	14	13
Above average	12	12	11	11
Average	10	8	7	6
Below average	7	6	5	4
Poor	4	3	2	1
Men				
Excellent	41	32	25	20
Above average	34	27	21	18
Average	27	21	16	12
Below average	21	16	12	9
Poor	16	11	8	6

Source: Fair, S. E. (2007b). *Wellness and Physical Therapy*. St. Augustine: Embury.

Table 6-4 Muscular Fitness: Abdominal Curl Test (Number of Curls)

	Age 18–25	*Age 26–35*	*Age 36–45*	*Age 46–55*	*Age 56–65*	*Age 65+*
Women						
Excellent	> 43	> 39	> 33	> 27	> 24	> 23
Above average	33–43	29–39	23–33	18–27	14–24	13–23
Average	29–28	21–24	19–22	14–17	10–12	11–13
Below average	25–28	21–24	15–18	10–13	7–9	5–10
Poor	< 25	< 21	< 15	< 10	< 7	< 5
Men						
Excellent	> 49	> 45	> 41	> 35	> 31	> 28
Above average	39–49	35–35	30–41	25–35	21–31	19–28
Average	35–38	31–34	27–29	22–24	17–20	15–18
Below average	31–34	29–30	23–26	18–21	13–16	11–14
Poor	< 30	< 29	< 23	< 18	< 13	< 11

Source: Fair, S. E. (2007b). *Wellness and Physical Therapy.* St. Augustine: Embury.

zero to 160 degrees can be assigned the value of within functional limits, and zero to 70 degrees can be assigned the value of maximally impaired.

Summary: Evaluation of Fitness and Fitness Wellness

If fitness and fitness wellness are examined in the tests and measures, the evaluation should include a section related to fitness and fitness wellness. The fitness and fitness wellness evaluation is an analysis of the fitness and fitness wellness information obtained in the history, systems review, and the tests and measures; particularly the information in the fitness and fitness wellness sections of the examination. If the fitness wellness survey is utilized as a test and measure, the evaluation should include an analysis of this instrument. In most cases, evaluation of the fitness tests can result in rating the patient/client by category using normative tables of excellent, above average, average, below average, or poor. In the case of flexibility, the categories are within normal limits, very minimally impaired, minimally impaired, moderately impaired, and maximally impaired.

While each client is unique, it is helpful to be familiar with the typical American's fitness and fitness wellness values because many physical therapy patients/clients may present with fitness and fitness wellness deficits that are similar to the reference client (see Chapters 1 and 2). The typical physical therapy patient/client will present with unsatisfactory fitness wellness and an impaired level of fitness.

SECTION 7: FITNESS WELLNESS CONDITION/DIAGNOSIS

If the patient/client does not engage in the recommended amount of aerobic capacity, strength training, or flexibility activity, you should assign a condition of "impaired aerobic capacity," "impaired muscular fitness," or "impaired flexibility," as the case may be. If the patient/client presents with a below average or poor $\dot{V}O_{2max}$, she or he should be assigned the condition of "impaired aerobic capacity wellness." For the patient/client presenting with a below average or poor strength, the condition should be "impaired muscular fitness wellness." A patient/client presenting with moderately or maximally impaired flexibility should be assigned the condition of "impaired flexibility wellness."

An appropriate diagnosis code for a patient/client with an impaired aerobic capacity wellness may be "780.9, decreased functional activity." Appropriate diagnoses for impaired aerobic capacity may be "785, symptoms involving cardiovascular system" and "V81.2, other and unspecified cardiovascular conditions." Certain diagnostic codes, such as "305.1, tobacco use disorder," may be associated with a decreased aerobic capacity.

An appropriate diagnosis for a patient/client with impaired muscular fitness wellness may be "780.9, decreased functional activity." An appropriate diagnosis for decreased muscular fitness may be "728.2 muscular weakness or wasting or disuse atrophy." Two APTA Preferred Practice Patterns are specifically relevant to muscular fitness wellness: "4A, primary prevention/risk reduction for skeletal demineralization" and "4C, impaired muscle performance."

The correct diagnosis code for a patient/client with an impaired flexibility wellness may be "780.9, decreased functional activity." Appropriate diagnoses for decreased flexibility may be "728.8, other disorders of muscle, ligament, and fascia," "727.81, tight tendon," "719.90, joint disorder," or "729.0, other disorders of soft tissue." Review the APTA Preferred Practice Pattern that is specifically relevant to flexibility wellness: "4D, impaired joint mobility, motor function, muscle performance, and range of motion associated with connective tissue dysfunction."

Summary: Fitness Wellness Condition/Diagnosis

A physical therapist may diagnose a patient/client with decreased aerobic capacity if she or he presents with a below average or poor $\dot{V}O_{2max}$ or a below average or poor aerobic capacity if a $\dot{V}O_{2max}$ cannot be directly or indirectly assessed. Note, however, that while the medical and insurance communities recognize a diagnosis (e.g., "780.9, decreased functional activity"), they do not yet recognize conditions (e.g., impaired aerobic capacity wellness or impaired aerobic capacity).

SECTION 8: FITNESS AND FITNESS WELLNESS PROGNOSIS, PLAN OF CARE, AND GOALS/OBJECTIVES

Prognosis

The fitness prognosis and the fitness wellness prognosis are subsets within the physical therapy prognosis. The template of fitness and fitness wellness prognosis is for the patient/client to demonstrate optimal fitness and fitness wellness, which thereby enhances her or his ability to function in the home, during leisure, active time in her or his occupation, and in community environments. During the length of time under the physical therapist's care, the goals described in the plan of care should be achieved.

Plan of Care and Goals/Objectives

The fitness plan of care and the fitness wellness plan of care (including goals) are components within the broader physical therapy plan of care. The fitness wellness plan of care and the fitness wellness plan of care that you devise for your patient/client should be in alignment with her/his examination, evaluation, and condition/diagnosis.

Plan of Care

"Physical therapists promote increased fitness to their patients by developing and implementing plans of care that incorporate exercise and physical activity as well as by providing education about the positive health benefits of an active lifestyle . . . . Development of a plan of care incorporating fitness principles . . . depends upon a physical therapist's understanding of contemporary concepts and terminology pertaining to fitness and of the elements of an exercise prescription" (Jewell, 2006, p. 47).

When developing a fitness wellness plan of care, consider the components of an exercise session, the variables of exercise, the principles of training, and the stages of conditioning.

Components of an Exercise Session The components of an exercise session are the warm-up, the exercise itself, and the cool-down. The warm-up occurs before the exercise and its purposes include but are not limited to preparing the body for exercise and helping to prevent delayed-onset muscle soreness. The exercise component can consist of physical activities to promote aerobic capacity, muscular fitness, body composition, and/or flexibility. The cool-down occurs after the exercise component and its purposes include but are not limited to safely returning the body to resting state, preventing pooling of the blood in the lower extremities, and helping to dissipate byproducts of the exercise, such as lactic acid.

Variables of Exercise The variables of exercise are intensity, duration, frequency, and mode. The following scenario exemplifies each of the variables of exercise. Joan is jogging on a treadmill at a speed of a 10-minute mile. (This denotes the intensity.) Joan jogs on the treadmill for 20 minutes. (This denotes the duration.) Joan exercises on a treadmill three times this week. (This denotes the frequency.) Joan utilizes a treadmill rather than a stationary bicycle or participating in a group exercise class. (The treadmill, bicycle, and group exercise class are all modes of exercise.)

Principles of Training The four principles of training are specificity, overload, reversibility, and individual differences. The acronym for the principles of training is "SORI" and a physical therapist will be "sorry" if she or he does not take the principles of training into account when developing a fitness plan of care for her or his patients/clients!

The individual differences principle recognizes that the baseline fitness level of an individual and the training response to a given exercise regimen are unique (McArdle et al., 2006). While rest, sleep, nutrition, illness/injury, motivation, maturity, and the environment influence a baseline fitness measurement and the response to a specific fitness protocol, the core determinants are genetics and habitual exercise patterns (modification of Seiler, 2006). An example of a genetic determinant is muscle fiber type. For example, while the fiber type distribution in a human's thigh muscles is roughly 50% slow and 50% fast twitch fibers, Simoneau and Bouchard (1989) found that the range of slow twitch fibers in the vastus lateralis range from 15% to 85% in different people. An illustration that captures the individual differences principle is

> On average, a 25-year-old untrained man will have a maximal oxygen consumption of 45 mL/min/kg. However, completely untrained people have walked into a lab, gotten on a treadmill and had a $\dot{V}O_{2max}$ of 70 mL/min/kg. I tested a fellow exactly like this myself once. I was teaching a class and he "volunteered" to perform a cycling max test. I predicted his max for the class based on his exercise history (little if any). Imagine my surprise as he kept cycling and his VO_2 kept climbing and climbing as I progressively increased the workload on the bike! He didn't bother to tell me his sister had rowed in the Olympics until after the test! There are equally "healthy" untrained young men whose max is only 35 mL/min/kg. That's a two times difference in aerobic capacity before they do their first workout! This is a physiological gap will not be closed, no matter how hard the "less endowed" fellow trains. If the high VO_2 guy trains very hard, he might reach 80 mL/kg·min, a 14% increase. The low VO_2 guy can train equally hard and possibly reach 50 mL/kg·min, a larger 42% increase. The gap can narrow (to 60% here), but it will not go away. Genetics place limitations on our body. (Seiler, 2006, para. 13)

Empirical evidence supports the individual differences principle. For example, Macková and colleagues (1986) examined the difference in skeletal muscle characteristics of sprint cyclists and nonathletes. They found that the ratio of fast to slow muscle fibers was 2:3 in the cyclists and 3:2 in the nonathletes, the mean diameter of each muscle fiber type was significantly higher in the athletes, and that (knee extension) maximum voluntary isometric strength was about 17% greater in cyclists than in the nonathletes. What these results indicate is that to be a sprint cyclist, one must be genetically predisposed with a high ratio of fast to slow twitch muscle fibers. They also indicate that because sprint cycling heavily uses the quadriceps, these muscles are hypertrophied and are stronger than the quadriceps in nonathletes. Thus, individuals who are genetically predisposed to cycling obtain the maximum benefit from engaging in the sport.

The overload principle is concerned with the concept that for improvement to occur, there must be an ever-increasing amount of stress. A simple example is a sedentary man who begins a walking program and gradually increases his aerobic capacity. In a relative short period of time, the previously sedentary man must increase the speed at which he walks, the duration of his walks, and/or the frequency of his walks to gain the same benefits of the exercise. The general adaptation syndrome (described by Hans Selye, and expanded by Yakovlev) is the basis of the overload principle, which states that "if the stress is too small in either intensity or duration, little or no adaptation growth is stimulated. On the other hand, if the stress is too severe, 'growth' is delayed or even prevented" (Seiler, 2006, para. 3).

The specificity principle acknowledges that metabolic and physiologic adaptations occur in response to the type of overload (McArdle et al., 2006). According to SONV

(Special Olympics Nevada [SONV], 2004, para. 5), "Specific training yields specific results. Train the desired muscles. The long distance runner trains by running not swimming or biking. Although the runner receives some training benefits from biking and swimming, specificity garners the greatest return on training investment." Empirical evidence supports the specificity principle. Verstappen, Huppertz, and Snoeckx (1982) examined the effect of training specificity on maximal treadmill and bicycle ergometer exercise. Their study focused on two groups: competitive long-distance running athletes and competitive cycle-racing athletes. Each athlete completed three sets of maximal exercise tests on a bicycle ergometer and three sets of maximal exercise tests on a treadmill. A comparison of the results demonstrated that the $\dot{V}O_{2max}$ of the long-distance runners was 14% higher on a treadmill, but equal in the cycle racers. The authors concluded that, "congruence between the mode of ergometer exercise and the sport activity improves the validity of the test result" (p. 43).

The reversibility principle recognizes that the effects of exercise are transient (McArdle et al., 2006). When a person stops regularly exercising, the training effect reduces at about one-third the rate of acquisition (Jenson & Fischer, 1972, as cited in SONV, 2004). Although there is a shortage of larger-scale studies related to the reversibility principle, a case study of an athlete was recently published. Godfrey, Ingham, Pedlar, and Whyte (2005) found that following 8 weeks of inactivity, the athlete's $\dot{V}O_{2max}$ declined by 8%. During the subsequent retraining period the athlete's $\dot{V}O_{2max}$ initially increased rapidly, but then the rate of improvement slowed. By week 20 of the retraining period, the athlete's $\dot{V}O_{2max}$ neared but did not reach his premorbid level. A conclusion of the study was that retraining takes considerably longer to achieve than detraining.

Seiler (2006) provides details of the concept of reversibility:

> The human body is nothing if not thrifty! The iron and protein in those millions of blood cells that die each day is almost completely re-used to build new blood cells! The body does not build proteins it doesn't need . . . , and it doesn't retain proteins that are no longer needed! For the athlete, the unfortunate consequence of this thriftiness is the rapid reversibility of training adaptations if training is stopped. In general, I think it is fair to say that those adaptations that occur fastest when we start training fade away fastest when we stop training. So, a week in bed with the flu will result in a substantial loss in blood plasma volume, but little change in mitochondrial enzyme concentration, and essentially no change in capillary density. Once over the virus, a couple of good training bouts will have blood volume back up to normal levels, and cardiac function back to normal as a result. However, take 3 months completely off from your training routine due to a big project at work and you will lose a lot of the adaptive foundation gained over the previous year of regular workouts. If you were highly fit before the break, it may take 6 months to come all the way back. What is clear is that training adaptations are always transient and dependent on chronic stress to the system. However, it does seem that people who have been really fit, and take a break, often seem to be able to return to high fitness levels FASTER then those who have not been highly trained before. Whether this is a function of good genetics for training responsiveness, a certain "muscle memory" in the brain or muscle cells of the detrained athlete, or just past knowledge of how to train is unclear, but it does seem to be real. (para. 10)

Fitness Stages of Conditioning The three stages of conditioning are the initial stage, the progression stage, and the maintenance stage. The goal of the initial conditioning stage is to gradually increase exercise stimulus and fitness while avoiding muscle discomfort, soreness, and injury (ACSM, 2006). The length of this first stage varies about the baseline status of the individual but may take an average of 4 weeks (ACSM, 2006).

The goal of the progression stage is to continue to enhance fitness (e.g., aerobic capacity, muscular fitness, flexibility; ACSM, 2006). Compared to the initial conditioning stage, however, the progression stage is more "assertive." The length of the progression stage varies upon the baseline fitness level and the goals of the individual, but typically lasts 4 to 5 months (ACSM, 2006).

When an individual achieved her or his fitness goal(s), she or he has entered into the maintenance stage. It is important to recognize that an individual may be in the maintenance stage in terms of one aspect of physical fitness; for example aerobic capacity, but be in a "lower" stage of conditioning in another aspect of physical fitness; for example, flexibility. An individual in the maintenance stage in the stages of conditioning would be in the maintenance stage or the permanent maintenance stage in the wellness model. (Note: See Chapter 2.)

Goals

The fitness and fitness wellness goals are a subset within the physical therapy goals section. It is often indicated to develop one or more fitness goals as well as one or more fitness wellness goals. The fitness goals and fitness wellness goals should be guided by the patient's/client's evaluation (including the diagnosis and/or condition), normative fitness guidelines or fitness wellness guidelines (as applicable), the patient's/client's personal goals, realistic expectations, and the physical therapist's clinical judgment. Factors that contribute to a patient's/client's fitness and fitness wellness goals and plan of care are her/his fitness and fitness wellness baseline status and history, medical and health status, personal goals, age, gender, her/his motivation, and the physical therapist's expertise in fitness and fitness wellness.

Fitness A fitness goal is related to the patient's/client's level of fitness and can be specific or generalized. An example of a specific aerobic capacity (as opposed to an aerobic capacity wellness) goal is: Within 6 months, the patient's/client's $\dot{V}O_{2max}$ will be in the above average category (i.e., between 34 and 37 mL/kg·min). An example of a generalized aerobic capacity goal is: In 3 months, the patient's/client's $\dot{V}O_{2max}$ will be increased from its current value of 30 mL/kg·min.

Fitness Wellness A fitness wellness goal is related to the patient's/client's fitness wellness, which includes the frequency, duration, intensity, and mode of activities that promote aerobic capacity. Fitness wellness goals also may be specific or generalized. Examples of generalized fitness wellness goals are improved aerobic capacity wellness, improved muscular fitness wellness, and improved flexibility wellness. An example of a specific fitness wellness goal is: Within 3 months, the patient/client will be exercising at a moderate intensity (e.g., 70% to 75% of her or his MHR, or 125 to 135 BPM) five times per week at 30 minutes per session. Typically, a fitness wellness goal should be very specific because the patient/client uses it as a guide in her/his weekly exercise regimen.

Each fitness wellness goal should fully consider the stages of the wellness model: primordial, pre-contemplation, contemplation, assessment, action, maintenance, and permanent maintenance. Although as part of the examination you already would have assessed the patient's/client's fitness wellness, the patient/client may in fact be in a "lower" wellness stage (i.e., primordial or pre-contemplation stage). If this is the case, then the immediate fitness wellness goal(s) should be to achieve the contemplative stage in each area of fitness wellness in which the patient/client has not achieved the contemplative stage. For example, if the physical therapist determines that the patient/client is in the contemplation stage for aerobic capacity wellness, the pre-contemplation stage for body composition wellness, and the primordial stage for flexibility wellness, the initial fitness wellness goals should be to increase the patient's/client's body composition and flexibility wellness to the contemplation stage.

A physical therapist should always develop weekly short-term goals related to the wellness long-term goal(s) because it is these goals that will relay to the client what she or he is supposed to be doing in each successive week. Moreover, the progress toward each weekly wellness goal can be objectively measured with ease and precision. In some cases, a particular weekly goal will be equivalent to the previous week's goal. For example, the aerobic capacity wellness goal for week 2 might be to "walk on a treadmill 20 minutes three times per week at 75% of maximum heart rate" and the goal for week 3 might be exactly the same. Then in week 4, the goal is modestly increased (e.g., to walk on the treadmill 25 minutes three times per week at 75% of maximum heart rate.)

It is critical that upon—if not before—discharge (or discontinuance), each long-term fitness and fitness wellness goal be addressed. For example, if a goal was discharged/discontinued, the incident should be documented. No goal should slip through the cracks.

Prognosis of Goals/Objectives The prognosis is a qualitative descriptor (e.g., excellent, above average, below average, or poor) of the likelihood that the patient/client will achieve a specific goal or a group of goals. It is helpful to determine the individual prognosis for each goal, including each fitness wellness goal rather than assign a global prognosis for all of the goals. For example, the prognosis to achieve the goal of "above average aerobic capacity" might be excellent but the prognosis to achieve the goal of "above average muscular fitness" might be average. In addition to each specific prognosis, a more global prognosis also may be identified.

Plan of Care Related to Exercise Adherence

According to the U.S. Department of Health and Human Services (2006), numerous factors increase the risk of noncompliance with exercise.

1. Inconvenient location (e.g., health club is too far away)
2. Inconvenient time (e.g., aerobics class begins before you get off work)
3. Safety (e.g., you are concerned about exercising outdoors in your neighborhood)
4. Cost (e.g., the health club monthly dues are too expensive)

5. Increased exercise intensity (e.g., the patient/client tries to keep up with her or his more fit exercise buddy)
6. Decreased exercise variety (e.g., the individual enjoys variety, but only owns a stationary bicycle and is bored with it)
7. Exercising alone
8. Lack of positive feedback (e.g., the individual responds well to external praise, but doesn't receive any)
9. Inflexible exercise goals (e.g., the individual's goal, either internally or externally, is rigid)
10. No spousal support (e.g., the individual's spouse complains that housework or whatever is more important than exercise)
11. Inclement weather (e.g., the individual prefers to exercise outdoors, but the weather is too cold or too hot)
12. Excessive job travel (e.g., the individual finds it challenging to maintain an exercise regimen because she or he travels every week)
13. Job change or move (e.g., the individual used to exercise with her coworkers, but has changed jobs)
14. Injury

Factors that are correlated with long-term exercise adherence are increasing the enjoyment relative to the mode of activity and thereby enhancing the participant's motivation; improving or deemphasizing body image; increasing ability to access support, facilitating the use of self-regulation strategies; and making exercise a high priority in the client's life (Huberty et al., 2008).

It is important to appreciate that every individual has certain risk factors. For example, some individuals prefer to exercise alone rather than with someone else and others like to only engage in one mode of exercise rather than varying their activities. The bottom line is that each patient/client is a unique individual and what works for some does not work for others. Our job, as physical therapists, is to help our patients/clients identify and address their unique barriers to exercise adherence and facilitate their progression (in terms of the wellness model) to at least the maintenance stage of fitness wellness.

Summary: Prognosis, Plan of Care, and Goals

The fitness and fitness wellness prognosis, plan of care, and goals are integrated into the patient's/client's prognosis, plan of care, and goals, respectively. The fitness goals and fitness wellness goals should be guided by the patient's/client's evaluation, diagnosis and/or condition, normative fitness guidelines or fitness wellness guidelines (as applicable), the patient's/client's personal goals, realistic expectations, and the physical therapist's clinical judgment. Factors that contribute to a patient's/client's fitness and fitness wellness goals and plan of care are her/his fitness and fitness wellness baseline status and history, medical and health status, personal goals, age, gender, the patient's/client's motivation, and the physical therapist's expertise in fitness and fitness wellness. Fitness and fitness wellness goals may be general or specific. A physical therapist always should develop weekly short-term goals related to the long-term goal(s).

SECTION 9: AEROBIC CAPACITY WELLNESS AND AEROBIC CAPACITY PLAN OF CARE AND GOALS/OBJECTIVES

Variables of Aerobic Capacity

The mode, frequency, duration, and intensity of exercise are the variables of aerobic capacity wellness and the aerobic capacity plan of care and goals. Modes of aerobic capacity exercise include (but are not necessarily limited to) traditional cardiovascular/ aerobic capacity exercise, sporting activities, calisthenics, strength training exercise, and daily activities. Examples of traditional exercise are jogging and swimming laps; examples of sporting activities are soccer and lacrosse; an example of a calisthenic is jumping jacks; a strength training exercise example is circuit weight training; and examples of daily activities are raking leaves and vacuuming floors. The frequency of aerobic exercise is defined as the number of sessions per week. The duration of aerobic exercise is the number of minutes per exercise session. The intensity of aerobic exercise refers to how vigorously the aerobic exercise is performed. There are several methods to determine the intensity of an aerobic capacity exercise session; the two most popular are heart rate (HR) and rating of perceived exertion (RPE).

Heart Rate Method to Determine Aerobic Intensity

The HR method can be used to determine the intensity of an aerobic capacity exercise session if the patient/client is not taking a medication that affects blood pressure, such as a beta blocker.

There are two methods to determine an aerobic capacity HR training range: the straight method and the Karvonen method. To utilize either method, you need to know the patient's/client's maximum heart rate (MHR). Maximum heart rate can be obtained through a maximal stress test or age predicted. The original formula for an age-predicted MHR is 220 minus the individual's age. For example, the age-predicted MHR of an individual who is 40 years old is 180 beats per minute (BPM). Be aware that the MHR of all of the people who are 40 years old resemble the numbers along a bell-shaped curve. Most 40-year-olds will have a MHR that is truly 180 BPM, many will have a MHR that is 182 or 178 BPM, a few will have a MHR of 185 or 175 beats per minute, and so on.

Tanaka, Monahan, and Seals (2001) used published studies involving 18,712 healthy people and data from 514 healthy people they recruited to devise a new formula for MHR. Using their formula, MHR is 108 minus 0.7 times the individual's age. For example, the age-predicted MHR of an individual who is 40 years old is 180 BPM. The revised formula gives a higher average MHR for older people, with the original and revised heart rate curves starting to diverge at age 40. For example, the age-predicted MHR of a patient/client who is 60 years of age is 160 BPM using the original formula versus 166 BPM using the revised formula. At age 80, an individual's age-predicted MHR is 140 BPM using the original formula and 152 BPM using the revised formula.

Straight Method To employ the straight method to determine the "broad" aerobic capacity HR training range for a patient/client, multiply the MHR by 65% and by 85%.

For example, the broad training range of a 20-year-old client (with an age-predicted MHR of 200 BPM) would be 130 BPM (i.e., 65% of 200) to 170 BPM (i.e., 85% of 200). To determine the individualized aerobic capacity HR training range of a patient/client, take into account her/his medical status, recent history of aerobic capacity (i.e., $\dot{V}O_{2max}$), and goals. For example, if your 20-year-old patient/client had been extremely sedentary, you might initially prescribe a 65% to 75% MHR, or 130 to 150 BPM. However, if your 20-year-old client has been physically active and has a goal to run faster, you might prescribe a 75% to 85% MHR, or 150 to 170 BPM.

Karvonen Method In addition to knowing the patient's/client's estimated MHR, you also need to know her/his resting heart rate (RHR) to determine her/his HR training range with the Karvonen method. The Karvonen method to determine the "broad" aerobic capacity HR training range for a patient/client is:

$$[(MHR - RHR) \times 50\%] + RHR = \text{lower target HR}$$
$$[(MHR - RHR) \times 80\%] + RHR = \text{higher target HR}$$

To illustrate the Karvonen method, consider a patient/client who is 40 years of age and has a RHR of 70 BPM. The patient's/client's lower target HR is 125 BPM ([(180 − 70) × 50%] + 70 = 125) and the patient's/client's higher target HR is 158 BPM ([(180 − 70) × 80%] + 70 = 158). As with the straight method, however, you would want to individualize your patient's/client's aerobic capacity HR training range by considering her/his medical status, recent history of aerobic activity, aerobic capacity ($\dot{V}O_{2max}$), and goals.

Precautions and Contraindications for the Heart Rate Method

If your patient/client is a smoker, be aware that smoking cigarettes increases the HR. Within 1 minute after a person begins to smoke, her/his heart rate begins to increase (DeCesaris, Ranieri, Filitti, Bonfantino, & Andriani, 1992). During the first 10 minutes of smoking, the HR may increase up to 30% (e.g., 75 BPM to 98 BPM; DeCesaris et al., 1992). Minami, Toshihiko, and Matsuoka (1999) found that in habitual smokers the 24-hour HR was 7.3 ± 1.0 BPM (P < 0.0001) lower in a nonsmoking period than in a smoking period.

If your patient/client is taking a medication that affects her or his HR (e.g., a beta blocker or other antihypertensive medication), you cannot determine your client's aerobic capacity heart rate range. The reason is because the medication not only suppresses the patient's/client's blood pressure, but also suppresses her or his MHR, RHR, and exercise HR. To illustrate, the maximum RHR of a 40-year-old patient/client taking a beta-blocker is more likely to be 140 BPM rather than 180 BPM, the RHR is more likely to be 45 BPM rather than 75 BPM, and aerobic capacity HR range is more likely to be 90 to 95 BPM rather than 120 to 140 BPM. The only healthcare professional who can determine the aerobic capacity HR range of patient/client taking medication that affects the HR is a cardiologist.

Alternative Methods to Determine Exercise Intensity

When it is contraindicated for you to assess a patient's/client's aerobic capacity intensity with a HR method (e.g., she or he is taking a medication that affects HR and her or his cardiologist does not provide a prescriptive HR training range), you may assess the patient's/client's perception of her/his intensity.

The most widely recognized alternative method is the rating perceived exertion (RPE) method, which Gunnar Borg developed in 1970 (CDC, 2009b). The numbers on Borg's scale range from 6 to 19 and "practitioners generally agree that perceived exertion ratings between 12 to 14 on the Borg Scale suggests that physical activity is being performed at a moderate level of intensity" (CDC, 2009b, para. 2). Borg later revised the RPE scale with numbers that ranged from 0 to 10. According to Borg (as cited in CDC, 2009b, para. 4), "a high correlation exists between a person's perceived exertion rating times 10 and the actual heart rate during physical activity; so a person's exertion rating may provide a fairly good estimate of the actual heart rate during physical activity; so a person's exertion rating may provide a fairly good estimate of the actual heart rate during activity."

Although physical therapists may not freely borrow Borg's RPE because it has a copyright, they may utilize a 0 to 10 physical exertion scale that is analogous to the 0 to 10 pain scale that is often utilized by physical therapists to quantify pain. To utilize this type of physical exertion scale, you instruct a patient/client to consider a scale of 0 to 10 with 0 being equivalent to rest and 10 being equivalent to the most intense exercise.

For my fitness wellness practice, I developed and utilized the perceived activity scale (PAS) (**Table 6-5**). To utilize the PAS, show your patient/client the scale (before she or he begins to exercise) and explain the level of exertion at various thresholds, such as 0, 5, 7, and 10. For example, 0 is equivalent to resting, such as lying in a bed; 5 is equivalent to an activity that can theoretically be performed for hours, such as a slow walk; 7 is an activity that can be performed for at least 20 to 30 minutes, such as a moderate intensity bicycle ride; and a 10 is equivalent to a maximum activity that can only be performed for a minute or so, such as lifting or carrying something really heavy. Next, instruct the patient/client to exercise at an intensity that she or he can theoretically perform for hours (e.g., a slow walk

Table 6-5 Perceived Activity Scale

10	Activity I can't do for more than a minute or so
9	Activity I can do for about 10–15 minutes or maybe more, but it's very hard
8	
7	Activity I can do for at least 20–30 minutes; it's hard, but not too hard
6	
5	Activity I can do for hours (e.g., easy walk)
4	
3	Very light activity
2	
1	
0	Resting

on a treadmill) and then facilitate her/his feelings of physical exertion to the number 5 on the scale. As advanced by the Centers for Disease Control (2009c) when assessing perceived exertion, instruct the patient/client to consider all feelings and sensations of physical effort, stress, and fatigue, but disregard other feelings, such as leg pain or shortness of breath. Assist the patient/client in her/his practice with the scale to ensure that her/his perception of exertion is "objective" as possible. When you are confident that the patient/client's perception of her/his exertion is valid at lower intensity exercises, then utilize the scale at a higher intensity. Once the patient/client is familiar with the scale, you may simply ask her or him at what level she or he is exercising.

Whether you prescribe an aerobic capacity HR training range to your patient, or utilize the RPE scale, it is important that you individualize the patient's aerobic capacity HR training range to take into account the client's medical status, recent history of aerobic capacity exercise, aerobic capacity (i.e., $\dot{V}O_{2max}$), goals, and, if indicated, age.

Aerobic Capacity Wellness Preferred Practice Pattern

Because the most recent edition of the *Guide to Physical Therapist Practice* (APTA, 2001b) does not include an Aerobic Capacity Wellness Preferred Practice Pattern, I have incorporated these components into my Wellness Preferred Practice Pattern, which is presented in Chapter 9.

Aerobic Capacity Wellness Goals/Objectives

To adequately address a patient's/client's aerobic capacity wellness deficits, you will establish goals related to the psychomotor, cognitive, and/or affective dimensions of aerobic capacity wellness, as indicated. It is likely that you should establish one or more short-term goals for each long-term goal.

Cognitive Goals

The cognitive aerobic capacity wellness goals focus on the patient's/client's level of knowledge about aerobic capacity wellness. For example, a long-term goal might be for the patient/client to, within 1 month, verbalize the contraindications and precautions for aerobic capacity exercise; a short-term goal might be for her or him to, within 1 week, verbalize the contraindications and one precaution for aerobic capacity exercise. (Note: Because engaging in a functional task activities program was not found to enhance self-reported physical activity; that is, fitness wellness [de Vreede et al., 2007], even among physical therapists [Fair, 2007], patient/client education should include the cognitive understanding that daily activities can "count" as exercise.) For example, raking leaves or cleaning the house can at least maintain or even enhance aerobic capacity. A long-term goal might be for the patient/client to, within 1 month, verbalize 10 daily activities she or he performs and estimate their respective effects on her or his aerobic capacity. A related short-term goal might be for the patient/client to, within 1 week, verbalize five daily activities she or he performs and estimate their respective effects on her or his aerobic capacity.

Psychomotor Goals

The psychomotor aerobic capacity wellness goals address the mode, frequency, duration, and intensity of aerobic capacity exercise. Because the U.S. DHHS (2000) recommends moderate intensity aerobic exercise five times per week at 30 minutes per exercise session, it is appropriate to consider whether this is a realistic goal for your patient/client. If it is, then establish it as a long-term goal. If this amount of exercise is not a realistic long-term goal, then determine whether it is realistic for your patient/client to exercise three times per week at 30 minutes per session at 70% to 85% of MHR, which is the amount of exercise that the ACSM (2006) deems is adequate to maintain if not improve aerobic capacity. If this exercise protocol is realistic, establish it as the long-term goal. If not, determine whether it is realistic for your patient/client to engage in adequately intense aerobic capacity activities three times per week (nonconsecutive days) for 15 minutes each session, which is the amount of activity to maintain aerobic capacity health (Lukaski & Bolonchuk, 1989). An example of a psychomotor aerobic capacity wellness long-term goal is for a patient/client to, in 2 months, strength train with a combination of calisthenics and weight equipment 3 days per week and perform three sets of 10 to 12 repetitions of 70% to 85% of the respective one repetition maximum of the eight major muscle groups. A short-term goal linked to this long-term goal might be for the patient/client to, in 1 month, strength train with a combination of calisthenics and weight equipment 3 days per week and perform three sets of 10 to 12 repetitions of 60% to 70% of the respective one repetition maximum of the eight major groups.

Affective Goals

The affective aerobic capacity wellness goal examines the patient's/client's level of commitment to aerobic capacity wellness. For example, a long-term goal might be for the patient/client, in 3 months, to indicate via a self-report survey that her/his commitment to aerobic capacity wellness is at least an 8 on a scale of 1 to 10. A related short-term goal might be for the patient/client to, within 2 months, indicate on a self-report survey that her/his commitment to aerobic capacity wellness is at least a 6 on a scale of 1 to 10.

Aerobic Capacity Preferred Practice Patterns

The *Guide to Physical Therapist Practice* (APTA, 2001b) includes two Preferred Practice Patterns related to aerobic capacity: "6A, primary prevention/risk reduction for cardiovascular/pulmonary disorders" and "6B, impaired aerobic capacity/endurance associated with deconditioning." By way of inference, both Preferred Practice Patterns approximate the length of time under the care of a physical therapist. The estimated lengths of care are deliberately broad to accommodate individual differences between patients/clients. The APTA appreciates that some patients/clients will require more than the maximum number of visits and others will not need even the minimum number of visits. According to the Preferred Practice Pattern 6A in the *Guide to Physical Therapist Practice* (APTA, 2001b), approximately 80% of the patients/clients that present at risk for an aerobic capacity disorder will achieve their objectives and goals within one and six sessions. The implication of this stance is that to achieve their objectives and goals, approximately 20% of patients/clients who present at risk for aerobic capacity disorders will not require physical therapy or will require greater than six physical therapy visits. The *Guide to Physical Therapist Practice* also states that patients/clients who present with impaired aerobic capacity will require physical therapy for 6 to 12 weeks, during which time approximately 80% of the patients/clients will achieve their objectives and goals within 6 to 30 sessions. The implication of this position is that to achieve their objectives and goals, approximately 20% of patients/clients who present at risk for aerobic capacity disorders will require fewer than 6 or greater than 30 physical therapy visits.

Both Preferred Practice Patterns related to aerobic capacity identify factors that may modify the duration of the episode of care. These include: "accessibility and availability of resources, adherence to the intervention program, age, anatomical and physiological changes related to growth and development, caregiver consistency or expertise, chronicity or severity of the current condition, cognitive status, co-morbidities, complications, or secondary impairments; concurrent medical, surgical, and therapeutic interventions; decline in functional independence; level of impairment; level of physical function; living environment; multi-site or multi-system involvement, nutritional status, overall health status, potential discharge destinations, pre-morbid conditions, probability of prolonged impairment, functional limitation, or disability; psychological and socioeconomic factors, psychomotor abilities, social support, stability of the condition" (APTA, 2001b, p. 477, 488). For example, if a patient/client is diagnosed with hypertension and coronary artery disease, it will likely take longer to achieve a satisfactory level of aerobic capacity fitness. In addition, poor socioeconomic factors and social networks probably will impede their progress toward a fitness wellness goal.

Aerobic Capacity Goals/Objectives

The aerobic capacity goals will address the mode, frequency, duration, and intensity of aerobic capacity exercise. An aerobic capacity goal may be more general or more specific. A generalized aerobic capacity goal would be to improve aerobic capacity within the next 3 months. A more specific goal identifies the desired aerobic capacity category: excellent, above average, average, below average, poor. A very specific goal identifies the desired $\dot{V}O_{2max}$. When establishing a specific goal, the physical therapist considers the patient's/client's baseline $\dot{V}O_{2max}$; her/his medical status and history, including age, gender, and history of exercise; the patient's/client's input about factors related to her/his aerobic activity, including, but not limited to, exercise preferences, available resources, support from others, personal goals related to aerobic capacity, the patient's/client's motivation to engage in activities that promote aerobic capacity; and reasonable expectations. It is likely that you should establish one or more short-term goals for each long-term goal.

When developing an aerobic capacity plan of care for a patient/client, you may consider anecdotal data but also should take into account guidelines from reputable organizations such as the ACSM and peer-reviewed evidence. While it is typically necessary to extrapolate the results from a study because most investigate a narrow population (e.g., young men, older women), there are numerous peer-reviewed articles you may find useful when developing an aerobic capacity plan of care.

Gettman et al. (1976) found that deconditioned men may improve aerobic capacity with only twice-weekly exercise, greater improvements result from a frequency of 3 to 5 days per week, and improvements generally plateau within the 3 to 5 day frequency. Although an analogous study has not been conducted with women, it is reasonable to venture the same holds true for women. Hickson and associates investigated the effect of a reduced exercise regime on the aerobic capacity gains obtained through a longer duration frequent exercise regimen (i.e., 40 minutes per day, 6 days per week), and while the gains were maintained when the frequency was reduced to 2 to 4 days per week (Hickson, Kanakis, Davis, Moore, & Rich, 1982) or the duration was reduced to 26 minutes per session, they were significantly reduced when the duration was reduced to 13 minutes per session (Hickson & Rosenkoetter, 1981). Other investigations require a higher level of analysis. For example, O'Donovan et al. (2005) investigated the effect of 44 minutes of moderate intensity (60% $\dot{V}O_{2max}$) exercise three times per week to 33 minutes of high intensity (80% $\dot{V}O_{2max}$) three times per week on 30- to 45-year-old sedentary, nonsmoking, randomly assigned men. [Note: Both protocols equated to a 400 caloric output per exercise session.] The study found that the moderate intensity protocol produced a 4.85 mL/kg·min increase in $\dot{V}O_{2max}$ (range, 30.97 ± 5.7 to 35.82 ± 6.28 mL/kg·min), while the higher intensity protocol produced a 7.3 mL/kg·min increase in $\dot{V}O_{2max}$ (31.76 ± 5.99 to 38.90 ± 8.08 mL/kg·min). In another study, Findlay and associates (1987) investigated the effects of a 30 week (~ 7 months) exercise program on a group of randomly assigned sedentary men ages 35 to 50 who were training for their first marathon, and found that their mean $\dot{V}O_{2max}$ values increased 5.0 mL/kg·min (33.9 to 39.0 mL/kg·min).

In another study, Ayse, Fusan, Ozgen, Topuz, and Semez (2006) found that a 3-month aerobic capacity program increased the $\dot{V}O_{2max}$ of sedentary, noncalorie restricted, randomly assigned obese women by 7.21 ± 4.76 mL/kg·min (27.19 ± 5.6 to 34.40 ± 7.14 mL/kg·min). Their training program consisted of 12 to 15 minutes 3 days per week during the first month, 20 to 30 minutes 4 days per week during the second month, and 30 to 45 minutes per day 4 days per week during the third month. During each exercise session, the women exercised at 50% to 85% of their heart rate reserve (as calculated with the Karvonen method) and as individually prescribed by the researchers. Ayse et al. also found that 3 months of thrice weekly strength training (of the quadriceps, pectoral major, biceps, triceps, abdominals, and hip abductors/gluteus medius) increased the $\dot{V}O_{2max}$ of another group of sedentary, noncalorie-restricted obese women by 6.14 ± 5.68 mL/kg·min (27.09 ± 5.13 to 33.23 ± 6.3 mL/kg·min). (The strength-training protocol was one set of 10 repetitions of 40% to 60% one-repetition maximum during the first week; two sets during the second week; three sets during the third week; and three sets of 10 repetitions of 75% to 85% of one-repetition maximum during the third through the twelfth weeks; there were 15- to 30-second rest periods between each exercise). A conclusion of this research is that both an aerobic capacity exercise protocol and a strength-training exercise protocol increases $\dot{V}O_{2max}$ in obese women.

Summary: Aerobic Capacity and Aerobic Capacity Wellness

Variables of aerobic capacity wellness are the frequency (of the exercise sessions), duration of an exercise session, and the intensity of exercise. The heart rate method and the rating of the perceived exertion method can be used to estimate the intensity of aerobic capacity exercise. While the *Guide to Physical Therapist Practice* (APTA, 2001b) has Preferred Practice Patterns related to aerobic capacity, it does not contain any Preferred Practice Patterns related to aerobic capacity wellness. My Wellness Preferred Practice Pattern (Chapter 9) includes an aerobic capacity wellness component. Aerobic capacity and aerobic capacity wellness goals and objectives can be general or specific. Aerobic capacity wellness goals/objectives may involve the cognitive, psychomotor, and/or affective dimensions.

SECTION 10: MUSCULAR FITNESS AND MUSCULAR FITNESS WELLNESS PLAN OF CARE AND GOALS

Variables

The mode, frequency, duration, and intensity of exercise are variables of the muscular fitness wellness plan of care and goals. Modes of muscular fitness exercise include (but are not necessarily limited to) strength training with weights, calisthenics, sporting activities, cardiovascular/aerobic capacity exercise, and daily activities. Examples of strength training with weights are free weights and exercising on a Nautilus machine; examples of calisthenics are push-ups and abdominal curls; an example of a sporting activity is competitive swimming; examples of cardiovascular/aerobic capacity exercises are recreational soccer and bicycling; examples of daily activities are digging a ditch and carrying boxes. The frequency of muscular fitness exercise is the number of sessions per week. The duration of muscular fitness exercise is the number of minutes per exercise session. When strength training or doing calisthenics, the number of sets of the various exercises is sometimes considered in addition to or instead of the minutes of duration of the exercise session. For example, a patient/client might perform three sets of eight different strength-training exercises for a total of 24 sets. The intensity of a strengthening exercise is determined by the weight of the equipment and the number of repetitions. For example, the intensity of a bicep curl exercise might can be expressed as 10 repetitions of 20 pounds. The intensity of a calisthenic exercise is determined by the number of repetitions. For example, the intensity of push-ups can be expressed as 20 repetitions.

Reputable resources agree that muscular fitness is developed via the overload principles, that is, the increase in resistance, frequency, or duration of an activity (ACSM, 2006; Williams 2008). By definition, an individual can perform one repetition of her or his one-repetition maximum (1RM). Further, it is supported that the typical client/patient can perform five repetitions of 90% of her or his 1RM; eight repetitions of 80% of her or his IRM; 12 repetitions of 70% of her or his 1RM; and 17 repetitions of 60% of her or his 1RM (Williams, 2008). In fact, it is widely supported that it is appropriate to perform six or fewer repetitions with high-intensity strength training, 8 to 15 repetitions with moderate intensity strength training, and more than 15 repetitions with low-intensity strength training because "a lower repetition range with a heavier weight may better optimize strength and power, whereas a higher repetition range with a lighter weight may better enhance muscular endurance" (Williams et al., 2007, p. 579).

Muscular Fitness Wellness Preferred Practice Pattern

Because the most recent edition of the *Guide to Physical Therapist Practice* (APTA, 2001b) does not include a Muscular Fitness Wellness Preferred Practice Pattern, I have incorporated the components of one into my Wellness Preferred Practice Pattern, presented in Chapter 9.

Muscular Fitness Wellness Goals/Objectives

To adequately address a patient's/client's muscular fitness wellness deficits, you will establish goals related to the psychomotor, cognitive, and/or affective dimensions of muscular fitness wellness, as indicated. It is likely that you should establish one or more short-term goals for each long-term goal.

Cognitive Goals

The cognitive muscular fitness wellness goals are focused on the patient's/client's level of knowledge about muscular fitness wellness. For example, a long-term goal might be for the patient/client to, within 1 month, verbalize the contraindications and precautions for strength-training activities, and a short-term goal might be for her or him to, within 1 week, verbalize the contraindications and one precaution for strength training. (Note: Because engaging in a functional task activities program was not found to enhance self-reported physical activity; that is, fitness wellness [de Vreede et al, 2007] even among physical therapists [Fair, 2005], the patient/client education should include the cognitive understanding that daily activities can "count" as muscular fitness exercise). For example, raking leaves or cleaning the house can at least maintain or enhance muscular fitness. A long-term goal might be for the patient/client to, within 1 month, verbalize 10 of the daily activities she or he performs and estimate their respective effects on her/his muscular fitness. A related short-term goal might be for the patient/client to, within 1 week, verbalize five of the daily activities she or he performs and estimate their respective effects on her or his muscular fitness.

Psychomotor Goals

The psychomotor muscular fitness wellness goals will focus on the mode, frequency, duration, and intensity of muscular fitness exercise. Because it is recommended that people perform at least one set of 8 to 12 repetitions of 8 to 10 strength training exercises for 2 to 3 days per week (ACSM, 2006), it is appropriate for you to consider whether this is a realistic goal for your patient/client. If so, then establish it as her or his long-term goal. If this amount of exercise it not a realistic goal, determine what level of muscular fitness wellness exercise is realistic. For example, if your patient/client is 60 years old, it may be more appropriate to reduce the weight and set the repetition goal to 10 to 15. If this amount of exercise is too modest, determine a higher-level goal. If your patient/client is young, healthy, has been regularly engaging in strength training, and wishes to enhance the routine, it may be appropriate for him or her to perform three sets of 12 strength-training exercises 4 days per week. In any event, it is prudent to keep the duration of a strength-training session to 1 hour because programs lasting longer than 1 hour are associated with higher dropout rates (ACSM, 2006).

An example of a psychomotor muscular fitness wellness long-term goal is for a patient/client to, in 2 months, strength train with a combination of calisthenics and weight equipment 3 days per week and perform three sets of 10 to 12 repetitions of 70% to 85% of the respective one-repetition maximum of the eight major muscle groups. A short-term goal linked to this long-term goal would be for the patient/client to, in 1 month, strength train with a combination of calisthenics and weight equipment 3 days per week and perform three sets of 10 to 12 repetitions of 60% to 70% of the respective one-repetition maximum of the eight major groups.

Although the *Guide to Physical Therapist Practice* (APTA, 2001b) suggests the concept of muscular fitness wellness, it does not present muscular fitness wellness prescriptive guidelines. Accordingly, it is helpful to consider the guidelines of the ACSM (2006), which are

- Perform a minimum of 8 to 10 separate exercises that train the major muscle groups (arms, shoulders, chest, abdomen, back, hips, and legs). A primary goal of the program should be to develop totally body strength and endurance in a relatively time-efficient manner. Programs lasting longer than one hour per session are associated with higher dropout rates.
- Perform a minimum of one set of 8 to 12 repetitions of each of these exercises to the point of volitional fatigues. This is for individuals who are primarily interested in developing muscular endurance as well as older (~ 50 to 60 years of age) or more frail persons, for whom 10 to 15 repetitions may be more appropriate.
- Perform these exercises two to three [days per week]. Although more frequent training and additional sets or combinations of sets and repetitions may elicit larger strength gains, the additional improvement is relatively small for previously sedentary individual training in the typical fitness setting.
- Adhere as closely as possible to the specific techniques for performing a given exercise.
- Perform every exercise through a full range of motion.
- Perform both the lifting (concentric phase) and lowering (eccentric phase) portion of the resistance exercises in a controlled manner.
- Maintain a normal breathing pattern: breath-holding can induce excessive increases in blood pressure.
- If possible, exercise with a training partner who can provide feedback, assistance, and motivation. (p. 160)

The instructions on how to perform a muscular fitness should be extensive enough to enable the patient/client to perform it safely and effectively. For example, the instructions for performing curls might be (Figure 6-5):

- Starting Position: Lie on your back with one knee bent with the foot flat on the floor and the other leg extended. Cross your arms over your chest or place them, unclasped, behind your head with your elbows out to the side. Maintain a neutral alignment in the cervical spine (neck).

- Action: Engage your abdominals and exhale while curling up. Initiate the movement by gently flexing your cervical spine by dropping your chin slightly. Next, activate your abdominals by raising your shoulders and upper back off the floor toward the pelvis. Contract at the top of the movement. Pause, and then slowly return to the starting position.
- Common Errors:
  - Error: Forward neck position
    Correction: Imagine an orange tucked between your chin and neck and maintain this position throughout the exercise.
  - Error: Moving the elbows forward while curling up
    Correction: Keep your elbows out of vision and remain open through the chest and shoulders.
  - Error: Holding the breath
    Correction: Emphasize exhaling during the exertion phase.
- Repetitions/Sets/Frequency: Perform two sets of 25 repetitions three times per week.

Affective Goals

The affective muscular fitness wellness goal focuses on the patient's/client's level of commitment to muscular fitness wellness. For example, a long-term goal might be for the patient/client to, in 3 months, indicate via a self-report survey that her or his commitment to muscular fitness wellness is at least an 8 on a scale of 1 to 10. A related short-term goal might be for the patient/client to, within 2 months, indicate via a self-report survey that her/his commitment to muscular fitness wellness is at least a 6 on a scale of 1 to 10.

Muscular Fitness Preferred Practice Pattern

The *Guide to Physical Therapist Practice* (APTA, 2001b) includes one Preferred Practice Pattern related to muscular fitness: "4-C, impaired muscle performance." This Preferred Practice Pattern states that the patient/client history may include general demographics, social history, employment/work/school/play, growth and development, general health status, social/health habits (past and current), family history, medical/surgical history, current condition(s)/chief complaint(s), functional status and activity level, medications, and other clinical tests. It also states the systems review may include (1) the anatomical and physiological status of the cardiovascular/pulmonary, integumentary, musculoskeletal, and neuromuscular system; and (2) communication, affect, cognition, language and learning style. Tests and measures may include: aerobic capacity and endurance, assistive and adaptive devices, anthropometric characteristics, arousal, attention, and cognition; circulation; cranial and peripheral nerve integrity; environmental, home, and work; ergonomics and body mechanics; gait, locomotion, and balance; motor function; muscle performance (including endurance, strength, and power); orthotic, protective, and supportive devices; pain; posture, self-care and home management (including activities of daily living and instrumental activities of daily living), ventilation and respiration; and work (work/play/school), leisure, and community integration or reintegration.

The *Guide to Physical Therapist Practice* (APTA, 2001b) states that patients/clients within the "impaired muscle performance" Preferred Practice Pattern generally require 2 to 6 months of physical therapy. It further states that approximately 80% of the patients/clients will require 6 to 30 sessions of physical therapy to achieve their individualized objectives and goals. The implication of this statement is that approximately 20% of physical therapy patients/clients who present with impaired muscle performance will require fewer than 6 or greater than 30 physical therapy visits to achieve their objectives and goals. According to the *Guide to Physical Therapist Practice*, the same factors that can modify the duration of the episode of care of an aerobic capacity condition can modify the duration of care of the muscular fitness condition. For example, if a patient/client has access to a health club or owns home strength-training equipment, she or he may achieve the goals related to muscular fitness in a more timely fashion. However, if a patient/client has an impaired mental status, a longer duration of care may be required secondary to the need for extended patient/client instruction.

Muscular Fitness Goals/Objectives

The muscular fitness goals address the mode, frequency, duration, and intensity of muscular fitness exercise. A muscular fitness goal may be more general or more specific. A generalized muscular fitness goal is to improve muscular fitness within the next 3 months. A more specific goal identifies the desired muscular fitness category: excellent, above average, average, below average, poor. A very specific goal identifies the desired one-repetition maximum (1RM) or five-repetition maximum (5RM) of a specific muscle group or other specific measure of muscular fitness. When establishing a specific goal, the physical therapist needs to consider the patient's/client's baseline muscular fitness; her/his medical status and history, including age, gender, and history of exercise; the patient's/client's input about factors related to her/his strengthening activity, including, but not limited to, exercise preferences, available resources, support from others, personal goals related to muscular fitness, the patient's/client's motivation to engage in activities that promote muscular fitness; and reasonable expectations. It is likely that you should establish one or more short-term goals for each long-term goal.

Ayse et al. (2006) found 3 months of thrice weekly, moderate-intensity strength training (of the quadriceps, pectoral major, biceps, triceps, abdominals, and hip abductors/gluteus medius) increased the muscular fitness of sedentary, noncalorie-restricted obese women. The strength-training protocol consisted of exercising each of six tested muscle groups three times per week. The specifics were one set of 10 repetitions of 40% to 60% one-repetition maximum (1RM) during the first week; two sets during the second week; three sets during the third week; and three sets of 10 repetitions of 75% to 85% of 1RM during the third through the twelfth weeks; there were 15- to 30-second rest periods between each exercise. Following the 3 months of moderate-intensity strength training, the increases in 1RM were quadriceps 14.0 lbs $\pm$ 7.18 (18.75 $\pm$ 7.58 to 32.75 $\pm$ 9.24 lbs), pectoral major 8.75 ± 5.09 lbs (14.75 ± 4.72 to 23.5 ± 6.5 lbs), biceps 3.37 ± 2.84 lbs (18.0 ± 4.1 to 21.37 ± 4.09 lbs), triceps 5.4 lbs ± 3.97 (18.3 ± 3.75 to 23.7 ± 4.78 lbs), abdominals 10.6 ± 3.05 lbs (15.25 ± 5.25 to 25.85 ± 4.94 lbs), and hip abductors/gluteus medius 7.95 ± 3.58 lbs (9.77 ± 2.94 to 17.72 ± 3.88).

In another study, 25 minutes of high-intensity resistance exercises (for hip abduction, quadriceps, pectorals, biceps, triceps, and abdominals) two times per week for 6 weeks significantly increased muscular strength (as measured by 1RM tests; Taylor, 2007). The strength-training protocol was: Week 1, session 1—six sets of three repetitions of 80% of 1RM; Week 1, session 2—six sets of two repetitions of 80% of 1RM; Week 2, session 1—six sets of four repetitions of 80% of 1RM; Week 2, session 2—six sets of two repetitions of 80% of 1RM; Week 3, session 1—six sets of five repetitions of 80% of 1RM; Week 3, session 2—six sets of two repetitions of 80% of 1RM; Week 4, session 1—six sets of six repetitions of 80% of 1RM; Week 4, session 2—six sets of two repetitions of 80% of 1RM; Week 5, session 1—five sets of five repetitions of 85% of 1RM; Week 5, session 2—six sets of two repetitions of 80% of 1RM; Week 6, session 1—four sets of four repetitions of 90% of 1RM; Week 6, session 2—six sets of two repetitions of 80% of 1RM. Following the 6 weeks of high-intensity strength training, the increases in 1RM were hip abduction increased by 5.5 pounds, quadriceps increased by 9 pounds, pectorals increased by 6.5 pounds, biceps increased by 1.5 pounds, triceps increased by 3 pounds, and abdominal curls increased by 7 repetitions (from 15 to 22).

It is important to appreciate that research data found in these and other studies should not be used to formulate a "cook book" muscular fitness goal, but assist the physical therapist to determine realistic muscular fitness goals for a given patient/client.

Summary: Muscular Fitness and Muscular Fitness Wellness

Variables of muscular fitness wellness are the frequency (of the exercise sessions), the amount of weight, the number of repetitions, and the number of sets. While the *Guide to Physical Therapist Practice* (APTA, 2001b) has Preferred Practice Patterns related to muscular fitness, it does not contain any related to muscular fitness wellness. My Wellness Preferred Practice Pattern (Chapter 9) includes a muscular fitness wellness component. Muscular fitness goals can be either general or specific and involve the cognitive, psychomotor, and/or affective dimensions.

SECTION 11: FLEXIBILITY AND FLEXIBILITY WELLNESS PLAN OF CARE AND GOALS

Variables

The mode, frequency, duration, and intensity of exercise are factors of flexibility wellness and flexibility goals and plan of care. Modes of flexibility exercise include (but are not limited to) traditional stretching, proprioceptive neuromuscular facilitation (PNF), yoga, tai chi, sporting activities, strength training with weights, calisthenics, cardiovascular/aerobic capacity exercise, and daily activities. An example of a stretch is a 30-second static stretch; an example of a yoga exercise is the lotus pose; an example of strength training with weight is circuit weight training; an example of a calisthenic is jumping jacks; an example of a sporting activity is gymnastics; an example of cardiovascular/aerobic capacity exercise is swimming; examples of daily activities are gardening and washing windows. The frequency of a flexibility exercise is the number of sessions per week. The duration of a flexibility exercise is the number of minutes per exercise session. An alternate consideration of the duration is the number of sets. The intensity of a static stretch is determined by the "degree" of the stretch and the duration that the stretch is held. For example, the intensity of a shoulder flexion stretch might be expressed as 160 degrees for 30 seconds.

Flexibility Wellness Preferred Practice Pattern

Because the most recent edition of the *Guide to Physical Therapist Practice* (APTA, 2001b) does not include a Flexibility Wellness Preferred Practice Pattern, I have incorporated these components into my Wellness Preferred Practice Pattern found in Chapter 9.

Flexibility Wellness Goals

To adequately address a patient's/client's flexibility wellness deficits, you should establish goals related to the psychomotor, cognitive, and/or affective dimensions of flexibility wellness, as indicated. It is likely that it will be indicated to establish one or more short-term goals for each long-term goal.

Cognitive Goals

The cognitive flexibility wellness goals focus on the patient's/client's level of knowledge about flexibility wellness. For example, a long-term goal might be for the patient/client to, within 1 month, verbalize the contraindications and precautions for flexibility exercise and a short-term goal might be for her or him to, within 1 week, verbalize the contraindications and one precaution for flexibility exercise. Because engaging in a functional task activities program was not found to enhance self-reported physical activity; that is, fitness wellness (Vreede et al, 2007)—even among physical therapists (Fair, 2005); patient/client education should include the cognitive understanding that daily activities can "count" as exercise. For example, raking leaves or cleaning the house can at least maintain or enhance flexibility. A long-term goal might be for the patient/client to, within 1 month, verbalize 10 of the daily activities she or he performs and estimate their respective effects on her or his flexibility. A related short-term goal might be for the patient/client to, within 1 week, verbalize 5 of the daily activities she or he performs and estimate their respective effects on her or his flexibility.

Psychomotor Goals

To determine a patient's/client's flexibility long-term goal, consider the patient's/client's baseline flexibility; her or his medical status and history, including the age, gender, and history of exercise; the patient's/client's input about factors related to her or his flexibility, including, but not limited to, exercise preferences, available resources, support from others, personal goals related to flexibility; and the patient's/client's motivation to engage in activities that promote flexibility.

Although the *Guide to Physical Therapist Practice* (APTA, 2001b) suggests the concept of flexibility wellness, it does not present flexibility wellness prescriptive guidelines. Accordingly, it is helpful to consider the guidelines of the American College of Sport Medicine (2006, p. 158):

> Stretching exercises can be effectively included in the warm-up and/or cool-down periods that precede and follow the . . . exercise session. It is recommended that an active warm-up precede vigorous stretching exercises. Some commonly employed stretching exercises may not be appropriate for some participants who may—through prior injury, joint insufficiency, or other conditions—be at greater risk for musculoskeletal injuries. Although research evidence concerning the risks of specific exercise is lacking, those activities that require substantial flexibility and/or skills are not recommended for older, less flexible, and less experienced participants.

According to the ACSM (2006), the stretching guidelines for apparently healthy individuals are

- Type: A general stretching routine that exercises the major muscle and/or tendon groups using static or proprioceptive neuromuscular facilitation (PNF) techniques
- Frequency: A minimum of 2 to 3 days per week
- Intensity: To a position of mild discomfort
- Duration: 10 to 30 seconds for static; 6-second contraction followed by 10 to 30 second assisted stretch for PNF
- Repetitions: 3 to 4 for each stretch (p. 158)

While the ACSM (2006) states that stretches be held for a 10- to 30-second period, holding stretches for longer than 30 seconds provides greater benefit (Feland, 2001; Manzari et al., 2001). In fact, the physical therapy profession appears to support the recommendation that the duration of stretches be greater than 30 seconds. For example, Feland concluded that a stretch of 1 minute duration provided significantly greater benefit than a 30-second stretch. Research by Manzari et al. (2001) also supported stretching durations of longer than 30 seconds.

An important consideration in developing the plan of care, including the selection of the mode of intervention, is the broad-based goal of the participant. Is the patient/client interested in general flexibility or participation in a sport that requires a specific degree of flexibility? For example, does your female client want to maintain her flexibility so that she can comfortably continue to perform her daily activities or would she like to participate in recreational jazz dancing?

Affective Goals

The affective flexibility wellness goal focuses on the patient's/client's level of commitment to flexibility wellness. For example, a long-term goal might be for the patient/client to, in

3 months, indicate via a self-report survey that her or his commitment to aerobic capacity wellness is at least an 8 on a scale of 1 to 10. A related short-term goal might be for the patient/client to, within 2 months, indicate via a self-report survey that her or his commitment to flexibility wellness is at least a 6 on a scale of 1 to 10.

Flexibility Plan of Care

APTA Preferred Practice Patterns

As detailed in the history section of this chapter, the *Guide to Physical Therapist Practice* (APTA, 2001b) includes several Preferred Practice Patterns related to flexibility and range of motion. However, these Preferred Practice Patterns were designed for restorative patients and address range of motion only in combination with a diagnosis; that is, a connective tissue dysfunction, localized inflammation, spinal disorders, fracture, joint arthroplasty, bony or soft tissue surgery, and amputation. Nonetheless, by way of inference, these Preferred Practice Patterns approximate the duration of care. The estimated lengths of care are deliberately broad to accommodate the individual differences between patients/clients. The APTA (2001b) appreciates that some patients/clients will require more than the maximum number of visits and other patients/clients will not need even the minimum number of visits. According to the Preferred Practice Patterns 4D through 4J, approximately 80% of the patients/clients who present with impairments including, but not limited to, range of motion will generally achieve their objectives and goals within 6 months. The estimated range of the number of sessions vary considerably: 4D, connective tissue estimate is between 3 and 36; 4E, inflammation estimate is between 6 and 24; 4F, spine estimate is within 8 and 24 sessions; 4G, fracture estimate is within 6 and 18; 4H, arthroplasty estimate is within 12 and 60; 4I, surgical estimate is within 6 and 70; and 4J, amputation estimate is 15 to 45.

Each of the Preferred Practice Patterns related to range of motion/flexibility identify factors that may modify the duration of the episode of care: "accessibility and availability of resources, adherence to the intervention program, age, anatomical and physiological changes related to growth and development, caregiver consistency or expertise, chronicity or severity of the current condition, cognitive status, co-morbidities, complications, or secondary impairments; concurrent medical, surgical, and therapeutic interventions; decline in functional independence; level of impairment; level of physical function; living environment; multi-site or multi-system involvement, nutritional status, overall health status, potential discharge destinations, pre-morbid conditions, probability of prolonged impairment, functional limitation, or disability; psychological and socioeconomic factors, psychomotor abilities, social support, stability of the condition" (APTA, 2001b, p. 193, 211, 229, 247, 265, 284, 301).

Flexibility Goals/Objectives

The flexibility goals address the mode, frequency, duration, and intensity of flexibility exercise. A flexibility goal may be more general or more specific. A generalized flexibility goal is to improve range of motion within the next 3 months. A more specific goal identifies the desired flexibility/range of motion category: within normal limits, very minimally impaired, minimally impaired, moderately impaired, and maximally impaired. (Note: Very minimally impaired and minimally impaired are within functional limits but moderately impaired and maximally impaired are not.) A very specific goal identifies the desired range of motion or muscle length of a specific joint or muscle group, or another specific measure of flexibility. When establishing a specific goal, the physical therapist needs to consider the patient's/client's baseline flexibility/range of motion; her/his medical status and history, including age, gender, and history of exercise; the patient's/client's input about factors related to her/his flexibility activity, including, but not limited to, exercise preferences, available resources, support from others, personal goals related to flexibility, the patient's/client's motivation to engage in activities that promote flexibility; and reasonable expectations. It is likely that you will establish one or more short-term goals for each long-term goal.

When developing a muscular fitness plan of care for a patient/client, you may consider anecdotal data but you should also take into account guidelines from reputable organizations such as the ACSM and peer-reviewed evidence. While it is typically necessary to extrapolate the results from a study because most investigate a narrow population (e.g., young men, older women), there are numerous peer-reviewed articles you may find useful when developing a muscular fitness plan of care.

Research indicates that static stretching produces a greater acute improvement in flexibility compared with ballistic stretching (Bacurau et al., 2009) and suggests that PNF isometric contraction stretching produces greater increases in flexibility than static or ballistic stretching (Bonnar, Deivert, & Gould, 2004). Fasen et al. (2009) recently compared the efficacy of active stretching, passive stretching, PNF, and neuromobilization (i.e., integration of manipulation and stabilization procedures). After 4 weeks of stretching, Fasen et al. found that there was a statistically significant improvement in hamstring length using active stretches as compared with passive stretches. After 8 weeks of stretching, the straight leg raise (SLR) passive stretch group had the greatest improvement in hamstring length. There was no correlation between hamstring flexibility and initial tightness, age, or frequency of sessions per week.

Particulars of PNF stretching have also been investigated. For example, Bonnar et al. (2004) investigated the effects of three PNF isometric contraction hold times (i.e., 3 seconds, 6 seconds, and 10 seconds) on hamstring flexibility and found that the three protocols were equally effective.

There is also research related to the effect of stretching on the upper extremity. For example, Borstad and Ludewig (2006) found that of three stretching techniques for the pectoralis minor muscle, a unilateral standing self-stretch (e.g., corner stretch) was the most effective, the supine manual stretch was the second most effective, and the sitting manual stretch was the least effective.

While there is limited information about when to stretch during an exercise session (ACSM, 2006), Beedle, Leydig, and Carnucci (2007) investigated the effect of static stretching before versus after an exercise session on flexibility. The subjects were college-age women and men that differed in their level of training (i.e., highly trained, moderately trained, and sedentary). All subjects completed both protocols and were randomly assigned. Each protocol included three sets of a 15-second static stretch for the quadriceps, hamstrings, and calf muscles. One treatment included a 5-minute warm-up walking on a treadmill followed by stretching and the other treatment included a 20-minute moderate-intensity exercise bout followed by the stretching. The results indicated that the placement of stretching, before or after a workout, does not make a difference in its effect on flexibility.

Summary: Flexibility and Flexibility Wellness

Variables of flexibility wellness are the frequency (of the exercise sessions), the intensity of the stretch, the duration of the stretch, and the number of sets. While the *Guide to Physical Therapist Practice* (APTA, 2001b) has Preferred Practice Patterns related to range of motion and flexibility, it does not contain any Preferred Practice Patterns related to flexibility wellness. My Wellness Preferred Practice Pattern (Chapter 9) includes a flexibility wellness component. Flexibility wellness goals can be general or specific and can involve the cognitive, psychomotor, and/or affective dimensions.

SECTION 12: FITNESS AND FITNESS WELLNESS INTERVENTIONS AND GLOBAL OUTCOMES

Interventions

The fitness and fitness wellness interventions are identified in the same section as any other physical therapy interventions. These fitness and fitness wellness interventions are in accordance with the fitness and fitness wellness plan of care.

Fitness interventions include traditional exercise (e.g., swimming, lifting weights, static stretching) and leisure activities (e.g., playing basketball, tai chi, yoga, and cleaning house). When prescribing a fitness intervention, you should specify the mode, frequency, duration, and intensity. An example of a simplified aerobic capacity exercise prescription is to bicycle 20 minutes three times per week at a level 7 or 8 on the PAS. When prescribing traditional muscle fitness activities, the duration and intensity is often substituted with the weight, number of repetitions, and number of sets. For example, one exercise in a strength training regimen might be to curl a 5-pound dumbbell 10 to 12 times a total of three sets (30-second rest periods between each set). When prescribing a flexibility exercise, the intensity may be quantified by a feeling of discomfort at a certain degree or position. For example, one exercise in a flexibility regimen might be to perform two sets of a 30-second door stretch (for the pectoralis muscle) and hold each stretch at the point of mild discomfort. When prescribing a leisure activity, the intensity may be described in a manner befitting the activity. Examples of simplified leisure activity prescriptions are (1) play ½ to 1 hour of singles tennis two or three times per week; (2) participate in the 1-hour tai chi class the two times per week that it is offered at your fitness club; (3) once per week, do your harder housecleaning chores one right after the other and do not take a break for at least 20 minutes (e.g., vacuum all the carpets and sweep and/or mop the tile floors).

A primary fitness wellness intervention is patient/client education. This intervention is broad in scope and can include education in the cognitive domain (e.g., the benefits of exercise and activity and how to assess exercise and activity intensity), psychomotor domain (e.g., the appropriate execution of an abdominal curl with a return demonstration), and/or the affective domain (e.g., the integration of strategies to enhance motivation and compliance).

A home program is also a primary fitness wellness intervention. The intervention of a home program involves patient/client education and the added component of instructing the patient/client to actually practice the prescribed activities in her/his home or other suitable environment (e.g., a fitness club or outdoors at a park). When you prescribe a home program to a patient/client, you must also educate her or him about certain related topics, such as the parameters of the activity (i.e., frequency, duration, intensity) and precautions and contraindications. For example, if you are instructing a patient/client to utilize housecleaning as a leisure activity, then you would contemporaneously teach her or him when she or he would abort the task (e.g., if she or he becomes significantly short of breath). Instruction in a home program directly addresses the cognitive and psychomotor domains and can also impact the affective domain. The impact of a home program on the affective domain should not be undervalued. For example, if the home program is too intense, then the patient/client may become overwhelmed and quit the home program and perhaps not even return for another physical therapy wellness session. An example of a simplified home program is to educate a patient/client about the importance of abdominal curls, instruct her or him how to perform abdominal curls, and then direct the patient/client to perform 10 additional curls each day until she or he returns in 3 days for her or his next physical therapy session.

A referral is also an intervention. In some cases, the physical therapist informs that patient/client that a referral may be appropriate and, if there is a physician affiliated with the case, the physical therapist notifies the physician. In these cases, it is the physician who will decide whether a referral (order) is indicated. An example is a referral to a licensed mental health counselor (LMHC). If there is not a physician affiliated with the patient/client, then the physical therapist advises her or him to seek out the indicated services. If the patient/client does not obtain the recommended services, then the physical therapist must determine whether the wellness services she or he is providing to the patient/client should be continued or discontinued. In some cases, a referral is appropriate and the patient/client has a physician, but the recommendation is made directly to the patient/client and, as a courtesy, the patient's/client's physician can be notified. An example is a referral to a group yoga class.

Global Outcomes

Fitness and fitness wellness global outcomes are the cumulative effects that physical therapy has upon the fitness and fitness wellness of the patient/client. As a goal is achieved, an outcome is realized. Upon discharge from physical therapy, each of the goals that have been met contributes to the fitness outcome and the fitness wellness outcome of the patient/client.

Summary: Fitness Interventions and Global Outcomes

The fitness and fitness wellness interventions are a subset of the physical therapy interventions. The predominant interventions related to fitness wellness are patient/client education and a home program. An intervention also can be a referral. Fitness and fitness wellness outcomes are the cumulative effects that physical therapy has upon the fitness and fitness wellness of the patient/client.

chapter seven

Physical Wellness and Body Composition

I guess I don't so much mind being old,
as I mind being fat and old.

▪ ▪ ▪ ▪ ▪ ▪ ▪ ▪ ▪ ▪

Benjamin Franklin

OBJECTIVES

Upon completion of this chapter, you should be able to:

1. Discuss the provision of body composition wellness by physical therapists, including the concepts of an expertise and scope of care.
2. Define and discuss terms and concepts related to body composition and body composition wellness.
3. Explore the body composition and body composition wellness components of a history, systems review, and tests and measures.
4. Examine, apply, and critique templates assessing body composition.
5. Explore the body composition and body composition wellness components of an evaluation, diagnoses and conditions, and goals and plans of care.
6. Discuss the variables that may affect a prognosis related to a body composition and/or body composition wellness problem.
7. Discuss body composition and body composition wellness interventions and outcomes.

SECTION 1: SCOPE OF PHYSICAL THERAPY PRACTICE

Body composition refers to the quality of body weight; that is, fat weight versus muscle weight. *Body composition wellness* refers to the habits and practices related to body composition, including nutritional wellness, aerobic capacity wellness, muscular fitness wellness, and mental wellness.

Addressing body composition and body composition wellness is well within the scope of physical therapy. However, to provide appropriate care of patients/clients, the physical therapist should possess some expertise in these areas. This degree of expertise is similar to what a physical therapist should possess to provide manual physical therapy to the orthopedic patient, neurological physical therapy to the brain-injured patient, home health to the geriatric home-bound patient, women's physical therapy to the female patient with incontinence, or aquatic physical therapy to the obese patient with osteoarthritis. Not all physical therapists will be expert in body composition and body composition wellness, just as not all physical therapists are expert in the subfields of manual therapy, neurology, home health, women's therapy, or aquatic therapy.

As discussed in Chapter 5, restorative physical therapy patients who are classified in any American Physical Therapy Preferred Practice Pattern (APTA, 2006b) also may present with impaired body composition and/or body composition wellness. For this reason alone, all physical therapists should possess at least a minimum understanding of these factors, just as they should possess at least a minimum understanding of each of the specialties of physical therapy. This basic understanding can vary from a minimum competence in a discipline (e.g., manual therapy) that would enable the physical therapist to provide basic treatments (e.g., stretching) to a full knowledge about a specific discipline (e.g., women's therapy), which would enable the physical therapist to screen and treat or refer the patient/client. Possessing at least an awareness of body composition and body composition wellness is necessary to each physical therapist because obesity is a worldwide epidemic and contributes to early mortality (Kushner, 1993; Simopoulous, & Van Itallie, 1984). Other adverse health consequences of obesity include: cardiovascular disease (Hubert, Feinleib, McNamara, & Castelli, 1983); stroke; diabetes mellitus type 2 (Hu, Manson, Stampfer, Colditz, & Liu, 2001); hypertension; dyslipidemis cancers of the breast, colon, endometrium, and prostrate (Stoll, 1999); gallbladder disease; osteoarthritis (Hartz et al., 1986); respiratory problems, including sleep apnea (Young, Peppard, & Gottlieb, 2002); asthma (in women) (Chen, Dales, Tang, & Krewski, 2002); depression (Roberts, Kaplan, Shema, & Strawbridge, 2000), and psychological distress (Friedman, Reichmann, Costanzo, & Musante, 2002). Furthermore, obesity may hinder aerobic capacity and the ability to perform physical activities (Tsuritani et al., 2002), which may impact a patient's/client's ability to participate in physical therapy.

Summary: Scope of Physical Therapy Practice

Body composition and body composition wellness is well within the scope of physical therapy. All physical therapists should possess an adequate amount of knowledge about body composition and body composition wellness to examine them during the systems review and analyze the results of the screen. If the results indicate there is a body composition and/or body composition wellness problem, the physical therapist who possesses the necessary expertise should address the problem, or if not, refer the patient/client to a physical therapist who does.

SECTION 2: BASIC TERMS AND CONCEPTS

Basal and Resting Metabolic Rate

Basal metabolic rate (BMR) is the energy needed to sustain the body in the postabsorptive state, defined as no food for at least the previous 12 hours and no exercise for at least several hours, in a thermoneutral environment (McArdle et al., 2006). The *resting metabolic rate (RMR)*, or the body's energy requirement at rest, is typically only slightly higher than an individual's BMR and is measured under less rigid conditions (McArdle et al., 2006).

Independent of a person's gender, age, activity level, and so on, his or her BMR accounts for approximately 60% to 75% of total caloric input (McArdle et al., 2006). While the BMR is always the largest component of total caloric output, numerous factors can significantly affect this rate, including, but not limited to, lean body mass, total body mass, history of "crash" dieting, age, and gender. Generally speaking, the larger the lean body mass, the higher the BMR (Bachko, 2007). However, the more precise predictor of BMR is lean body mass rather than total body mass, because lean body mass is significantly more active metabolically than fat mass.

Body Composition

Body composition is determined by the percent of fat mass (or fat weight) and fat-free mass (or lean body weight).

Body Mass Index

Body mass index (BMI) is a numerical value derived from an individual's height and weight. The metric equation for body mass index is

> body weight in kilograms divided by the height (in meters) squared.

For example, if a woman weighs 63.6 kilograms and is 1.6764 meters tall, then her body mass index is 22.6. The American equation for body mass index is: Body weight in pounds divided by the height (in inches) squared. For example, if a woman weighs 140 pounds and is 5 feet 6 inches tall (or 66 inches), then her BMI is 22.6. BMI does not assess body composition or percent of body fat.

Body Classification: Ectomorph, Endomorph, Mesomorph

Sometime in the early 1900s, William Sheldon developed a human body classification system consisting of the ectomorph, the endomorph, and the mesomorph. According to *Taber's Cyclopedic Dictionary* (Venes, 2001, p. 663), an *ectomorph* is "a person with a body build marked by predominance of tissues derived from the ectoderm. The body is linear with sparse muscular development," or the outermost layer in the embryo that gives rise to the skin structures, nervous system, and parts of certain glands. In lay terms, the ectomorph has been described as "lanky," but a more contemporary description is a person with lower lean muscle mass and lower-to-average fat mass. An *endomorph* is a "person with a body build marked by a predominance of tissue derived from the endoderm," or the innermost layer in the embryo that gives rise to the digestive track, bladder, urethra, respiratory organs, and vagina (Venes, 2001, p. 704). The endomorph has been described as being "round," but a more contemporary description is someone with average-to-higher lean muscle mass and higher body fat. A *mesomorph* is "a body build characterized by predominance of tissues from the mesoderm (i.e., muscle, bone, connective tissue; a well-proportioned individual" (Venes, 2001, p. 1337). The mesomorph can be described as someone with a higher lean muscle mass and lower-to-average body fat. A humorous way to remember the difference between the three is that M (in mesomorph) is for muscle and D (in endomorph) is for doughnut.

Body Type: Android and Gynoid

According to *Taber's Cyclopedic Dictionary* (Venes, 2001, p. 106), the definition of an android is "resembling a male; manlike," whereas a gynoid resembles a woman. The android body type is more prevalent in males and implies that more of the adipose tissue is deposited in the abdominal region (McArdle et al., 2006). An android body type is commonly referred to as "apple" shaped. The gynoid body type is more prevalent in females and implies that more of the adipose tissue is deposited in the hip and thigh region (McArdle et al., 2006). The gynoid body type is commonly referred to as "pear" shaped. Evidence shows that there is greater risk of cardiovascular disease with the android (apple) body shape (ACSM, 2000). Newell-Morris, Moceri, and Fujimoto (2005) promote more "progressive" definitions of these two terms as follows: android, compared to average, a greater percentage of total body fat on the trunk; gynoid, compared to average, a greater percentage of total body fat on the extremities.

Caloric Input and Caloric Output

Body weight is stable when calories in equals calories out. However, while the components of caloric input are fairly obvious (i.e., food and drink), the components of caloric output are more complex and consist of the BMR, dietary-induced thermogenesis, and physical activity (McArdle et al., 2006). Contrary to what some may think, BMR—not physical activity—is the primary component of total caloric output. Still, physical activity typically burns between 500 and 1000 calories per day. Additional factors that affect total caloric output include the thermogenic effect of drugs, climate, and pregnancy (McArdle et al., 2006).

Dietary-Induced Thermogenesis

Dietary-induced thermogenesis (DIT) consists of the energy to digest, absorb, and assimilate nutrients (i.e., obligatory thermogenesis) and the stimulating effect of this process on metabolism (i.e., facultative thermogenesis) (McArdle et al., 2006). Typically, DIT accounts for approximately 10% of the total caloric output (McArdle et al., 2006). DIT is increased if there is a higher protein or alcohol intake and lower if there is a higher fat consumption (Westerterp, 2004).

Examination of Body Composition Wellness

While it is appropriate and feasible to directly estimate body composition (e.g., by using a skinfold caliper, hydrostatic weighing), it is not viable to directly assess body composition wellness. It is impractical because, by definition, these are the habits and practices related to body composition. In other words, to directly examine body composition wellness, the physical therapist would have to monitor the patient/client throughout her/his daily activities (e.g., dietary intake, exercise) and record the observed data. An appropriate alternative to the prohibitive task of directly monitoring a patient's/client's body composition-related activities over the course of days, weeks, or longer is the survey method. Chapter 3 has a detailed discussion of surveys.

Fat Mass

Fat mass (FM) equals the total body mass multiplied by the percent of body fat. FM is also referred to as fat weight (FW). For example, if a woman weighs 140 pounds and her percent body fat is 30%, then her fat weight is 42 pounds.

Hyperplasia and Hypertrophy of Fat Cells

Hyperplasia of fat cells (i.e., an increase in the number of fat cells) occurs normally in three stages in life: the last trimester prior to birth, the first year of life, and during adolescence (Hirsch, 1987). However, if an individual gains too much fat tissue and each fat cell size is maximized, the individual will undergo hyperplasia. An individual initially having a significant hyperplasia of fat cells who loses fat actually only reduces the size of the fat cells to lower than "normal" for the individual to obtain an optimal body composition. The fat cell number remains the same. In theory, the "shrunken" fat cells send signals to the body that they are "too small," which triggers the body to gain body fat to restore them to their "normal" size. The problem, of course, is that there are simply too many of them!

Lean Body Mass

Total body mass minus fat mass is lean body mass (LBM), also referred to as lean body weight (LBW). For example, if a woman weighs 140 pounds and her fat weight is 42 pounds, her LBW is 98 pounds.

Obese

A woman is classified as obese if she has 40% or more body fat. A man is classified as obese if he has 30% or more body fat.

Overfat

A woman is classified as overfat if she has 30 to 39.9% body fat. A man is classified as obese if he has 20 to 29.9% body fat.

Overweight

Adults are classified as overweight if their BMI is 25 or more.

Set Point Theory

Bennet and Gurin (1982) and Keesey (1986) initially proposed the set point theory. According to this theory, humans, like other animals, have a "set point" at which weight is held within a particular range (Frankle & Yang, 1988). The more developed set point theory contends that humans have a set point at which body composition is held within a particular range. This revised theory is based upon research results showing that body fat has a large genetic component (Stunkard, Sorensen, & Hanis, 1984). The set point mechanism receives input from the body, including, but not limited to, the fat cells, enzymes, and hormones (Frankle & Yang, 1998). The set point weight and/or body composition is what is comfortable to the body. While an individual's set point can be changed, it is difficult and slow to do so. Research related to changes in BMR support the set point theory. One study investigated the effects of an increased caloric consumption in confined male prisoners who were provided appealing, high-calorie meals instead of regular prison food (Frankle & Yang, 1998). The subjects gained weight but did not gain as much weight as they should have considering their increased caloric consumption and estimated caloric output. The rationale for the suppressed weight gain was an increased metabolic rate. Most of us have experienced opposite results. We have gone on a strict diet and calculated that we should lose 2 pounds per week. Although indeed we did lose 2 pounds during each of the first few weeks, our weight loss slowed and several weeks into the diet only 1 pound per week or less was lost. In these instances, our basal metabolic rates were slowing down in response to the decreased caloric consumption.

Summary: Basic Terms and Concepts

Many concepts are pertinent to body composition and body composition wellness, including basal metabolic rate, caloric input and caloric output, body classification (i.e., ectomorph, endomorph, mesomorph), body type (i.e., android, gynoid), dietary-induced thermogenesis, examination of body composition wellness, fat mass, hyperplasia and hypertrophy of fat cells, lean body mass, obese, overfat, overweight, and set point.

SECTION 3: EXAMINATION: HISTORY

During the completion of the history of a patient/client, the physical therapist should examine the history of her or his body composition and body composition wellness. This historical data may be obtained through patient/client self-report, family report, caregiver report, and/or the patient's/client's medical record. A patient/client self-report also can be obtained through using open and closed questions. Information from the external sources (e.g., family report, caregiver report) should be viewed as complementary rather than alternative. While the history can include data from as early as childhood, it is often most important to include data from the past year.

While the history of a patient's/client's body composition wellness is available to the extent to which she or he accurately self-reports it, the history of her/his body composition will often be limited or nonexistent. In some cases, the patient/client may have had a body composition test at some point in the past. A record of this, even if verbal from the patient's/client's memory, is a useful item to include in her/his body composition history. It is unlikely that the patient's/client's medical record (if available) will provide any information about her/his body composition or body composition wellness.

The *Guide to Physical Therapist Practice* (APTA, 2001b) does not include a Preferred Practice Pattern related to body composition. Nonetheless, APTA's Preferred Practice Patterns state that the history may include general demographics, social history, employment/work/ school/play, growth and development, living environment, general health status, social/health habits (past and current), family history, medical/surgical history, current condition(s)/chief complaint(s), functional status and activity level, medications, and other clinical tests.

A body composition and body composition wellness history also should include—and indeed emphasize—the patient's/client's perception of her or his own body composition status and body composition wellness during the course of her or his life and during the past 5 years. My proposal for a survey to examine a patient's/client's body composition and body composition wellness history is provided in **Figure 7-1**. Whether you choose to utilize this instrument, it is important to complete a body composition and body composition wellness history and perform an analysis of that examination.

Analysis of History of Body Composition and Body Composition Wellness

If you utilized the Body Composition History Form (Figure 7-1) to examine a patient's/client's body composition and body composition wellness history, you can use the information in this section to analyze the results. Item #1 (Figure 7-1) will be compared to the current weight that is assessed in the systems review. Item #2 will be compared to the current clothing size. If the patient/client has had a body composition test, information about that test can be useful in the future examination and planning.

Summary: History

During the history portion of a physical therapist's examination of a patient/client, the therapist should complete a history of her or his body composition and body composition wellness. This history is often largely obtained through self-report and should detail the past weight, body size (i.e., clothing size), and body composition, if known. To assess the history of a patient's/client's body composition and body composition wellness, you can utilize the form in Figure 7-1.

SECTION 4: EXAMINATION: SYSTEMS REVIEW

As discussed in the previous section, the *Guide to Physical Therapist Practice* (APTA, 2001b) does not include a Preferred Practice Pattern related to body composition. However, each Preferred Practice Pattern states that the systems review may include the anatomical and physiological status of the cardiovascular/pulmonary, integumentary, musculoskeletal, and neuromuscular system; and communication, affect, cognition, language, and learning style. While the systems review recommendations in the *Guide to*

Physical Therapist Practice are certainly helpful for a patient/client who presents with impaired body composition and body composition wellness, it also should include—and indeed emphasize—screens related to body composition and body composition wellness. The body composition systems review typically should include measurements of height

---

Body Composition History
(To be completed by the patient/client)

Surname: _____ First: _____ Date: ___/___/_____

1. About how much did you weigh **5 years ago**? _____ lbs _____ I don't know

2. About how much do you weigh **now**? _____ lbs _____ I don't know

3. During the **course of your life**, how would you describe yourself? (check one)
   - ❑ morbidly obese
   - ❑ very fat/obese
   - ❑ somewhat overfat
   - ❑ not too fat or too thin
   - ❑ somewhat underfat/thin but with good muscle mass
   - ❑ somewhat underfat/thin with average muscle mass
   - ❑ very underweight/thin with poor muscle mass (i.e., frail)

4. During the **past 5 years**, how would you describe yourself?
   - ❑ morbidly obese
   - ❑ very fat/obese
   - ❑ somewhat overfat
   - ❑ not too fat or too thin
   - ❑ somewhat underfat/thin but with good muscle mass
   - ❑ somewhat underfat/thin with average muscle mass
   - ❑ very underweight/thin with poor muscle mass (i.e., frail)

5. Have you ever had a test to measure your percent of body fat?
   - ❑ Yes ❑ No ❑ I don't know

6. If you have had a body fat test, provide as much information about it as you can about the following:
   - Approximate date of the test: _____
   - The result of the test: _____% body fat
   - Your approximate body weight on the date of the test: _____ lbs
   - The type of test: ❑ underwater weighing ❑ skinfold calipers ❑ BOD POD
     ❑ handheld device or scale ❑ other: _____

NOTE: As part of this "Body Composition History" survey, you also should complete the "Fitness History" survey and the "Nutrition History" survey.

Figure 7-1 History of Body Composition Wellness

and weight, calculation of BMI, a visual estimate of the patient's/client's body fat category, and questions to determine whether the patient/client is currently on a diet to lose fat and/or gain muscle. The body composition wellness systems review should screen the patient's/client's habits and practices related to nutrition and exercise, because these components of caloric balance are two important factors affecting body composition.

To complete a systems review of the patient's/client's body composition, you can utilize my Body Composition Systems Review provided in **Figure 7-2**. To complete a systems review of the patient's/client's body composition wellness, you can utilize my Nutritional Wellness Screen (Chapter 5) and Fitness and Fitness Wellness Screen (provided in Chapter 6). Combined, the three screens enable a complete picture of a patient's/client's body composition and body composition wellness. Whether you utilize my screen or another, it is important to complete a body composition and body composition wellness systems review and analyze that screen.

Body Composition Screen

(To be completed by the patient/client)

Surname: _____ First: _____ Date: ___/___/_____

Name of the Physical Therapist (PT): _____

1. Height: _____ feet _____ inches

2. Weight: _____ lbs

3. Body Mass Index (BMI): _____ (m^2/kg) (e.g., per http://www.bmi-calculator.net/)

4. The physical therapist's visual estimate of patient's/client's fat mass category:
   - ❏ Extremely underfat (i.e., less than 18% body fat for female; less than 5% body fat for male)
     Note: This person may appear healthy or frail, depending on her/his muscle mass.
   - ❏ Moderately underfat (i.e., about 18% to 21% fat for female; about 5% to 9% for male)
   - ❏ Average body fat level (i.e., about 22% to 29% fat for female; about 10% to 19% for male)
   - ❏ Moderately overfat (i.e., about 30% to 39% fat for female; about 20% to 29% body fat for male)
   - ❏ Obese (i.e., greater than 40% fat for female, greater than 30% for male)
   - ❏ Morbidly obese (i.e., greater than 50% fat for female, greater than 40% fat for male)

5. The physical therapist's visual estimate of the patient's/client's muscle mass category:
   - ❏ Little muscle mass. *Note: This person may appear frail, average, or overfat depending upon her/his amount of body fat mass.*
   - ❏ Adequate muscle mass
   - ❏ Significant muscle mass (e.g., she or he appears as though she or he regularly strength trains)
   - ❏ Extremely significant muscle mass (e.g., she or he resembles or almost resembles a bodybuilder)

6. Ask the patient/client: Are you on a diet to lose fat mass (fat weight)? ❏ Yes ❏ No

7. Ask the patient/client: Are you on a specific diet to gain muscle? ❏ Yes ❏ No

Figure 7-2 Systems Review of Body Composition

Analysis of the Body Composition Screen and Body Composition Wellness Screens

The body composition screen will yield measurements of height and weight, the calculated BMI, an estimate of the patient's/client's body fat category (i.e., extremely underfat, moderately underfat, average body fat level, moderately overfat, or obese), and indicates whether the patient/client is on a diet to lose fat and/or gain muscle. It is important to note that a physical therapist with more expertise in body composition will be better able to visually estimate a patient's/client's body fat category.

The nutritional wellness and the fitness and fitness wellness screens also will help screen for body composition wellness and serve as an adjunct to the body composition screen.

Summary: Systems Review

During the systems review portion of a physical therapist's examination of a patient/client, she or he should complete a screen of the patient's/client's body composition and body composition wellness. This screen is accomplished through a combination of self-report and direct screening. The systems review of the patient's/client's body composition and body composition wellness should include the weight, BMI, an estimate of the patient's/client's body fat category, and whether the patient/client is currently on a diet to lose fat and/or gain muscle. To assess the history of a patient's/client's body composition and body composition wellness, you can utilize the "Body Composition Screen."

SECTION 5: EXAMINATION: TESTS AND MEASURES

If the body composition wellness component of the systems review suggests that an aspect of the patient's/client's body composition wellness is unsatisfactory, it is appropriate for the physical therapist to examine the patient's/client's body composition wellness during the Tests and Measures section of the physical therapy examination. As discussed in Chapter 3, it is appropriate to use a survey to test and measure an aspect of wellness. The survey should fully examine the patient's/client's habits and practices related to body composition wellness, including her/his (psychomotor) body composition wellness, her/his cognitive knowledge of body composition wellness, and her/his affective commitment to body composition wellness. As discussed in the previous section, the *Guide to Physical Therapist Practice* (APTA, 2001b) does not include a Preferred Practice Pattern related to body composition. However, it does include one Preferred Practice Pattern related to impaired aerobic capacity and numerous Preferred Practice Patterns that focus on a group of related restorative disorders (e.g., fracture) and may involve impaired aerobic capacity and/or muscular fitness. Generally, these Preferred Practice Patterns state that the tests and measures may include: aerobic capacity and endurance; anthropometric characteristics; arousal, attention, and cognition; circulation; ergonomics and body mechanics; muscle performance (including endurance, strength, and power); posture; self-care and home management (including activities of daily living and instrumental activities of daily living); ventilation and respiration; environment, home, and work (job/play/school); leisure; and community integration or reintegration. In addition, the "impaired aerobic capacity" Preferred Practice Pattern states that the tests and measures may include assistive and adaptive devices; environmental, home, and work barriers; gait, balance, and locomotion; motor function (motor learning and motor control); range of motion (including muscle length); and sensory integration.

Of the tests and measures identified in the *Guide to Physical Therapist Practice* (APTA, 2001b), the most relevant to impaired body composition and body composition wellness are aerobic capacity and endurance, anthropometric characteristics, muscle performance; work (job/play/school); and leisure activities. These are relevant because the caloric output-enhancing aspect of body composition is achieved through physical activity. The additional tests and measures most relevant to impaired body composition and body composition wellness are the actual examinations of body composition and body composition wellness. One method of testing body composition is by measuring anthropometric characteristics (e.g., girth measurements). Additional methods to assess body composition are discussed later in this section. We will now discuss body composition wellness, which consists of nutritional wellness, aerobic capacity wellness, and muscular fitness wellness.

Body Composition Wellness Tests and Measures

As discussed in Chapter 1, it is appropriate to utilize a survey to test and measure body composition wellness. The survey should fully examine the patient's/client's habits and practices related to body composition, including her or his (psychomotor) fitness and nutritional wellness, cognitive knowledge of body composition wellness, and affective commitment to body composition wellness. The written survey should fully examine the patient's/client's body composition wellness; for example, her or his habits and practices related to aerobic capacity and muscular fitness exercise, caloric output, and caloric input as compared to caloric output.

The Body Composition Wellness Survey, a modification of a survey developed as part of my Philosophy Doctorate (PhD) coursework, is provided in **Figure 7-3**. The purpose of the survey is to test and measure the body composition wellness of physical therapy patients/clients. In conjunction with the Body Composition Wellness Survey, the examining physical therapist should employ sections C, D, E, and F of the Nutrition Wellness Survey (Figure 5-4), the Food Journal (Figure 5-5), and Sections A, B-1, B-2, B-4, B-5, and C of the Fitness Wellness Survey (Figure 6-3). As necessary, the examining physical therapist should facilitate the understanding of any questions that are unclear to the patient/client. Whether you utilize the surveys I propose, it is important to complete a body composition wellness examination and analyze that examination.

Body Composition Tests

When asked, "What is the direct method to examine body composition?" those familiar with the term *body composition* will reply that the only method to directly assess body composition is postmortem (in a cadaver lab). Therefore, the only means by which we can assess the body composition of a live human being is through indirect assessment, which, of course, is subject to an increased margin of error. Accordingly, when assessing body composition by whatever technique, you must interpret the result with clinical reasoning

Body Composition Wellness Survey

(PT to examine patient/client and fill in this survey)

Surname: _____   First: _____   Date: ___/___/_____

Name of the Physical Therapist (PT): _____

Note to the PT: Dialog with the patient/client to complete these tests and measures. Utilize lay terminology unless there is direct evidence that more clinical terminology is indicated.

For the PT to state to the patient/client: I will be asking you numerous questions to obtain information about your habits that affect body composition (i.e., body fat and muscle.) Please answer as honestly, accurately, and completely as possible. This will enable me to help you meet any goals you may have related to your body composition. At the end of this survey, you will have the opportunity to ask me questions. Are you ready to start?

Section A: Cognitive Aspect of Body Composition Wellness

  1. What is a good diet for a person who wants to lose weight/body fat?

  _____

  _____

  2. What exercises should a person do to lose body fat?

  _____

  _____

  3. What exercises should a person do to gain muscle?

  _____

  _____

  4. Can leisure activities (such as cleaning the house, playing basketball, and shoveling snow) help you to lose body fat and gain muscle?   ❑ Yes   ❑ No   ❑ I don't know

If the patient/client replies yes, ask him or her how.

  _____

  _____

  _____

Section B: Psychomotor Aspect of Body Composition Wellness

  1. Weight, Clothing Sizes, and Percent Body Fat

	Current	1 month ago	3 months ago	6 months ago	1 year ago
Weight in lbs.	_____	_____	_____	_____	_____
Dress (if woman) Shirt (if man)	_____	_____	_____	_____	_____
Pants Size	_____	_____	_____	_____	_____
% Body Fat (if known)	_____	_____	_____	_____	_____

Figure 7-3 Body Composition Wellness Tests and Measures

2. Tell me about how your clothes have fit you over the past year.

_____

_____

3. Self-Weighing Habits:
   - About how often do you weigh yourself on a scale? _____

   If the patient/client weighs her/himself **at least once a month**, ask her/him the following questions:
   - What time of the day do you typically weigh yourself? _____
   - Do you typically weigh yourself before or after your first meal of the day (e.g., breakfast)?
     ❑ before ❑ after ❑ varies ❑ I don't know
   - Typically, do you weigh yourself before or after a bowel movement?
     ❑ before ❑ after ❑ varies ❑ I don't know
   - Do you typically use the same scale every time that you weigh yourself?
     ❑ yes ❑ no ❑ varies ❑ I don't know
   - Do you typically you use a medical or calibrated scale?
     ❑ yes ❑ no ❑ varies ❑ I don't know

4. If the Systems Review revealed the patient/client is on a diet to lose fat and/or gain muscle, ask her/him to describe the diet.

_____

_____

_____

_____

Section C: Affective Aspect of Body Composition Wellness

Note to the PT: Rephrase these questions as appropriate to the specific patient/client. For example, if the patient/client is a young man and the goal is to gain muscle, substitute "gain muscle mass" for "lose fat and/or gain muscle mass." If the patient/client understands the phrase "improved body composition," you may use that as the substitute at the end of each question.

On a scale of 1 to 10, with 1 being no commitment and 10 being total commitment, how committed are you to:

1. Participating in cardiovascular (endurance/aerobic capacity) exercise to lose fat and/or gain muscle mass? _____

2. Participating in strength training (muscular fitness) exercise to maintain or increase your muscle mass? _____

3. Participating in leisure activities (such as taking stairs instead of elevators, washing your own car instead of going to a car wash) that will help you to lose fat and/or maintain or increase your muscle mass? _____

4. Eating (consuming) the types of foods (e.g., vegetables; foods high in fiber, low in sugar, or low in fat) that will help you to lose fat and/or gain muscle mass? _____

5. Practicing mental and/or social activities to help you to lose fat and/or gain muscle mass? _____

Figure 7-3 Body Composition Wellness Tests and Measures (continued)

Section D: Body Composition and Body Composition Wellness Goal(s)
What is/are your body composition (fat/muscle) goal(s)?

_____

_____

_____

_____

_____

_____

This Body Composition Wellness Survey includes the tests in Sections A, C, D, E, F, and G of the Nutritional Wellness Survey and the tests in Sections A, B-1, B-2, B-3, B-4, B-5, C, and E of the Fitness and Fitness Wellness Survey. If these tests have not already been completed, complete them now. The Food Journal is a part of this Body Composition Survey.

- _If the patient/client has not completed at least 1 day of the Food Journal:_ Provide the Food Journal to her/him and instruct her/him to record the items she or he has eaten so far that day and take the journal home and complete the remainder of it at the end of the day. Also instruct the patient/client to complete the rest of the Food Journal over the next 2 days.

- _If the patient/client has completed only 1 or 2 days of the Food Journal:_ Collect what has been completed and instruct her/him to complete the remainder.

- _If the patient/client has completed 3 days of the Food Journal by the first PT session:_ Collect it.

Figure 7-3 Body Composition Wellness Tests and Measures (continued)

and not accept the results at face value. Not only is the assessment subject to human error, but the method may not be valid and reliable for your particular patient/client.

There are numerous indirect examinations to estimate percent body fat including, but not limited to, underwater densitometry, air densitometry, dual energy x-ray, fat fold, anthropometric measurements, bioelectrical impedence, and near-infrared interactance.

Densitometry

The densitometry method of assessing body composition is based upon the principle of tissue density. Body density (BD) is the ratio of body mass (weight) to body volume (displacement) (McArdle et al., 2006). In simplistic terms, muscle tissue is more dense and thus takes up less space than fat tissue. Body density is determined by comparing body mass to body volume; for example, scale weight to underwater weight. The Siri equation is then used to determine percent body fat from body density (Siri, 1956; 1961): Percent body fat = [(4.95 ÷ BD) − 4.5] × 100. Two body composition methods that are based upon the principle of tissue density are underwater densitometry (i.e., hydrostatic weighing) and air densitometry (i.e., plethysmography).

Underwater Densitometry (Hydrostatic Weighing)

Underwater densitometry, commonly known as underwater weighing, is often considered the "gold standard" to assess body composition because it is based upon principles advanced by

Archimedes. Archimedes' principle states a body submerged "in a fluid is buoyed up by a force equal to the weight of the fluid displaced" (Office of Naval Research, n.d., para. 1). Because lean body mass is more dense than fat mass, a more muscled individual will weigh more in the water and tends to "sink," but a less muscled and more obese individual will weigh less in the water and tends to "float." Underwater densitometry remains a valid, reliable, and rather common clinical method to assess body composition (McArdle et al., 2006).

The primary disadvantage of this method is that some people, such as the elderly or otherwise deconditioned, may find it difficult if not impossible to perform. Additional considerations include the cost of the equipment, which is high. An individual body composition analysis cost using underwater densitometry is about $100 (University of Maryland at College Park lab personnel, personal communication, April 12, 2007).

Air Densitometry (Plethysmography)

Another densitometry method is air densitometry, also known as plethysmography. Like underwater densitometry, plethysmography utilizes the Siri equation to convert the body density into percent body fat. In contrast to underwater densitometry, which uses water to assess body density, plethysmography uses air. An example of a plethysmography device is the BOD POD. Research indicates that the validity between the BOD POD and underwater densitometry is strong ($r = 0.96$) (Ball, 2005; Frisard, Greenway, & Delany, 2005; Ginde et al., 2005). However, research suggests that the BOD underestimated body density, and therefore body composition, in athletes, African Americans, and children ages 10 to 18 (Collins & McCarthy, 2003: Collins et al., 2004; Dioum, Gartner, Maire, Delpeuch, & Wade, 2005).

Compared to underwater densitometry, a primary advantage of plethysmography like the BOD POD is that it is significantly less demanding and uncomfortable. However, the cost is very high. According to the manufacturer, the price of a new unit is $42,675 (Becky Keehn, sales representative, LMI, personal communication, April 6, 2009). The cost of an individual body composition analysis with a BOD POD varies, but is typically about $50 to $100 (University of Florida lab personnel, personal communication, April 12, 2007).

Dual Energy X-Ray Absorptiometry

A highly valid method to predict percent body fat is dual energy x-ray absorptiometry (DXA) (Frisard et al., 2005; Kohrt, 1995; Maddalozzo, Cardinal, & Snow, 2002; Miyatake, Takename, Kawasaki, & Fujii, 2005). Dual x-ray absorptiometry has replaced underwater densitometry as the gold standard for body composition (Fields, Higgins, & Radley, 2005).

In addition to assessing body composition, perhaps the primary use of the DXA is to measure total bone mineral (Albanese, 2003). Advantages of DXA in the measurement of body composition, in addition to its validity and reliability, is that is comfortable and only requires a brief period (Greg Dudra, sales representative, LMI, personal communication, April 12, 2007). A primary disadvantage of the DXA is the cost of the machine. According to the manufacturer, DXA models vary in price from $40,000 to over $100,000 (Greg Dudra, sales representative, LMI, personal communication, April 12, 2007). Another significant disadvantage of the DXA is that a physical therapist cannot utilize it to examine body composition without additional certification and physician supervision. In the state of Florida, one must be certified as a basic x-ray machine operator and a physician must provide onsite supervision during the assessment of body composition with DXA (Ben Register, Technicians Investigations Coordinator, University of Florida, personal communication, April 12, 2007). The cost of an individual body composition analysis with the DXA is about $100 (at the University of Gainesville, Florida).

Fatfold/Skinfold Technique

To assess the thickness of a fatfold (e.g., triceps fatfold), the device known as the caliper is used. There are several brands of calipers, but perhaps Lange (Beta Technology, Santa Cruz, CA) is the most widely known and used. Common fatfold sites are abdominal, triceps, biceps, pectoral, medial calf, midaxiallary, subscapular, suprailiac, and thigh. The *fatfold technique*, more commonly referred to as the *skinfold technique*, is based upon the principle that the amount of subcutaneous body fat is proportional to the total amount of body fat (ACSM, 2000). In the "reference" man, approximately 50% of total body fat is subcutaneous in nature. There are regression equation formulas as the exact proportion of subcutaneous fat to total fat is influenced by age, gender, and ethnicity (Roche, as cited by ACSM, 2000). Research suggests that the validity of the fatfold technique to estimate body fat is high ($r = 0.85$; Bentzur, Kravitz, & Lockner, 2008). However, due to improper technique (e.g., handling of the caliper, grasping of the fatfold) and/or obesity in the client, the error in predicting body fat can be as much as 200% (McArdle et al., 2006). In short, unless you possess an expertise in caliper use, it is probably wise to use another technique. If you have limited resources, your best option may be the circumference technique.

Anthropometric Measurements

The circumference technique to assess body fat, though considered by many to be less sophisticated than the fatfold technique, has strong validity (2.5% to 4.0% of hydrostatic weighing) (McArdle et al., 2006). Unlike the fatfold technique, the circumference technique does not take much training to perform. The disadvantage of the circumference technique is that, because of the inherent nature of the test, it will likely overestimate body fat in a muscled client and underestimate body fat in a client with lower lean body mass.

Bioelectrical Impedence

According to McArdle and colleagues (2006):

> A small alternating current flowing between two electrodes passes more rapidly through hydrated fat-free body tissues and extracellular water than through fat or bone tissues because of the greater electrolyte content . . . of the fat-free component. Impedance to electric current flow relates to the quantity of total body water; this in turn relates to FFM [fat free mass or lean body weight], body density, and percentage of body fat. (p. 776)

In other words, because muscle is a good conductor and fat is a poor conductor, a current travels more slowly through an obese individual than through a person with low body fat. Research has found that bioelectrical impedance technique is less reliable than either the fatfold/skinfold technique or the circumference technique (Broeder, Burrhus, Svanevik,

Volpe, & Wilmore, 1997; Eliakim, Ish-Shalom, Giladi, Falk, & Constantini, 2000; Stolar-cyzyk et al., 1997). Hydration levels can dramatically impact test results, specifically, moderate dehydration will cause body fat to be underestimated and hyperhydration will cause body fat to be overestimated (McArdle et al., 2006). Bioelectrical impedence is commonly integrated into a weight scale or a handheld device.

Near-Infrared Interactance

The near-infrared interactance (NIR) technique to assess body fat is based upon the principles of light absorption and reflection to estimate the chemical composition of the body (McArdle et al., 2006). Futrex manufactures several models of portable, lightweight, and safe analyzers (Hagerstown, Maryland) and requires very little training to operate. The NIR technique does not accurately predict body fat across a broad range of body fat levels, however, and is even less accurate than fatfolds/skinfolds (Broeder, et al., 1997; Clark, 1993; Hicks, 2000; Stout, 1994, 1996; Vehrs, 1998; all as cited in McArdle et al., 2006; McLean, 1992). The bottom line is that although the Futrex looks sophisticated and may be promoted at health fairs, it would be cheaper to invest in calipers or a tape measure!

Summary: Tests and Measures

The only direct method to assess body composition is postmortem. There are numerous methods to indirectly assess body composition. The three most valid and reliable methods are hydrostatic densitometry, air densitometry, and DXA. The densitometry method is based upon the principle that muscle tissue is more dense and takes up less space than fat tissue. Historically, water densitometry was the gold standard, but DXA is becoming increasingly recognized as the new gold standard.

Additional methods to assess body composition are fatfold/skinfold, circumference, bio-electrical impedance, and NIR interactance. The fatfold/skinfold method relies upon the measurement of subcutaneous fat and is valid if the examiner is skilled in the use of a caliper and the correct equation is selected for the given patient/client. The circumference technique is usually valid unless the subject possesses a very low or very high amount of muscle mass. The bioelectrical impedance and NIR interactance methods are less reliable than the fatfold/skinfold and circumference techniques. If cost is a prohibitive factor, the fatfold/skinfold and circumference techniques are the best options to assess body composition.

SECTION 6: EVALUATION OF BODY COMPOSITION AND BODY COMPOSITION WELLNESS

If the examination includes tests and measures related to body composition and body composition wellness, the evaluation must include a section related to body composition and body composition wellness. The body composition and body composition wellness evaluation is an analysis of the body composition and body composition wellness information obtained in the examination, including the history, the systems review, and the tests and measures. This evaluation may be influenced by other information obtained in the physical therapy examination. In terms of components of body composition wellness, it is important that the psychomotor, cognitive, and affective dimensions are assessed as well.

Evaluation of the Surveys Related to Body Composition Wellness

If you utilized the Body Composition Wellness Survey (Figure 7-3), the Food Journal (Figure 5-4), the Nutritional Wellness Survey (Figure 5-4), and/or the Fitness Wellness Survey (Figure 6-3) to examine a patient's/client's body composition, you may utilize the information in this subsection to evaluate her or his body composition wellness.

Evaluation of the Cognitive Aspect

To determine whether a patient/client possesses an adequate knowledge of body composition wellness, evaluate the results in Section A (Figure 7-3). A satisfactory response to an item could be an extremely abbreviated version of the elementary aspects (in lay terminology) of this textbook's discussions of that topic. If the patient/client accurately answers the items in Section A, then you may conclude that her/his cognitive aspect of body composition wellness is satisfactory.

Evaluation of the Psychomotor Aspect

To determine whether a patient's/client's psychomotor aspect of body composition wellness is satisfactory, evaluate the results in Section B (Figure 7-3). For item #1, compare the percent body fat of the various dates. If the body fat percentages are not available (which very likely will be the case), compare the clothing sizes of each of the different dates. For example, a steady increase in clothing size from 1 year ago to the current size indicates a gain in body mass. The type of mass gain (i.e., fat or muscle) then can be established by observation and additional questioning. The results of item #2 enable a closer evaluation of the clothing sizes on any given exam date.

The results of item #3 reveal whether the patient/client is a reliable candidate to self-monitor her/his weight. This is being evaluated because there is evidence that self-monitoring weight is positively correlated to maintaining lost weight (Wing & Phelan, 2005). Weight measurements deemed reliable should be measured in the morning before food is consumed and before a bowel movement, without clothing, and on a calibrated scale.

If the systems review indicated the patient/client is on a diet, the details of that diet are available for analysis. Important factors to analyze include the caloric input and the nutrient intake. For example, if the caloric intake is too low (e.g., less than 1200 calories per day), the diet may be depressing the patient's/client's basal metabolic rate.

The results of the Food Journal should be used and analyzed from the perspectives of nutritional and mental wellness. Refer to Chapters 6 and 9 for details.

Evaluation of the Affective Aspect

To determine whether a patient/client possesses an adequate commitment to body composition wellness, evaluate the results to item #2 in Section C (Figure 7-3). If her/his commitment level is at least a 7 on the scale of 1 to 10, then you can conclude that the affective aspect of her/his body composition wellness is satisfactory.

Evaluation of the Patient's/Client's Goals

Evaluate the patient's/client's response to Section D (Figure 7-3). Given the patient's/client's comprehensive status, determine which goals are realistic and which are not. Begin to consider the tentative time frame to achieve each reasonable goal. Also analyze each realistic goal in terms of its compatibility with other goals the patient/client has verbalized, including body composition goals and non-body composition goals.

The Typical Patient's/Client's Body Composition and Body Composition Wellness

While each patient/client is unique, it is helpful to be familiar with the typical American's body composition and body composition wellness because many will present with similar body composition wellness deficits. As a reminder, the components of body composition wellness are nutritional wellness, aerobic capacity wellness, and muscular fitness wellness.

In terms of nutritional wellness, the typical American diet is low in complex carbohydrates (Briefel & Johnson, 2004), low in fiber (Lanza, 1987), and high in fat (Briefel & Johnson, 2004). Additionally, low-nutrient, energy-dense foods account for almost one-third of the daily diet (Briefel & Johnson, 2004). Sixteen percent of Americans consume a poor diet and an additional 74% need an improvement in their diet (Briefel & Johnson, 2004).

In terms of aerobic capacity wellness, the prevalence of regular physical activity is 47% among women and 50% among men (Kruger, 2007). While muscular fitness wellness has not been studied on a broad scale, I investigated the muscular fitness of physical therapist members of the APTA and found that nearly 75% had an unsatisfactory level (Fair, 2004b).

In terms of body composition, approximately 65% of the adult population is overweight, including the 31% who are obese (Flegal, Carroll, Ogden, & Johnson, 2002). In terms of nutritional wellness, most adult Americans practice poor eating habits. About 26% of their intake is in the form of energy-dense, nutrient-poor foods, an additional 4% of their intake is alcohol, their caloric intake is increased but micronutrients are marginal, and their compliance with nutrient dietary guidelines and food group-related guidelines is poor (Kant, 2000). In terms of physical activity, in 2005 only 47% of women and 50% of men accomplished regular physical activity (Kruger, 2007). The primary cause of weight gain is an energy intake that constantly exceeds the amount of physical activity or energy expenditure of an individual. However, it is the decrease in regular physical activity and not the increase in energy intake that is responsible for the recent increase in obesity (Blair & Nichaman, 2002). The typical physical therapy patient/client will present with unsatisfactory body composition wellness and overweight/overfat, if not obese.

In terms of strategies to lose fat mass, an analysis of a nationally representative sample of the U.S. population found that the top four strategies are eating less food, eating less fat, switching to lower-calorie foods, and exercising (Weiss, Galuska, Khan, & Serdula, 2006). Of those who were trying to lose fat mass, Weiss et al. found that 65% ate less food, 51% exercised, 46% ate less fat, and 37% switched to lower-calorie foods.

In terms of weight regain following a substantial weight loss, an analysis of a nationally representative sample of the U.S. population found that compared to their weight

1 year prior, 7.6% continued to lose weight, 58.9% had maintained their weight, and 33.5% had regained weight (Weiss et al., 2006). Factors associated with weight regain included losing a greater amount of weight, reported daily screen (i.e., television) time, and a Mexican American ethnicity. Consciously attempting to control weight was negatively correlated with weight regain. Not surprisingly, weight regain was higher in those who were sedentary or did not meet the public health recommendations for physical activity.

Body Composition and Gender

While both men and women require about 3% essential body fat, women require an additional 12% for child bearing purposes, including at menses. A woman is classified as overfat if she has 30% to 39% body fat. A man is classified as obese if he has 20% to 29% body fat. A woman is classified as obese if she has 40% or more body fat. A man is classified as obese if he has 30% or more body fat.

Body Composition and Age

Body composition tends to degrade with age. While LBW decreases, fat weight increases. This change can be thwarted, but not extinguished, by proper nutrition and exercise.

Summary: Evaluation of Body Composition

If body composition and body composition wellness are examined in the tests and measures, the evaluation should include a section related to body composition and body composition wellness. This analysis is from information obtained in the examination, including the history, the systems review, and the tests and measures, particularly the information in the body composition and body composition wellness sections of the examination. If the Body Composition Wellness Survey (Figure 7-3) is utilized as a test and measure, the evaluation should include an analysis of this instrument.

While each patient/client is unique, it is helpful to be familiar with the typical American's body composition wellness because many will present with deficits that are similar to the reference patient/client. The typical physical therapy patient/client will present with unsatisfactory nutritional wellness, aerobic capacity wellness, muscular fitness wellness, and body composition wellness, as well as be defined as overweight/overfat, if not obese.

SECTION 7: BODY COMPOSITION WELLNESS CONDITION AND/OR DIAGNOSIS

When indicated, the physical therapist should assign a body composition wellness diagnosis and/or condition. The body composition wellness condition/diagnosis is based upon information obtained in the examination, including the history, the systems review, and the tests and measures, particularly the information in the body composition sections of the examination. The body composition wellness conditions and diagnoses also serve as one-word summations of the body composition wellness evaluation, and are used to help guide the goals and plan of care, which impact the interventions and outcomes.

Diagnoses

It is becoming increasingly acceptable for a physical therapist to assign diagnoses related to body composition that are within her/his expertise in body composition. Examples of such diagnoses are obesity (278.00); morbid obesity (278.01); other symptoms concerning body composition, metabolism, and development—hypometabolism (783.9); loss of weight (783.21); abnormal basal metabolic rate (794.7); (V85.0) body mass index (BMI) less than 19, adult; (V85.1) BMI between 19 and 24, adult; (V85.2) BMI between 25 and 29, adult; (V85.3) BMI between 30 and 39, adult; (V85.4) BMI 40 and over, adult. (Note: V85 codes are Supplementary Classification of Factors Influencing Health Status and Contact with Health Services [*CPT-Plus!*, 2009]).

Conditions

Body composition wellness conditions may be broad or specific. Generally, it is more appropriate to indicate a specific condition (or conditions) rather then rely upon a broad condition, unless, of course, the client's condition is truly broad. An example of a broad condition is impaired body composition. An example of a specific condition includes, but is not limited to overfat (32% body fat). These conditions are not diagnoses but—like diagnoses—succinctly capture the body composition findings in the examination, serve as a one-word summation of the body composition wellness evaluation, and are used to guide the goals and plan of care, which impact the interventions and outcomes.

Summary: Condition and/or Diagnosis

When indicated, the physical therapist should assign a body composition wellness condition and/or diagnosis. It is based upon information obtained in the examination, particularly the information in the body composition sections of the examination. It is becoming increasingly acceptable for a physical therapist to assign diagnoses related to body composition that are within her/his expertise. Body composition wellness conditions may be broad or specific.

SECTION 8: BODY COMPOSITION WELLNESS PROGNOSIS, PLAN OF CARE, AND GOALS

Prognosis

The body composition wellness prognosis is a subset within the physical therapy prognosis. The template wellness prognosis is for the patient/client to demonstrate optimal body composition wellness and thereby enhance functioning in the home, leisure, occupation, and community environments. During the episode of care, the goals described in the plan of care will be achieved.

Plan of Care

The body composition wellness plan of care is an aspect of the total physical therapy plan of care. The body composition wellness plan of care that you devise for your patient/client should be in alignment with the patient's/client's examination, evaluation, condition/ diagnosis, goals, and prognosis. Like the goals and the prognosis, the plan of care should be realistic.

Goals

The body composition wellness goals are a subset within the physical therapy goals. These goals should be based upon the patient's/client's evaluation and the diagnosis and/or condition, and be guided by optimal body composition guidelines and the patient's/client's personal goals. Ultimately, the body composition wellness goals should be based upon realistic expectations and your clinical judgment. Body composition wellness goals may be defined as broad (general), specific, or very specific. Generally, it is more appropriate to indicate specific goals rather then relying upon broad goals. A broad body composition wellness goal would be to improve body composition. Specific body composition wellness goals include but are not limited to: increase caloric output and decrease caloric intake; increase activities that promote lean body mass; and increase activities that increase caloric output.

Prognosis of Goals

The body composition wellness prognosis is a subset within the physical therapy prognosis. The prognosis is a qualitative descriptor (such as excellent, good, fair, or poor) of the likelihood that the patient/client will achieve a specific goal or a group of goals. It is helpful to determine the individual prognosis for each goal, including each body composition wellness goal rather than assigning a global prognosis. For example, the prognosis to achieve the goal to "decrease body fat to 28% within 4 weeks" might be excellent but the prognosis to achieve the goal of a "decrease in body fat to 22% within 8 weeks" might be fair. In addition to the specific prognoses, the more global prognosis also may be identified.

Like the body composition wellness goals, the body composition wellness plan of care should fully consider the stages of the wellness model (primordial, pre-contemplation, contemplation, assessment, action, maintenance, and permanent maintenance). If a given patient's/client's wellness stage is less than contemplation, interventions to raise the patient's/client's wellness stage to at least contemplation should be initiated during the initial session. To raise the patient's/client's awareness of the importance of body composition wellness and her/his current deficits, you could directly and/or indirectly educate the patient/client by asking her or him to complete a "homework assignment." Other goals related to body composition should be deferred until the client achieves the stage of contemplation insofar as body composition wellness is concerned. Once the patient/client has achieved the contemplation stage, you should advance her or him to the action stage. In terms of body composition wellness, this might mean that you direct the patient/client to begin to practice the healthier body composition patterns that you have discussed. For example, you might instruct the patient/client to limit the intake of candy and other sweets to no more than one to two pieces per day and no more than 10 pieces per week.

It is important that the body composition wellness plan of care be flexible because rigid diet and exercise regimes increase the risk of noncompliance (United States Department of Health and Human Services, 2000; Vincent, 2008). A body composition wellness plan of care may be coupled with a complementary intervention. For example, you might instruct the patient/client to engage in yoga or tai chi.

Plan of Care and Goals Related to Caloric Input

According to the Food and Nutrition Board (2005, p. 110), "the energy requirement of an individual is a level of energy intake from food that will balance energy expenditure when the individual has a body size and composition, and level of physical activity, consistent with long-term good health; and that would allow for the maintenance of economically necessary and socially desirable physical activity." This applies to weight loss, weight maintenance, and weight gain. For example, if a woman expends a total of 1800 calories per day (i.e., adding the calories she burns through her resting metabolism, dietary-induced thermogenesis, and physical activity) and her body weight is stable, she is necessarily consuming those 1800 calories.

Body composition wellness goals related to calories typically involve increasing or decreasing caloric input. A goal to increase caloric input is appropriate if the patient's/client's caloric intake is too low in relation to her/his caloric output and the client is underweight and/or losing weight but there is no indication for losing weight. (If a patient/client presents with anorexia or anorexia nervosa, she or he should be referred to a medical doctor and a dietician.) A goal to increase caloric input is also appropriate if the patient/client will be increasing her/his caloric output (through exercise, such as strength training), does not want to lose weight, and in fact wants to gain muscle mass. If there is a goal to increase caloric input and a coexisting goal to enhance muscle mass, the extra calories consumed should include additional protein.

While it is indicated to increase caloric input in some cases, it is much more likely that your patient's/client's goal is to reduce caloric input because about 65% of Americans are overweight (i.e., overfat or obese; CDC, 2008). When reducing caloric intake to reduce fat mass, it is generally advisable to reduce it by no more than about 500 calories below caloric output. Caloric intake should not be severely decreased because it can unduly depress resting metabolism and it is difficult to obtain an adequate amount of certain nutrients. The amount of the maximum decrease will vary from person to person, however, and is based upon the patient's/client's medical status, history of dieting (especially crash dieting), resting metabolism, activity level, body weight, body composition, age, and gender.

If it is indicated for a patient/client to maintain her/his body weight and body composition, the patient's/client's caloric input and physical activity level (i.e., caloric output) may or may not need to be modified. For example, if the patient's/client's physical activity level should be increased because she or he is currently sedentary (and there is no indication to gain body weight or reduce body fat), the patient/client should increase her/his caloric input in proportion to her/his increase in caloric output.

If it is indicated for a patient/client to decrease her/his body weight by losing fat, the patient's/client's current caloric input and physical activity level (i.e., caloric output) will need to be altered. For example, a woman who is overfat because her caloric input is 2000 calories/day and she is sedentary has a goal to lose a small amount of body fat (e.g., reduce her body composition from 32% to 28%), then a goal might be to decrease her caloric daily intake by 500 calories/day to about 1500 calories/day and increase her caloric output by 300 calories per day.

If it is indicated for a patient/client to increase her/his body weight by adding muscle (and/or even some fat), the client's current caloric input and physical activity level (i.e., caloric output) may need to be altered. For example, if a man wants to gain a moderate amount of lean body weight (e.g., 10 pounds of muscle and thereby decrease his level of body fat from 18% to 14%), his current caloric input is in proportion to his current caloric output (e.g., balance of 2800 calories per day), and his physical activity will be moderately increased after beginning a strength-training protocol, then his caloric input should be increased by an amount that is sufficient to allow him to gain muscle mass.

Plan of Care Related to Reducing Fat Mass

The success of reducing fat mass is influenced by professional support (Vincent, 2008). Although the National Institutes of Health recommend that healthcare professionals advise obese patients to lose weight, the proportion of obese persons so counseled is slightly declining (Abid et al., 2005). One study found that of those who had received advice to lose weight from a healthcare professional, 64.2% were instructed to change their diet, 85.7% to increase their physical activity, and 58.5% to use both strategies (Ko et al., 2008).

General nutritional strategies to reduce fat mass include reducing calories, decreasing fat intake, and increasing fiber intake. There are also a number of specific nutritional strategies that enhance fat weight loss, including eating breakfast (Schlundt, Hill, Sbrocco, Pope-Cordle, & Sharp, 1992), eating regular meals (Masheb & Grilo, 2006), using ready-to-eat cereals as a meal replacement (Mattes, 2002) or evening snack (Waller et al., 2004), and consuming 1.5 grams of protein per kilogram of body weight (Layman, 2004).

It is important to address a patient's/client's mental wellness when developing a body composition wellness plan of care. Eating is linked to stress, meeting external demands of effort and time, maintaining a routine, and other emotional and social needs (Vue, Degen-effe, & Reicks, 2008). Because overeating and the selection of "comfort" and/or higher fat foods can be caused by stress (Gibson, 2006; Low & Kral, 2006; Zellner et al., 2006) or depression (Gibson, 2006; Vaidya, 2006), a physical therapist should consider a patient's/client's level of stress and depression when developing her/his body composition wellness plan of care. Options range from advising the patient/client to engage in stress-reduction activities (such as exercise or meditation) to referring her or him to a mental health specialist.

Plan of Care Related to Long-Term Weight Loss Maintenance

Each patient/client having a goal to lose fat will also have a goal to maintain lost fat weight. The statistics for maintaining lost weight are grim, however. Approximately 20% of overweight individuals are able to lose 10% of their initial body weight and maintain their weight loss for at least 1 year (Wing & Phelan, 2005). Accordingly, it is essential to incorporate strategies that will enhance the patient's/client's ability to maintain her/his lost weight. According to Wing and Phelan, individuals who lost an average of 70 pounds and maintained their weight loss for more than 5 years attributed their weight maintenance to: engaging in approximately 1 hour of physical activity per day; eating a low-fat, low-calorie diet; eating breakfast on a regular basis; self-monitoring their weight; and maintaining a consistent eating pattern over both weekdays and weekends. Additional factors positively correlated with maintaining lost weight are reaching a self-determined goal weight; an internal motivation to lose weight and assuming responsibility in life (i.e., an internal locus of control); social support; better coping strategies and the ability to handle life stress; self-efficacy; autonomy; an overall higher level of psychological strength and stability; a greater initial weight loss (Elfhag & Rössner, 2005); and a protein intake of 18% of total caloric input, as opposed to 15% of total caloric input (Lejeune, Kovacs, & Westerterp-Plantenga, 2005). Factors that increase the risk for weight re-gain include reacting to problems more passively, eating in response to stress and negative emotions, and binge eating (Elfhag & Rössner, 2005).

Summary: Plan of Care and Goals

The body composition and body composition wellness prognoses, goals, and plans of care are subsets of the overall physical therapy prognosis, plan of care, and interventions. The body composition and body composition wellness prognoses, goals, and plans of care should be realistic and be in alignment with the examination, evaluation, and condition and/or diagnosis. Body composition and body composition wellness outcomes are the cumulative effects that physical therapy has upon the body composition and body composition wellness of the patient/client.

SECTION 9: BODY COMPOSITION WELLNESS INTERVENTIONS AND OUTCOMES

Interventions

The body composition and body composition wellness interventions are identified in the same section as the other physical therapy interventions. These body composition and body composition wellness interventions are in accordance with the body composition and body composition wellness plan of care.

The predominant interventions related to body composition and body composition wellness are patient/client education and a home program. The educational intervention includes teaching the patient/client about aspects of body composition and body composition wellness. A body composition wellness home program is also an educational intervention but includes the added component of instructing the patient/client to practice an aspect of the body composition wellness program, such as a lower-calorie diet, an exercise program, and a stress-reduction technique to avoid emotional eating. Both the educational intervention and the home intervention can include cognitive education in body composition wellness, instruction in the psychomotor aspects of body composition wellness (e.g., exercise), and/or an affective component of body composition wellness (e.g., motivation).

A referral is also an intervention. In some cases, the physical therapist informs the patient/client that a referral may be appropriate and the physician is being notified. In this case, it is the physician who decides whether a referral (order) is indicated. An example is a referral to a licensed mental health counselor (LMHC). In other cases, a recommendation is made directly to the patient/client. An example is a referral to a stress-reduction class at the local community college.

Global Outcomes

Body composition wellness global outcomes are the cumulative effects that physical therapy has upon the body composition wellness of the patient/client. As a goal is achieved, an outcome is realized. Upon discharge from physical therapy, each of the goals that have been met contributes to the body composition wellness outcome of the patient/client.

Summary: Interventions and Outcomes

The body composition wellness interventions is a subset of the physical therapy interventions. The predominant interventions related to body composition wellness are patient/client education and a home program. An intervention also can be a referral. Body composition wellness outcomes are the cumulative effects that physical therapy has upon the body composition wellness of the patient/client.

chapter eight

Mental and Social Wellness

You must not lose faith in humanity. Humanity is an ocean;
if a few drops of the ocean are dirty, the ocean does not become dirty.

■ ■ ■ ■ ■ ■ ■ ■ ■ ■ ■ ■

Mahatma Gandhi

OBJECTIVES

Upon successful completion of this chapter, you should be able to:

1. Discuss the provision of mental and social wellness by physical therapists, including the concepts of scope of care, empathy, and respect.
2. Define and discuss terms and concepts related to mental wellness and social wellness.
3. Explore the mental and social wellness components of a physical therapy examination.
4. Examine, apply, and critique templates for a mental and social wellness history, systems review, and tests and measures.
5. Explore the mental and social wellness components of an evaluation of a physical therapy patient/client.
6. Identify and discuss mental diagnoses that are pertinent to physical therapy.
7. Discuss the mental and social wellness aspects of the physical therapy goals, prognosis, plan of care, interventions, and outcomes.

SECTION 1: SCOPE OF CARE

According to Healthy People 2010 (U.S. DHHS, 2000), in any given year, 20% of persons in the United States are affected by mental illness. While there are no statistics on the incidence of a mental comorbidity in the physical therapy census, throughout our careers, we will encounter a substantial number of patients/clients who present with an impaired mental and/or social wellness in addition to their diagnoses. While mental and social health practitioners (e.g., psychiatrists, psychologists, licensed mental health counselors [LMHC], and licensed clinical social workers [LCSW]) are the primary medical professionals who treat mental disorders, it is within the scope of physical therapists to address aspects of mental and social wellness.

As a routine matter, physical therapists should model appropriate mental and social wellness behaviors and demonstrate empathy and respect when discussing mental health. Sensitivity to mental health in our profession is critical because study results strongly indicate that there is a stigma associated with mental health, even among medical professionals (e.g., Alonso et al., 2008; Kanter, Rusch, & Brondino, 2008; McAllister, 2008). Physical therapists should also screen aspects of the mental and social habits of their patients/clients (APTA, 2001b). As indicated, physical therapists should perform mental and social wellness tests and measures, evaluate those examinations, assign a mental and/or social condition as well as a prognosis, develop goals and a plan of care related to mental and social wellness, and otherwise integrate mental and social wellness into their provision of physical therapy. Physical therapists should not discount the importance of the mental and social disorders of their patients because these may significantly impact the course of physical therapy. For example, a patient/client with impaired mental wellness may refuse or otherwise be inappropriate for physical therapy, and may require a referral through a physician to a mental health practitioner.

Several publications of the American Physical Therapy Association (APTA) support the importance of mental and social health and wellness in the provision of physical therapy. However, while the current *Evaluative Criteria for Accreditation Programs for the Preparation of Physical Therapists* (CAPTE, 2000b) requires physical therapy programs to prepare graduates to develop minimum competencies in mental and social health and wellness, the purpose of the publication is not to be a learning tool to accomplish this objective. The *Guide to Physical Therapist Practice* (APTA, 2001b) speaks to practicing physical therapists in a similar manner. Given the impact of the mental and social realms on the provision of physical therapy and the relationship between physical therapy and mental/social wellness, including the ability of physical therapists to render at least basic care, there is a need to explore this aspect.

Because there tends to be a stigma associated with mental disorders, especially when compared to physical disorders (e.g., Alonso et al., 2008; Kanter, et al., 2008; McAllister, 2008), it is crucial to demonstrate empathy and respect when questioning a patient/client about her/his mental health. (Note: When talking with a fellow physical therapy professor one day at a university, I was dismayed when she made condescending comments about another physical therapist's alleged mental health condition when she stated, "He's off his meds." Had I not had this one conversation with this academic colleague, I would have argued that her character was above reproach.)

Summary: Scope of Care

Many physical therapy patients/clients present with a mental disorder or social condition upon arrival for treatment. All physical therapists should possess a fundamental under-standing of mental and social wellness and be able to screen these areas during the systems review. If the results indicate that there might be a mental and/or social wellness problem, the physical therapist should examine the patient's/client's mental and social wellness in the tests and measures. If the physical therapist does not possess the necessary expertise, then she or he should refer the patient/client to an expert physical therapist and/or mental healthcare provider, as applicable.

Because of the stigma associated with mental disorders (e.g., Alonso et al., 2008; Kanter et al., 2008; McAllister, 2008), it is critical to demonstrate empathy and respect when questioning a patient/client about her/his mental health.

SECTION 2: BASIC TERMS AND CONCEPTS

Behavior and Personality Patterns

Human behavior and personality have been intensely studied for the last 50 years. According to the theories developed by researchers such as Meyer Friedman, Carl Jung, Elizabeth Briggs, and Isobel Meyer, we experience the entire range of responses to stimuli, but more often express our verbal and action behaviors within four specific categories. How we receive information (from internal to external sources), how we judge the validity of the information received (through our five senses or intuitively), how we make decisions (using logical and objective consideration [thinking] or subjective internal rationalization [feeling]), and how we cope daily with our environment (i.e., are we more comfortable in an organized, structured, and purposeful environment or in a flexible and diverse environment?) determines our general *personality type*. The four personality types are Type A, Type B, Type C, and Type D.

People with a Type A behavior/personality pattern are very achievement-motivated and dominant (Ray & Bozek, 1980). According to Sarafino (2008), people with a Type A behavior pattern tend to have a competitive achievement orientation, be very self-critical, strive toward goals without feeling a sense of joy in their efforts or accomplishments, have time urgency issues and seem to be in a constant struggle against the clock, become impatient with delays and unproductive time, schedule commitments too tightly, try to do more than one thing at a time (such as reading while eating or watching television), and tend to be easily aroused to anger or hostility (which they may or may not overtly express). Type A's also are bossy or dominating, are usually pressed for time, have a strong need to excel in most things, eat too quickly, and are hard-driving and competitive (Sarafino, 2008). Friedman (1996) has stated that Type A's drive to achieve is motivated by an underlying sense of insecurity and low self-esteem.

It has long been known that those with a Type A behavior personality pattern have an increased risk of coronary heart disease (Blumenthal, Williams, Kong, Sohanberg, & Thompson, 1978).

Historically, Type B behavior personality pattern is defined as the relative absence of Type A characteristics (Matthews & Krantz, 1976). Less driven and free from pressure, individuals characterized as Type B have a low level of competitiveness, a low time urgency, and a low level of anger and hostility (Sarafino, 2008). In other words, they tend to "stop and smell the roses."

Between the 1960s and the 1990s, it was suggested that there was a Type C personality behavior pattern that linked personality dispositions to the development of cancer (Blatny & Adam, 2008). This cancer-prone personality was characterized by being inhibited, uptight, emotionally inexpressive, and otherwise constrained (Sarafino, 2008). Because of inconsistent and contradictory research findings, however, the current view is that the relationship, if any, between personality dispositions and cancer is unconfirmed (Blatny & Adam, 2008).

A person with a Type D personality behavior pattern has a joint tendency toward social inhibition and negative affectivity (Denollett, 2005). Miller (2005) studied Type D survivors of a heart attack and found that they approached their health crisis with a rigid "doom and gloom" attitude, maintained a state of worry or depression, felt insecure and were less willing to participate in post-therapy, had a lower quality of life, and died prematurely.

No one can be squeezed into any single personality type because we use different levels of all four sets of behavioral traits when coping with stresses of daily living. Understanding these personality types is very useful for the physical therapist when tailoring her or his communication style to help the patient/client learn new strategies to gain better health. A Type B personality might simply want to know that an exercise will be beneficial, while a Type A personality might respect strong, authoritative leadership. A Type D personality would need coaxing and praise with instruction in thinking positively about her or his healing process.

Emotional Wellness

An integral aspect of mental wellness is emotional wellness, which has been defined as self-esteem (Adams et al., 1997). Self-esteem is the way we feel about ourselves. The two types of self-esteem are situational and characterological. Situational self-esteem is when a person has a positive or negative opinion of him- or herself and his or her abilities in a specific area (Freeman, Mahoney, Devito, & Martin, 2004). For example, a person may have a low self-esteem when playing a sport but a high self-esteem in academics. Characterological low self-esteem is when a person has global low or high self-esteem (Freeman et al., 2004).

Self-Worth, Self-Concept, Self-Confidence, Self-Efficacy

Self-esteem is an important component of self-worth, which consists of self-concept, self-confidence, and self-efficacy (Wilson & Wilson, 1989). Self-concept is an individual's evaluation and appraisal of her- or himself and is comprised of personal feelings about abilities, limitations, strengths, and weaknesses (Freeman et al., 2004). Self-concept develops from the image that others reveal to us, the comparisons we make between ourselves and others, and the way we interpret and assess our behaviors and thoughts (Chaplin,

1985, as cited in Wilson & Wilson, 1989). Self-confidence is the belief that we can successfully execute a specific activity or task (Anshel, 1988, as cited in Wilson & Wilson, 1989). It is a global trait accounting for overall optimism and is thus clearly a component of mental health. Self-efficacy is a specific form of self-confidence based on a situation (Carron, 1984, as cited in Wilson & Wilson, 1989).

Emotional Wellness: Self-Esteem and Well-Being

Adams et al. (1997) contends that self-esteem is one of the strongest predictors of general well-being. To support their claim, they cite research that supported the influence of emotional well-being on wellness in the elderly (Kozma & Stone, 1978), those with arthritis (Burckhardt, 1985), and cancer survivors (Dirksen, 1989). According to Diener (2004) and Diener, Lucas, & Schimmack (2008), subjective well-being is concerned with how and why people experience their lives in positive ways, including cognitive judgments, affective reactions, happiness, positive affect, and life satisfaction.

Environmental Wellness

Environmental wellness is concerned with an individual's relationship with the environmental or external world, including the enjoyment of nature as well as the conservation of the environment (Jonas, 2000).

Evolution of Environmental Wellness

To appreciate the evolution of environmental wellness, it is helpful to consider that in the early 1970s, a national advisory committee related to conservation was established, but when they met, the concept of conservation "was shrugged off by most members of the committee" and the consensus was that there was no need to conserve natural resources as "there would always be other things that we could invent and use" (Dunn, 1973, p. 186).

Although the world's population is still not as environmentally conscious as we need to be to preserve it for future generations, many individuals and organizations are very active in promoting environmental wellness. One of the more politically known figures in the current environmental scene is former Vice President Al Gore. His book (2006) explores a variety of topics, one of which is the environment. A popular excerpt is (Gore, 2006, p. 67):

> In Antarctica, measurements of CO_2 concentrations and temperatures go back 650,000 years. At no point in the last 650,000 years before the pre-industrial era did the CO_2 concentration go above 300 parts per million (ppm). Where CO_2 is now—350 ppm—is way above anything measured in the prior 650,000-year record.
>
> There is not a single part of this 650,000-year record—no fact, date, or number—that is controversial in any way or in dispute by anybody. To the extent that there is a controversy at all, it is that a few people in some of the less responsible coal, oil, and utility companies say, "So what? That's not going to cause any problem."
>
> [Does temperature follow CO_2 levels?] It's a complicated relationship, but when there is more CO_2 in the atmosphere, the temperature increases because more heat from the Sun is trapped.
>
> But if we allow this to happen, it would be deeply and unforgivably immoral. It would condemn coming generations to a catastrophically diminished future.

Incorporating Environmental Wellness into Your Life

As physical therapists, we apply environmental wellness to our practice when we encourage outdoor activities as part of the overall rehabilitation program, including creating psychological wellness and asking patients to spend time outside to promote synthesis of vitamin D (Guyton & Hall, 2005). "An environmentally well person aims toward a balance between human needs and environmental needs and takes action to protect and preserve the natural world" (Jonas, 2000, p. 54). According to California State University (*What Is Wellness?*, n.d.), we apply environmental wellness when we stop junk mail to reduce destruction of trees to produce paper; get involved in local recycling programs; conserve water by turning off the tap when not needed; use paper shopping bags instead of plastic ones (which aren't biodegradable); car pool, use mass transportation, or alternative transportation to minimize use of fuel. As physical therapists, we can apply environmental wellness to our practice when we properly dispose of pharmaceuticals to decrease medical waste (Daughton, 2007) and advise patients and employers on the hazards noise and air pollution pose to individuals and the environment (Franken & Page, 1972; Jacobs, 1979).

Family Wellness

Family wellness involves adult relations and marriage; children and parenting; family economics, family communication and conflict resolution, family stress and coping, family violence and safety; and family creation, restructuring, and dissolution (modification of Dunn, 1961, 1973). According to Dunn (1961), if a family is well, it has a future and the opportunity to develop to its full potential; the family is integrated "so that it can operate with wholeness in meeting its problems" (p. 168), and the direction of the family is forward and upright. A family is not well if "it is a collection of individuals held together by convenience" (Dunn, 1961, p. 168). Dunn considered family wellness to be the link between individual wellness and social wellness.

Feelings of love overlap and affect family wellness. Love also stimulates health and well-being (Esch & Stefano, 2005). Because of the mind/body connection, medical practice, including physical therapy, can make use of the concept of love through complementary medicine (Esch & Stefano, 2005).

Feelings of love deactivate a common set of regions associated with negative emotions, social judgment, and the logical assessment of other peoples' intentions and emotions, and they bond individuals through the involvement in the reward circuitry (Zeki, 2007). Because of these events, love also motivates and exhilarates (Zeki, 2007).

The primary types of love are maternal, romantic, sexual, and attachment (Esch & Stefano, 2005). Romantic love is a complex neurobiological phenomenon, relying on belief, trust, reward, and pleasure activities within the limbic processes of the brain (Esch & Stefano, 2005). It involves dopamine, serotonin, endorphins, endogenous morphinergic mechanisms, and the nitric oxide autoregulatory pathways (Esch & Stefano, 2005). Romantic and maternal love are mediated by regions of the brain specific to each (Beauregard, Courtemanche, Paquette, & St. Pierre, 2009; Zeki, 2007), as well as overlapping regions in the brain's reward system that coincide with areas rich in oxytocin and vasopressin receptors (Zeki, 2007). Beauregard et al. (2009) investigated unconditional love and found that it is mediated by a distinct neural network relative to that mediating other emotions.

In contrast to positive types of love, pathological love is characterized by involvement in an amorous relationship that emphasizes paying attention to and taking care of the partner in a way that is uncontrolled yet repetitive (Sophia, Tavares, & Zilberman, 2007). The risk of engaging in pathological love is increased if the person has a low self-esteem, has feelings of anger, is deprived of affection, is emotionally distressed, and has a family history of substance abuse or emotional negligence during childhood (Sophia et al., 2007).

Intellectual Wellness

Intellectual wellness has been defined as "the perception of being internally energized by an optimal amount of intellectually stimulating activity" (Adams et al., 1997, p. 211). To support their definition, the authors cited research (Antonovsky, 1987) suggesting that intellectual underload and overload can adversely affect health as well as research (Cohen, 1985; Lawton, 1990; Suedfeld, 1979) that concluded that moderate amounts of intellectual enrichment are optimal. Adams et al. also cited research findings by Langer and Rodin (1976) that, compared to a control group of elderly residents, elderly residents who were encouraged to make decisions involving their own care (e.g., caring for a plant in their room) were more sociable, vigorous, and interested in their environment. This research supports intellectual wellness as a component of mental wellness.

Domains of Learning

Intellectual wellness is linked to the domains of learning. For example, if you educate a patient/client about a particular exercise, you will ask her or him to verbalize the precautions, demonstrate that exercise, and make a commitment to practice it every day. This requires your patient/client to achieve a level of competence in each of three domains of learning: the cognitive, psychomotor, and affective domains.

The levels of cognitive learning, as developed by Bloom in 1956 (Bloom, 1984) are as follows:

1. Knowledge—the ability to recall previously learned material
2. Comprehension—the ability to grasp the meaning of and restate ideas
3. Application—the ability to apply information by using learned material in new situations
4. Analysis—the ability to separate information into component parts and show the relationships between those parts
5. Synthesis—the ability to integrate separate ideas to establish new relationships and form a new whole
6. Evaluation—the ability to judge/determine the worth of an idea against stated criteria

The levels of psychomotor learning, as proposed by Simpson (1972) are

1. Perception—awareness of situation or activity via the senses
2. Set—readiness for a specific experience or action
3. Guided Response—overt behavior of an activity under the guidance of another
4. Mechanism—overt behavior of an activity with a certain level of proficiency and confidence
5. Complex Overt Response—overt motor behavior of a complex activity

6. Adaptation—altering an overt motor activity to meet the demands of a problematic situation
7. Origination—creating and performing a new motor activity

The levels of affective learning are

1. Receiving—willingness to attend to something in the environment
2. Responding—as the result of an experience, illustrates a value by way of an observable behavior
3. Valuing—shows some commitment to a new value
4. Organization—prioritizing a new value within one's set of values
5. Characterization—internalize a value

The purpose of cognitive, psychomotor, and affective hierarchies is to classify educational objectives and goals. While a purpose of the social hierarchy also may be to classify education objectives and goals, a broader purpose is to enhance communication and socialization among people.

Learning Styles

Accommodator, Diverger, Assimilator, and Convergers A popular model of learning styles focuses on whether a particular person is more abstract or concrete and is more passive or active. According to David Kolb (as modified by Hunsaker, Alessandra, T., & Alessandra, A.J., 1986), the four categories within this model are the accommodator, the diverger, the assimilator, and the converger. The accommodator emphasizes concrete feelings and active doing. She or he gets things done, successfully adapts to new situations, is person and emotion oriented, and is impatient and spontaneous. Accommodators tend to have "action" professions, such as sales and management. The diverger has concrete feelings, but passively observes. She or he is imaginative and reflective, generates ideas, is person and emotion oriented, uses inductive reasoning, and has broad cultural interests. Divergers tend to be employed in the social sciences, including positions in counseling, organizational development, or personnel. The assimilator relies upon abstract thinking, but passively observes. She or he is patient and reflective, logical, unemotional, "thing" rather than people oriented, has broad scientific interests, and creates theories. Assimilators tend to be employed in the basic sciences, including research. The converger also relies upon abstract thinking, but is active in doing. She or he is unemotional, "thing" rather than people oriented, utilizes deductive reasoning, has a narrow technical focus, practically applies ideas, and is able to focus information to solve a problem. Convergers tend to be employed in the physical sciences and technical positions, such as an engineer. Accommodators and assimilators have opposite learning strengths and divergers and convergers have opposite learning strengths.

Sequential, Practical, and Intuitive Learners Another classification of learning styles was developed by Anthony F. Gregorc and Kathleen A. Butler and consists of the two perceptual qualities of concrete and abstract and the two ordering abilities of random and sequential (Mills, 2002). A modification of this theory consists of three learning styles:

Sequential, practical, and intuitive (Popescu, Badica, & Trigano, 2007). Sequential learners learn best when an overview is provided and information is presented in a highly organized and logical fashion: one step and then the next. Practical learners learn best if the purpose and application of the information is clearly delineated, and intuitive learners learn best if they use their intuition and take an active role in obtaining the information (Health Care Communication Group, 2001).

Common Learning Styles of Medical Professionals According to the Health Care Communication Group (2001), most medical professionals are intuitive learners. Accordingly, if you are providing an in-service or poster presentation, it is reasonable to expect that your audience will be largely comprised of intuitive learners, so you will strive to promote interaction. If it is not appropriate to have the audience answer a question, you may pause after asking a question, which allows the audience time to reflect, and then answer it yourself. If you are interacting with a medical colleague, it is preferable to ask him or her to consider your input, rather then demand acceptance.

Common Learning Style of Patients/Clients Learning styles of patients/clients vary. It is necessary to attempt to determine what type of learner she or he is and then tailor the way you present your information to best fit that learning style. While the ability to quickly and informally assess a patient's/client's learning style comes easily to some therapists, the task is quite challenging to others. Certain comorbidities and the use of certain medications can signal whether the patient/client will likely learn best via the sequential technique. If the patient/client is cognitively competent, a straightforward method to address that learning style is simply to ask her or him if she or he learns best if information is presented step-by-step, as an application, or through interactive dialog. Obviously, the exact verbiage can be altered to meet the approximate intellect of the patient, and one or two of the categories may be excluded as an option. For example, if a patient/client is cognitively impaired, the sequential learning style is likely the most appropriate. It is important to note, however, that even when the sequential learning style is most effective when working with a patient/client, it may not be the best method when educating the caregiver.

Mental Wellness

Mental wellness has been defined as, "a global orientation that expresses the extent to which one has a pervasive, enduring though dynamic feeling of confidence that one's internal and external environments are predictable and that there is a high probability that things will work out as well as can reasonably be expected" (Antonovsky, 1987, p. 19). Adams, Bezner, and Steinhardt (1997) defined psychological wellness as a "general perception that one will experience positive outcomes to the events and circumstances in life" (p. 210). According to Adams, Bezner, Drabbs, Zambarano, and Steinhardt (2000), the core of psychological wellness is optimism. Adams et al. (1997) stated that an individual who is dispositionally optimistic "believes that every situation and circumstance will ultimately produce positive outcomes" (p. 210). To support their claim, they cited research concluding that optimism was positively correlated with happiness (Broad,

1993), general well-being (Sweetman, Munz, & Wheeler, 1993), post-surgical recovery (Scheier, Matthews, & Owens, 1989), the quality of life in coronary artery bypass survivors (Fitzgerald et al., 1993), and the likelihood of alcoholics completing an intervention program (Sarafino, 2008). Adams et al. (1997) also stipulated that optimism is positively correlated with hardiness.

Hardiness

According to Kobasa, Maddi, and Zola (1983), hardiness is a personality style characterized by a perception of problems as challenges rather than as threats, a sense of commitment rather than alienation, and a sense of control rather than powerlessness. In women, hardiness is positively correlated with age, education level, and marital status (Schmied & Lawler, 1986). The characteristics of hardiness are challenge, commitment, and control (Kobasa, 1979).

Challenge is our tendency to view changes as incentives or opportunities for growth rather than as threats to our security (Kobasa, 1985). People who have a strong challenge orientation do not seek safety and stability as their main goals. They are likely to agree with the statement, "I would be willing to sacrifice financial security in my work if something really challenging comes along." They are likely to disagree with the statement, "I really enjoy those days at work when I have nothing to do."

Commitment is our sense of purpose or involvement in the events, activities, and people in our lives (Kobasa, Maddi, Puccetti, & Zola, 1985). When we are committed, we turn to others for assistance and resist giving up in stressful times. People who have a strong sense of commitment tend to agree with the statement, "I often wake up eager to start on the day's projects." They would not be inclined to agree with the statement, "Getting close to people puts me at risk of being obligated to them."

Control is the belief that we can influence events in our lives (Kobasa et al., 1985). This belief gives us a sense of personal control. Questionnaires that measure hardiness assess control by asking people to indicate agreement or disagreement with reactive and proactive statements. An example of a reactive statement is, "Most of my activities are determined by what society demands." An example of a proactive statement is, "I weigh the costs against the benefits of each activity before taking action." These items measure the locus of control.

Kobasa, Maddi, and Puccetti (1982) and Kobasa et al. (1985) found that people who are hardy (i.e., have a greater sense of control, commitment, and challenge) tend to remain healthier than those who are less hardy. Hardiness and regular exercise combined more favorably affect health than one or the other alone (Kobasa et al., 1982, 1985).

Locus of Control

Mental wellness is significantly influenced by locus of control. Locus of control refers to the tendency to believe whether the outcomes of our actions are contingent on what we do or on events outside our personal control, such as luck, fate, or other external circumstances (Rotter, 1982). Those who believe they have control over their successes and failures possess an internal locus of control (Rotter, 1982). This means that these individuals believe they are responsible for their successes and/or failures. Conversely, those persons who believe they are controlled by forces outside their control have an external locus of control (Rotter, 1982).

Having an internal locus of control is generally viewed as more desirable than having an external locus of control. Research suggests that some interventions, such as outdoor education programs, have been found to produce shifts toward internal locus of control (Hans, 2000; Hattie, Marsh, Neill, & Richards, 1997).

According to Neill (2006), males and the elderly tend to exhibit more of an internal locus of control. Neill also suggested that those people with an intrinsic internal locus of control require a realistic sense of their influence because if they lack opportunity, competence, and efficacy, they may become anxious and/or depressed.

Occupational Wellness

Occupation is not restricted to employment or job but also includes leisure activities. Occupational wellness involves achieving a balance between work and leisure in a way that promotes a sense of personal satisfaction and health (Anspaugh & Ezell, 2007).

Witmer and Sweeney (1992) coined the phrase "the life task of work" (p. 140) and believe that work includes employment, homemaking, childrearing, educational endeavors, and volunteer services. Witmer and Sweeney emphasized that occupation is a lifespan task and that there are economic, psychological, and social benefits of work. Witmer and Sweeney's "life task of work" premise was built upon concepts first proposed by Dunn (1961, 1973) and Ardell (1977, 1986b).

Incorporating Occupational Wellness into Your Life

According to Jones, Tanigawa, and Weiss (2003), you can incorporate occupational wellness into your daily life through yoga, guided imagery, exercise, and meditation. You also can enhance occupational wellness through volunteering. According to Smart and colleagues (2006, unpublished data), occupational wellness can promote stress management, a positive attitude, increased energy, efficient problem solving, and a decreased risk of anxiety and depression.

Purpose of Life

Purpose of Life Versus Spiritual Wellness

Research related to spiritual wellness is rooted in existential well-being; it supports the importance of a purpose for life and mental wellness but does not mandate a belief in a unifying force (i.e., a supreme being) (Adams et al., 1997). The life-purpose construct (i.e., the belief in a purpose for life) is positively correlated to feelings of connectedness (Bailey & Nava, 1989), coping beliefs (Fehring et al., 1987), and self-esteem and positive associations (Adams et al., 1997). It is negatively correlated with depression (Fehring et al., 1987) and loneliness (Ellis & Smith, 1991). Because purpose for life significantly impacts mental wellness, the subdiscipline of humanistic psychology continues to evolve and gain recognition (Miovic, 2004).

Belief in a Unifying Force and Atheism

Although there is a lack of empirical evidence that a belief in a unifying force or supreme being is necessary to the purpose of life wellness, the majority of the world's population are theists and believe in a higher power (BBC, 2004a). Less than 20% of the world's current population report that they are an atheist or free thinker, but the percentage varies among nations (e.g., in the United States, 12% are atheist or agnostic [Kosmin & Keysar, 2009]), with poorer nations having the lowest levels (BBC, 2004b). Free thinking has been discussed in scientific journals since the turn of the 20th century (Wenley, 1899), but the disbelief or doubt in the existence of God among scientists was first studied by Leuba in 1914 and has been increasing ever since (Larson & Witman, 1998). In a 1998 study of the members of the National Academy of Sciences, 93% were disbelievers (Larson & Witham, as cited in Larson & Witham, 1998).

The world's population is largely intolerant of people who categorize themselves as atheists and identified atheists may suffer from discrimination, social stigma, and/or persecution (Karpov, 2002). Atheism is associated with elitism and immorality, including extreme materialism and criminal behavior; atheists are the most distrusted of minorities, including gays and lesbians, recent immigrants, and Muslims (Edgill, 2006). America's increasing acceptance of religious diversity tends not to extend to atheists; however, the acceptance of atheists is higher among those who are more educated (Edgill, 2006). In his inaugural address, President Obama stated, "We are a nation of Christians and Muslims, Jews and Hindus, and nonbelievers" (New York Times, 2009, para. 20).

The extended dialog related to the belief in a unifying force is provided since a significant majority of the readers of this textbook are likely to be theists. It is important they recognize that spiritual wellness is an optional subset of mental and social wellness and that a belief in a higher power is not a requirement to well-being.

Social Wellness

Adams et al. (1997) defined social wellness as "the perception of having support available from family or friends in times of need and the perception of being a valued support provider" (p. 211). To support their impression, they cited numerous studies that linked social support to morbidity and mortality. However, although they cited several studies that concluded that social support was linked to morbidity and mortality in men (Blumenthal et al., 1987; House, Robbins, & Metzner, 1982; Kaplan et al., 1988; Reed et al., 1983; Ruberman et al., 1984), they acknowledged that research regarding women was contradictory. Research by Berkman and Lyme (1979) and Klein, Tatone, and Lindsay (1989) supported a link between social support to morbidity and mortality in women, but research by House, Robbins, and Metzner (1982) and Shumaker and Hill (1991) did not. Adams et al. (1997) also identified research concluding that social support was positively correlated with overall life satisfaction (Klein et al., 1989) and psychological and physical well-being (Manning & Fullerton, 1988), and negatively correlated with psychopathology and symptoms of distress (Procidano & Heller, 1983). In addition, Adams et al. (1997) cited literature to support their contentions that the most important protection of health is the perception of available support, quality is more important than quantity of available support, and reciprocal support relationships are healthier than unilateral ones. Although a recognition and appreciation of the link between social support and health is important, it is also valuable to recognize the importance of contributing to one's community, which the social dimension within Hettler's (1979) model espoused (National Wellness Institute [NWI], 2004).

Aspects of Social Wellness

The social aspect of wellness consists of a healthy relationship with others, including family, friends, colleagues, and society, as well as the environment (Dunn, 1961). Social wellness involves the importance of the society and contributing to one's community and involves a healthy relationship with others, including family, friends, colleagues, and society, as well as the environment (NWI, 2006).

Social Responsibility of Physical Therapists

According to the American Physical Therapy Association (APTA; 2008a, p. 7), "social responsibility is the promotion of a mutual trust between the [physical therapist] profession and the larger public that necessitates responding to societal needs for health and wellness" and sample indicators are

1. Advocating for the health and wellness needs of society including access to health care and physical therapy services
2. Promoting cultural competence within the profession and the larger public
3. Promoting social policy that affects function, health, and wellness needs of patients/clients
4. Ensuring that existing social policy is in the best interest of the patient/client
5. Advocating for changes in laws, regulations, standards, and guidelines that affect physical therapist service provision
6. Promoting community volunteerism
7. Participating in political activism
8. Participating in achievement of societal health goals
9. Understanding of current communitywide, nationwide, and worldwide issues and how they impact society's health and well-being and the delivery of physical therapy
10. Providing leadership in the community
11. Participating in collaborative relationships with other health practitioners and the public at large
12. Ensuring the blending of social justice and economic efficiency of services

Stress, Anxiety, Burn Out, Relaxation, and Antistress Wellness

Stress

Stress is the condition that results when person–environment transactions lead an individual to perceive a discrepancy—whether real or not—between the demands of a situation and the resources of the person's physiological, psychological, or social systems (Sarafino, 2008). The perception of whether there is a discrepancy between the demands of the situation and the person's resources are affected by many factors, including the individual's prior experiences and aspects of the current situation (Sarafino, 2008). Positive stress is eustress and negative stress is distress. Examples of stress are (1) a patient/client experiences eustress when the rehabilitation group claps for her when she completes a new goal; (2) a patient/client is bored and distressed by a lack of challenge in his home program.

Anxiety

Distress is often accompanied by anxiety. The predominant characteristic of anxiety is worry; associated features are the inability to relax, nervousness, fear of losing control, and physical symptoms reflecting an arousal of the sympathetic branch of the autonomic nervous system, such as trembling, sweating, tachycardia, and faintness (American Psychiatric Association [APA], 2004).

Response to Distress

While the experience of distress is an everyday occurrence, the ways in which persons perceive stress are unique and varied. Research indicates that Type A and Type B personalities respond differently to stress (Carver & Tamlyn, 1985; Glass, 1977). Type A's respond more quickly to stress, often interpreting stressors as threats to their personal control (Sarafino, 2008). Type A behavior may actually increase the person's likelihood of encountering stressful events (Byrne & Roseman, 1986). For example, people in a hurry have more accidents than people who are easygoing and patient. At the intrapersonal level (within the person) Glass (1977) proposed that Type A personality might represent an effort by individuals to control stressful experiences in their lives. On the interpersonal level (i.e., the relationship between two people), Type A behavior has been shown to have negative effects on social interaction because of the competitive rather than cooperative approach style of Type B individuals (Spiga, 1986). At the institutional level, research provides evidence that Type A's exhibit more stressful reactions to work demands, work longer hours, and are less supportive in relationships with coworkers (Sorensen et al., 1987).

Burnout

No matter the personality type, extreme and/or prolonged stress can lead to burnout. Girdin, Everly, and Dusek define burnout as "a state of mental and/or physical exhaustion caused by excessive and prolonged stress" (1996, para 2) and identify three stages: stress arousal, energy conservation, and exhaustion. During stage one, an individual presents with two or more signs/symptoms of persistent irritability, anxiety; decreased ability to concentrate, forgetfulness; headaches; insomnia; bruxism; or heart palpitations, arrhythmia, transient hypertension (Girdin et al., 1996). During stage two, an individual presents with two or more signs or symptoms of cynical, resentful, and/or apathetic attitude; persistent tiredness in the morning; lateness for school or work; procrastination or turning in work late; "I don't care" attitude; "unapproved" 3-day weekends; social withdrawal; increased alcohol, coffee, tea, or cola; or decreased sexual desire (Girdin et al., 1996). During stage three, an individual presents with two or more symptoms of chronic sadness or depression; chronic stomach or bowel problems; chronic mental and/or physical fatigue; chronic headaches; the desire to move away from work, friends, and/or perhaps even family; the desire to "drop out of society"; and perhaps even the desire to commit suicide (Girdin et al., 1996).

Relaxation

Relaxation is the relieving of distress, nervous tension, and anxiety (Pascal, 1949). Relaxation is accomplished in a variety of modes, including some that otherwise promote health, such as moderate amounts of physical exercise (Folkins, 1976; Juchmès-Férir et al., 1971; Naughton, 1978); and some that do not otherwise enhance health, such as alcohol (O'Connor, Farrow, & Colder, 2001) or significant intakes of chocolate (Dallard, Cathebras, Sauron, & Massoubre, 2001).

Antistress Wellness

Antistress wellness is a component of mental wellness and consists of the habits and practices to reduce or eliminate stress and anxiety, avoid burnout, and promote relaxation. As with other dimensions of wellness, antistress wellness is composed of the cognitive, psychomotor, and affective domains.

Summary: Basic Terms and Concepts

There are four personality type patterns: Types A, B, C, and D. A person may exhibit traits from more than one behavior/personality type pattern.

Emotional wellness is equivalent to self-esteem (Adams et al., 1997), which is the way we feel about ourselves.

Environmental wellness is concerned with an individual's relationship with the external world, including the enjoyment of nature as well as the conservation of the environment (Jonas, 2000).

Family wellness involves all aspects of the family. According to Dunn (1961, 1973), a family is well if their direction is forward and upright, and is not well if they're held together by convenience.

Intellectual wellness is "the perception of being internally energized by an optimal [or moderate] amount of intellectually stimulating activity" (Adams et al., 1997, p. 211). Intellectual wellness is linked to the cognitive, psychomotor, and affective domains of learning. People have different learning styles, but may possess more than one—and often do.

The core of "pure" mental wellness is optimism (Adams et al., 1997). Mental wellness is affected by hardiness, the characteristics of which are challenge, commitment, and control (Kobasa et al., 1985). Locus of control refers to the tendency to believe whether the outcomes of our actions are contingent on what we do or on external circumstances (Rotter, 1982).

Occupational wellness involves achieving a balance between work and leisure in a way that promotes a sense of personal satisfaction and health (Anspaugh & Ezell, 2007).

Research related to "spiritual wellness" supports the importance of a purpose for life and mental wellness, but does not mandate a belief in a unifying force or a supreme being (Adams et al., 1997). Thus, spiritual wellness is an optional subset of mental and social wellness. While the majority of the world's population believe in a unifying force (BBC,

2004a), 93% of the members of the National Academy of Sciences are disbelievers (Larson & Whitham, 1998).

Social wellness involves the importance of the society and contributing to one's community and involves a healthy relationship with others, including family, friends, colleagues, and society, as well as the environment (NWI, 2006). The APTA (2008d) advocates social responsibility for the profession.

Stress is the individual reaction to real or perceived positive or negative factors (Sarafino, 2008). Burnout is caused by excessive and prolonged stress" (Girdin et al., 1996). Anxiety is the worrying that accompanies distress (APA, 2004). Relaxation is the relieving of distress and anxiety (Pascal, 1949). Antistress wellness involves avoiding or minimizing stress and anxiety, avoiding burnout, and engaging in activities that promote relaxation.

SECTION 3: EXAMINATION: HISTORY

When completing the history of a patient/client, the physical therapist should also incorporate the history of her/his mental and social health and wellness. Historical data related to mental and social health and wellness may be obtained through self-report, family report, caregiver report, and/or the medical record. The self-report can be obtained through using open and closed questions.

The source from which the patient's/client's mental and social health is obtained varies but is often a combination of self-report and medical record. In any case, it is important to ask the patient/client whether she or he has been diagnosed with anxiety, depression, an eating disorder, or any other type of psychological condition. If the response is "Yes," follow-up questions should be asked, such as those pertaining to medications and other treatments (e.g., counseling).

Because it is unlikely that significant information related to the patient's/client's mental and social wellness will be available in the medical records, a self-report is critically important. The information from the external sources (e.g., family report, caregiver report) should be viewed as complementary rather than alternative. The depth of the mental and social wellness history should be based upon the patient's/client's chief complaints and preliminary goals (if offered).

The *Guide to Physical Therapist Practice* (APTA, 2001b) does not include a Preferred Practice Pattern related to mental and social wellness. Nonetheless, it states that a variety of past mental and social habits may be assessed; including, but not limited to, psychological history, history of depression, history of anxiety, history of social interactions, and history of social support (APTA, 2001b, p. 143). In addition to examining the history of the mental and social wellness of each physical therapy patient/client, I suggest that physical therapists also obtain the history of additional subdimensions of mental and social wellness. I developed a survey to examine a patient's/client's history of mental and social wellness and it is presented in **Figure 8-1**. Whether you choose to utilize this or another survey, it is important that you examine your physical therapy patient's/client's mental and social wellness history.

Mental and Social Wellness History

(To be completed by the patient/client)

Surname: _____ First: _____ Date: ___/___/_____

Please answer each of the questions honestly. Your honesty will help us to better assist you to meet any goals you may have related to your wellness.

1. During the **past 5 years,** have you been confident that **"things would work out"** as well as they reasonably could (i.e., have you been optimistic)?

   ❑ Yes ❑ Somewhat ❑ No

2. During the **past 5 years,** have you had a **strong self-esteem** (i.e., have you felt good about yourself)?

   ❑ Yes ❑ Somewhat ❑ No

3. During the **past 5 years,** have you **avoided activities that cause you stress?**

   ❑ Yes ❑ Somewhat ❑ No

4. During the **past 5 years,** has the **social support available to you been adequate?**

   ❑ Yes ❑ Somewhat ❑ No

5. During the **past 5 years,** have you **contributed to your community?**

   ❑ Yes ❑ Somewhat ❑ No

6. During the **past 5 years,** have you **taken time to enjoy nature?**

   ❑ Yes ❑ Somewhat ❑ No

7. During the **past 5 years,** have you helped to **conserve the environment?**

   ❑ Yes ❑ Somewhat ❑ No

Figure 8-1 History of Mental and Social Wellness

Analysis of the History of the Mental and Social Wellness Survey

If you utilized my survey (Figure 8-1) to examine a patient's/client's mental and social wellness history, you can use the information in this section to analyze the results. The focus of item #1 is (pure) mental wellness (i.e., confidence); item #2 is emotional wellness (i.e., self-esteem); item #3 is antistress wellness; items #4 and #5 are social wellness; and items #6 and #7 are environmental wellness. In each instance, a satisfactory (or well) response is "Yes"; an unsatisfactory (or unwell) response is "No."

Summary: History

During the history portion of a physical therapist's examination of a patient/client, the therapist also should obtain a history of the patient's/client's mental and social health and wellness. To assess the history a patient's/client's mental and social wellness, you can utilize my form in Figure 8-1.

SECTION 4: EXAMINATION AND SYSTEMS REVIEW

When completing the history of a patient/client, the physical therapist also should complete a systems review of her/his mental and social health and wellness. The data may be obtained through self-report, family report, caregiver report, and/or the medical record. A patient/client self-report can be obtained through using open and closed questions.

As mentioned in the previous section, the *Guide to Physical Therapist Practice* (APTA, 2001b) does not include a Preferred Practice Pattern related to mental and social wellness. Nonetheless, it states that a systems review may screen affect, cognition, and learning style, including but limited to expected emotional responses and expected behavioral responses. In addition to screening the mental and social wellness of each physical therapy patient/client, I suggest physical therapists also screen additional subdimensions of mental and social wellness. I developed a survey to screen the various aspects of mental and social wellness and it is presented in **Figure 8-2** (Mental and Social Wellness Screen).

Mental and Social Wellness Screen

(To be completed by the patient/client)

Surname: _____   First: _____   Date: ___/___/_____

Please answer each of the questions honestly. Your honesty will help us to better assist you to meet any goals you may have related to your wellness.

1. Do you believe **"things will work out"** as well as they reasonably can (i.e., are you optimistic)?
   ❑ Yes ❑ Somewhat ❑ No

2. Do you have a strong **self-esteem** (i.e., do you feel good about yourself)?
   ❑ Yes ❑ Somewhat ❑ No

3. Do you tend to **minimize (or avoid) activities that cause you stress**?
   ❑ Yes ❑ Somewhat ❑ No

4. Do you feel **"burned out"**?
   ❑ Yes ❑ Somewhat ❑ No

5. Do you feel you have **enough social support**?
   ❑ Yes ❑ Somewhat ❑ No

6. Do you adequately **contribute to your community**?
   ❑ Yes ❑ Somewhat ❑ No

7. Do you take time to **enjoy nature**?
   ❑ Yes ❑ Somewhat ❑ No

8. Do you **conserve the environment**?
   ❑ Yes ❑ Somewhat ❑ No

Figure 8-2 Mental and Social Wellness Screen

Whether you utilize this or another screen, it is important that you screen your physical therapy patient's/client's mental and social wellness.

Analysis of the Mental and Social Wellness Systems Review

If you used Figure 8-2 to screen a patient's/client's mental and social wellness, you can use the information in this section to analyze the results. Item #1 screens "pure" mental wellness; item #2 emotional wellness; items #3 and #4 antistress wellness; items #5 and #6 social wellness; and items #7 and #8 environmental wellness. For each item, except item #4, a satisfactory response is "Yes." For item #4, a satisfactory response is "No."

Summary: Systems Review

The mental and social wellness aspect of the Systems Review should screen the patient's/client's perception of her/his mental and social wellness. To complete a Systems Review of the client's mental and social wellness, you can utilize my Mental and Social Wellness Screen (Figure 8-2). Whether you utilize the screen I propose or another one, it is important to complete a mental and social wellness Systems Review and perform an analysis of that screen.

SECTION 5: EXAMINATION: TESTS AND MEASURES

In many cases (e.g., the Systems Review suggests an aspect of mental and/or social wellness is unsatisfactory), it is appropriate for a physical therapist to examine a patient's/client's mental and social wellness during the tests and measures section of the physical therapy examination. As discussed in Chapter 3, it is appropriate to utilize a survey to test and measure an aspect of wellness. The survey should fully examine the patient's/client's habits and practices related to mental and social wellness, including her/his (psychomotor) mental and social wellness, her/his cognitive knowledge of mental and social wellness, and her/his affective commitment to mental and social wellness.

As mentioned in the previous two sections, the *Guide to Physical Therapist Practice* (APTA, 2001b) does not include a Preferred Practice Pattern related to mental or social wellness. Of the tests and measures discussed in the various Preferred Practice Patterns in that resource, the most relevant to mental and social wellness are attention and cognition; environment, home, and work (job/play/school); leisure; and community integration or reintegration. While the list of examples of tests and measures related to mental and social wellness provided in the *Guide* is rather limited, the examination section also states that the history may include but is not limited to psychology, depression, anxiety, social interactions, and social support. Tests and measures of certain components of mental and social wellness will enable the physical therapist to identify a patient/client who is not appropriate for physical therapy because of a mental/social condition (e.g., a malingerer); or appropriately address presenting mental and/or social wellness deficiencies (e.g., impaired compliance); and should refer her or him to a mental health professional.

My proposal for a mental and social wellness survey is provided in **Figure 8-3**. (Note: A discussion of the analysis of this survey is provided in Section 6.) Because mental and social wellness is broad in scope, my survey examines a variety of facets of mental wellness

Mental and Social Wellness Survey

(PT to examine patient/client and fill in this survey)

Surname: _____ First: _____ Date: __/__/_____

Name of the Physical Therapist (PT): _____

Note to the PT: Dialog with the patient/client to complete these tests and measures. Utilize lay terminology unless there is direct evidence that more clinical terminology is indicated.

For the PT to state to the patient/client: I will be asking you numerous questions to obtain information about your nutritional habits. Please answer me as honestly, accurately, and as completely as possible. This will enable me to help you meet any goals you may have related to your mental wellness, social wellness, and other areas—such as body composition. At the end of this survey, you will have the opportunity to ask me questions. Are you ready to start?

Section A: Cognitive Aspect of Mental and Social Wellness

1. Tell me what you know about mental and emotional wellness:

   _____

   _____

2. Tell me what you know about stress and burn out:

   _____

   _____

3. Tell me what you know about social wellness:

   _____

   _____

4. Tell me what you know about environmental wellness:

   _____

   _____

Section B: Psychomotor Aspect of Mental and Social Wellness

Part 1: Mental Wellness (Define/discuss each term that is unfamiliar to the patient/client.)

1. As much as it is reasonably possible, are you confident that things will work out as well as they reasonably can?

   ❑ Yes ❑ Somewhat ❑ No

2. Do you believe that everything will probably work out the best that it can?

   ❑ Yes ❑ Somewhat ❑ No

3. Do you live your life as though everything will probably work out the best that it can?

   ❑ Yes ❑ Somewhat ❑ No

4. Do you believe that you tend to influence the events in your life?

   ❑ Yes ❑ To a certain extent ❑ No

Figure 8-3 Mental and Social Wellness Tests and Measures

5. When you have a problem that is causing you stress, do you tend to:
   ❏ turn to others for assistance *or*   ❏ attempt to handle the problem on your own?

6. When you face a difficult challenge, do you tend to:
   ❏ give up *or*   ❏ resist giving up?

7. At work, do you tend to:
   ❏ seek out challenges *or*   ❏ take the "easy route"?

8. At work, do you tend to prefer those days at work when you have:
   ❏ more to do *or*   ❏ nothing to do?

9. Do you believe that the outcomes of your actions are contingent upon:
   ❏ what you do *or*   ❏ events outside of your personal control?

10. Do you assume responsibility for your failures?
    ❏ Yes   ❏ Somewhat   ❏ No

Part 2: Emotional Wellness (Define/discuss each term that is unfamiliar to the patient/client.)

1. How do you feel about yourself?
   ❏ Good   ❏ Okay   ❏ Not so good

2. How do you rate your self-esteem?
   ❏ Low   ❏ Moderate   ❏ High

Part 3: Behavior/Personality Pattern (Define/discuss each term that is unfamiliar to the patient/client.)

1. Would you say that you are: ❏ very,   ❏ somewhat, *or*   ❏ not at all self-critical?
2. Are you: ❏ often,   ❏ sometimes, *or*   ❏ rarely impatient?
3. Do you: ❏ often,   ❏ sometimes, *or*   ❏ rarely try to do more one than thing at a time?
4. Are you: ❏ often,   ❏ sometimes, *or*   ❏ rarely easily angered?
5. Is your level of competitiveness: ❏ low   ❏ moderate, *or*   ❏ high?
6. Are you: ❏ rarely,   ❏ sometimes, *or*   ❏ often inhibited (or passive)?
7. Are you: ❏ rarely,   ❏ sometimes, *or*   ❏ often able to express yourself?

Part 4: Antistress Wellness (Define/discuss each term that is unfamiliar to the patient/client.)

1. Do you avoid and minimize activities/situations that cause you stress?
   ❏ Largely/yes   ❏ To a certain extent   ❏ Not really/no

2. When you feel stress, how often do you engage in relaxation activities (including "simple" stress-reduction techniques such as deep breathing)?
   ❏ Much of the time (or always)   ❏ Sometimes   ❏ Rarely or never

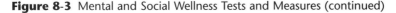

Figure 8-3 Mental and Social Wellness Tests and Measures (continued)

Part 5: Burn Out Secondary to Stress (Define/discuss each term that is unfamiliar to the patient/client. Check all symptoms that apply. Ensure the patient/client understands that the symptoms/signs must be linked to/caused from stress {rather than independent of stress}. If a patient/client acknowledges a symptom in #1, she or he may acknowledge a higher level of that symptom in #2 or #3. For example, she or he may report "headache" in #1 and then report "chronic headaches" in 3-A).

1. Stress in your life causes you to have which of the following, if any?
   - ❑ Irritability/anxiety   ❑ Decreased ability to concentrate/forgetfulness   ❑ Headaches
   - ❑ Insomnia/trouble sleeping   ❑ Bruxism/grinding your teeth
   - ❑ Heart palpitations/arrhythmia/transient hypertension   ❑ None

2. Stress in your life causes you to have which of the following, if any? (Check all that apply.)
   - ❑ Cynical attitude/resentful   ❑ Persistent tiredness in the morning
   - ❑ Lateness for work or school   ❑ Procrastination/turn in work late
   - ❑ "I don't care" attitude; frequently skipping work or school; social withdrawal
   - ❑ Increased alcohol, coffee, tea, or cola   ❑ Decreased sexual desire   ❑ None

3-A. Stress in your life causes you to have which of the following, if any?
   - ❑ Chronic sadness or depression   ❑ Chronic stomach or bowel problems
   - ❑ Chronic mental fatigue   ❑ Chronic physical fatigue   ❑ Chronic headaches   ❑ None

3-B. Which of the following, if any, are you considering?
   - ❑ Moving away from friends and/or family   ❑ Quitting your job or dropping out of school
   - ❑ Harming yourself   ❑ None

Part 6: Intellectual Wellness (Define/discuss each term that is unfamiliar to the patient/client.)

1. Is the amount of stimulating intellectual activity you have in your life:
   - ❑ Too much   ❑ Too little, *or*   ❑ Just about right?

2. Does the amount of intellectual activity in your life cause you to be: ❑ Overwhelmed
   - ❑ Bored, *or*   ❑ Appropriately engaged/challenged (i.e., neither overwhelmed nor bored)?

Part 7: Occupational Wellness (Define/discuss each term that is unfamiliar to the patient/client.)

1. Do you maintain a balance between your job and family time?
   - ❑ Yes   ❑ Somewhat   ❑ No

2. Do you maintain a balance between your job and personal time?
   - ❑ Yes   ❑ Somewhat   ❑ No

Part 8: Social Wellness (Define/discuss each term that is unfamiliar to the patient/client.)

1. Is the social support available to you adequate?
   - ❑ Yes   ❑ Somewhat   ❑ No

2. Do you adequately contribute to your community?
   - ❑ Yes   ❑ Somewhat   ❑ No

Figure 8-3 Mental and Social Wellness Tests and Measures (continued)

Part 9: Family Wellness (Define/discuss each term that is unfamiliar to the patient/client.)

Preface: Whom do you consider to be your immediate family members?

_____

1. How well does your family work together to solve its problems?

   ❑ Very well   ❑ Moderately well   ❑ Poorly

2. How would you describe the direction of your family?

   ❑ Forward/upward   ❑ Static   ❑ Backwards/downward

3. Is your family held together by positive emotions (such as caring) rather than convenience?

   ❑ Yes   ❑ To a certain extent   ❑ No

Part 10: Environmental Wellness (Define/discuss each term that is unfamiliar to the patient/client.)

1. How often do you take the time to enjoy nature?

   ❑ I enjoy nature on a regular basis.
   ❑ I occasionally take the time to enjoy nature.
   ❑ I rarely or never take the time to enjoy nature.

2. How well do you conserve the environment? (Consider if you stop junk mail; recycle, conserve water; conserve electricity; use paper shopping bags; use a fuel-efficient vehicle, car pool, or use mass transportation, etc.)

   ❑ I do a lot to conserve the environment.
   ❑ I do some things to conserve the environment.
   ❑ I do very little or nothing to conserve the environment.

Section C: Affective Aspects of Mental and Social Wellness

On a scale of 1 to 10, with 1 being no commitment and 10 being total commitment, how committed are you to:

1. telling yourself that "things will work out"? _____
2. accepting responsibility for your failures? _____
3. living a life that promotes your self-esteem? _____
4. avoiding or minimizing events that cause you stress? _____
5. choosing intellectual activities that do not cause you to be bored, but are not overwhelming either? _____
6. making sure that you have social support when you need it? _____
7. working with your family to solve problems and helping your family to move forward? _____
8. keeping a balance between your work and family/personal time? _____
9. enjoying nature? _____
10. preserving the environment? _____

Section D: Mental/Social Wellness Goal(s)

What is/are your mental and/or social wellness goal(s)?

_____

_____

_____

_____

_____

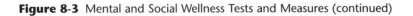

Figure 8-3 Mental and Social Wellness Tests and Measures (continued)

(i.e., optimism, hardiness, locus of control, emotional wellness [self-esteem], behavior/personality patterns, antistress wellness, stress secondary to burn-out, intellectual wellness, and occupational wellness) and social wellness (i.e., social support, contributing to one's community, family wellness, and environmental wellness). My survey also examines the cognitive, psychomotor, and affective domains because wellness is three dimensional. Whether you choose to utilize my survey or another one, it is important that you examine your physical therapy patient's/client's mental and social wellness.

Summary: Tests and Measures

In many cases, it is appropriate for a physical therapist to examine a patient's/client's mental and social wellness. Like other aspects of wellness, it is appropriate to examine mental and social wellness through a survey. The survey should measure the cognitive, psychomotor, and affective aspects of indicated aspects of mental wellness (e.g., "pure" mental wellness, including hardiness and locus of control; emotional wellness; antistress wellness; intellectual wellness; occupational wellness) and social wellness (e.g. "pure" social wellness, family wellness, environmental wellness). Whether you utilize the instrument I propose (Figure 8-3) or some other form, it is important to examine the mental and social wellness of indicated physical therapy patients/clients.

SECTION 6: EVALUATION OF MENTAL AND SOCIAL WELLNESS

If the examination includes tests and measures related to mental and social wellness, the evaluation must include a section related to mental and social wellness. The mental and social wellness evaluation is an analysis of the mental and social wellness information obtained in the examination, including the history, the systems review, and the tests and measures. This evaluation may also be influenced by other information obtained in the physical therapy examination.

Analysis of the Mental and Social Wellness Survey

To possess a satisfactory level of mental and social wellness, the patient/client must have an adequate knowledge of mental and social wellness, engage in activities that promote mental and social wellness, and possess an acceptable level of commitment to mental and social wellness. If you utilized the "Mental and Social Wellness Survey" (Figure 8-3) to examine a patient's/client's mental and social wellness, you can utilize the information in this subsection to evaluate her/his mental and social wellness.

Evaluation of the Cognitive Aspect

To evaluate the cognitive knowledge of a patient's/client's mental and social wellness, assess the feedback to the items in Section A (Figure 8-3). A satisfactory response to an item could be an extremely abbreviated version of the elementary aspects (in lay terminology) of this textbook's discussion of the topic. If the patient/client verbalized that mental wellness (item #1) is linked to optimism and/or "things working out" and emotional wellness is linked to a positive self-esteem, then her/his cognitive knowledge of the concept is satisfactory. Similarly, antistress wellness (item #2) should be linked to avoiding or minimizing stress and/or engaging in activities that promote relaxation and the patient/client should verbalize some of the signs or symptoms of burn out; social wellness (item #3) should be linked to the availability of support from family and friends, if not also providing valued support; and environmental wellness (item #4) should be linked to the conservation of the environment, if not also the enjoyment of nature.

Evaluation of the Psychomotor Aspect

To evaluate the psychomotor aspect of a patient's/client's mental and social wellness, assess the feedback to the items in Section B. Part 1 pertains to mental wellness. Numbers 1 through 3 examine "pure" mental wellness. For each item, a satisfactory response is "Yes," a moderate response is "Somewhat," and an unsatisfactory response is "No." If the patient/client scores a satisfactory in all three items, her/his "pure" mental wellness is likely satisfactory. If the patient/client scores an unsatisfactory in two or three of three items, her/his "pure" mental wellness is likely unsatisfactory.

Items #4 through #8 (in Part 1) evaluate the hardiness aspect of mental wellness. In response to #4, a satisfactory response is "Yes," a moderate response is "To a certain extent," and an unsatisfactory response is "No." In response to #5, a satisfactory response is "turn to others for assistance," and an unsatisfactory response is "attempt to handle the problem on your own." In response to #6, a satisfactory response is "resist giving up" and an unsatisfactory response is "give up." In response to #7, a satisfactory response is "seek out challenges" and an unsatisfactory response is "take the 'easy route.'" In response to #8, a satisfactory response is "more to do" and an unsatisfactory response is "nothing to do." If a patient/client scores a satisfactory in four out of the five items, her/his hardiness is likely satisfactory. If the patient/client scores an unsatisfactory in three out of the five items, her/his hardiness is likely unsatisfactory.

Items #9 and #10 (in Part 1) evaluate locus of control aspect of mental wellness. In response to #9, a satisfactory response is "what you do" and an unsatisfactory response is "events outside of your personal control." In response to #10, a satisfactory response is "Yes" and an unsatisfactory response is "No." If a patient/client scores a satisfactory in both items, then her/his locus of control is likely internal; if the patient/client scores an unsatisfactory in both items, then her/his locus of control is likely external.

To evaluate the psychomotor aspect of patient's/client's emotional wellness, assess her/his responses to Part 2 of Section B. In response to item #1, a satisfactory response is "Good," a moderate response is "Okay," and an unsatisfactory response is "Not so good." In response to item #2, a satisfactory response is "High," a moderate response is "Moderate," and an unsatisfactory response is "Low." (Note: The two items in this section are rather synonymous. The first is colloquial and the second is more formal.) If the patient/client scores an unsatisfactory in both items, her/his emotional wellness (self-esteem) is likely unsatisfactory. If a patient/client scores a satisfactory in both items, her/his emotional wellness is likely satisfactory.

To evaluate a patient's/client's behavior/personality pattern, assess her/his responses to Part 3 of Section B. In response to item #1, score one point for Type A if "very" is selected and one point for Type B if "not at all" is selected. In response to item #2, score one point for Type A if "often" is selected and one point for Type B if "rarely" is selected. In response to item #3, score one point for Type A if "often" is selected and one point for Type B if "rarely" is selected. In response to item #4, score one point for Type A if "often" is selected and one point for Type B if "rarely" is selected. In response to item #5, score one point for Type A if "high" is selected and one point for Type B if "low" is selected. In response to item #6, score one point for Type C if "often" is selected and one-half point if "sometimes" is selected. In response to item #7, score one point for Type C if "rarely" is selected and one-half point if "sometimes" is selected. If the patient/clients scores at least five Type A's, you may assign a Type A label; if she or he scores at least five Type B's, you may assign a Type B label; if she or he scores at least one and one-half Type C's, you may assign a Type C label. You may assign more than one personality-type label. In these cases, typically you should assign a primary personality type, a secondary personality type, and perhaps even a tertiary personality type. It is important to bear the personality type(s) in mind when you consider the patient's/client's level of distress and how it might impact physical therapy.

To evaluate a patient's/client's psychomotor aspect of antistress wellness, assess her/his responses to Part 4 in Section B. In response to item #1, a satisfactory response is "Largely/yes," a moderate response is "To a certain extent," and an unsatisfactory response is "Not really/no." In response to item #2, a satisfactory response is "Much of the time" or "Always," a moderate response is "Sometimes," and an unsatisfactory response is "Rarely or never." If a patient/client scores a satisfactory in both items, her/his antistress wellness is likely satisfactory. If a patient/client scores unsatisfactory in both items, then her/his antistress wellness is likely unsatisfactory.

To determine whether a patient/client has burn out, assess her/his responses to Part 5 in Section B. In response to item #1, a satisfactory response is "None" and an unsatisfactory response is one or more. The same criteria applies to items #2, #3-A, and #3-B. In the case of #3-B, if the patient/client considers self-harm, notify social services and, if applicable, your supervisor.

To evaluate a patient's/client's psychomotor aspect of intellectual wellness, assess her/his responses to Part 6 in Section B. In response to item #1, a satisfactory response is "just about right" and an unsatisfactory response is "too much" or "too little." In response to item #2, a satisfactory response is "appropriately engaged/challenged" and an unsatisfactory response is "overwhelmed" or "bored." If a patient/client scores a satisfactory in both items, her/his intellectual wellness is likely satisfactory. If a patient/client scores unsatisfactory in both items, her/his intellectual wellness is likely unsatisfactory.

To determine a patient's/client's psychomotor aspect of occupational wellness, assess her/his responses to Part 7 of Section B. In response to item #1, a satisfactory response is "Yes," a moderate response is "Somewhat," and an unsatisfactory response is "No." The same is the true for item #2. If a patient/client scores a satisfactory in both items, her/his occupational wellness is likely satisfactory. If the patient/client scores an unsatisfactory in both items, her/his occupational wellness is likely unsatisfactory.

To evaluate the psychomotor aspect of patient's/client's social wellness, assess her/his responses to Part 8 of Section B. In response to item #1, a satisfactory response is "Yes," a moderate response is "Somewhat," and an unsatisfactory response is "No." The same is true for item #2. If a patient/client scores a satisfactory in both items, then her/his social wellness is likely satisfactory. If the patient/client scores an unsatisfactory in both items, her/his social wellness is likely unsatisfactory.

To evaluate a patient's/client's psychomotor aspect of family wellness, assess her/his responses to Part 9 of Section B. In response to item #1, a satisfactory response is "Very well," a moderate response is "Moderately well," and an unsatisfactory response is "Poorly." In response to item #2, a satisfactory response is "Forward/upward," a moderate response is "Static," and an unsatisfactory response is "Backwards/downward." In response to item #3, a satisfactory response is "No," a moderate response is "To a certain extent," and an unsatisfactory response is "Yes." If a patient/client scores a satisfactory in each of the three items, then her/his family wellness is likely satisfactory; if the patient/client scores an unsatisfactory in two of the three items, her/his family wellness is likely unsatisfactory.

To evaluate the psychomotor aspect of a patient's/client's environmental wellness, assess her/his responses to Part 10 of Section B. In response to item #1, a satisfactory response is "I enjoy nature on a regular basis," a moderate response is "I occasionally take the time to enjoy nature," and an unsatisfactory response is "I rarely or never take the time to enjoy nature." In response to item #2, a satisfactory response is "I do a lot to conserve the environment," a moderate response is "I do some things to conserve the environment," and an unsatisfactory response is "I do very little or nothing to conserve the environment." If a patient/client scores a satisfactory in both items, her/his environmental wellness is likely satisfactory; if the scores are unsatisfactory in both items, then her/his environmental wellness is likely unsatisfactory.

Evaluation of the Affective Aspect

To evaluate a patient's/client's affective commitment to mental and social wellness (including various subcomponents), assess her/his feedback to the items in Section C (Figure 8-3). A satisfactory response is at least a 7 on the scale of 10. An unsatisfactory response is a 6 or less. Items #1 through #5 evaluate aspects of mental wellness; items #6 through #10 evaluate aspects of social wellness. Specifically, item #1 evaluates the affective commitment to "pure" mental wellness; item #2 the locus of control aspect of mental wellness; item #3 emotional wellness; item #4 antistress wellness; item #5 intellectual wellness; item #6 "pure" social wellness; item #7 family wellness; item #8 occupational wellness; and items #9 and #10 environmental wellness.

Summary: Mental and Social Wellness Evaluation

Each component of mental and social wellness examined during the tests and measures must be addressed in evaluation. This evaluation should speak to the cognitive, psychomotor, and affective aspects of mental wellness (i.e., "pure" mental wellness, including hardiness and locus of control; emotional wellness; antistress wellness; intellectual wellness; occupational wellness) and social wellness ("pure" social wellness, family wellness, and environmental wellness). An evaluation of the mental and social wellness of a patient/client may consist of an assessment of her/his feedback to the "Mental and Social Wellness Survey" example in Figure 8-3.

SECTION 7: MENTAL DIAGNOSES AND MENTAL AND SOCIAL WELLNESS CONDITIONS

Mental Diagnoses and Mental and Social Conditions

Although it is outside their scope of care for physical therapists to assign a mental health diagnosis, we should be aware of, and indeed versed in, mental health disorders. Mental diseases (i.e., diagnoses or V-Codes) that are pertinent to physical therapy include, but are not necessarily limited to, anxiety disorder, adjustment disorder, depression, body dysmorphic disorder, anorexia nervosa, bulimia nervosa, binge eating, malingering, factitious disorder, and noncompliance with treatment. (Note: Mental disorders are defined in the *Diagnostic and Statistical Manual of Mental Disorders* (DSM-4) of the American Psychiatric Association (APA, 1994). Neurological disorders, such as Alzheimer's disease and Parkinson's disease, are not mental disorders.)

If a patient/client presents with some of the symptoms of a particular diagnosis, but the symptoms are not clinically significant and/or all of the diagnostic criteria are not met, the patient/client may be assigned a corresponding condition. The conditions of impaired mental wellness–stress/anxiety, impaired mental wellness–depression, and impaired social wellness each are relevant to physical therapy.

Like a diagnosis, a mental and/or social wellness condition is based upon information obtained in the examination (history, systems review, and tests and measures), particularly the information in the mental and social wellness sections. The mental and social wellness conditions, if any, help guide the goals and plan of care, and impact the interventions and outcomes.

Diagnosis: Anxiety (300.02)

A generalized anxiety disorder is characterized by "excessive. . . worry (i.e., apprehensive expectation), occurring more days than not for a period of at least 6 months, about a number of events or activities," difficulty controlling the worry, and three of the following additional symptoms: difficulty concentrating, disturbed sleep, irritability, restlessness, muscle tension, and easily fatigued (APA, 2004, p. 432). The duration, frequency, and intensity of the worry is significantly out of proportion to the actual likelihood or impact of the feared event (APA, 2004). Examples of worries (of adults) include routine life circumstances such as finances, job responsibilities, and health of their family members (APA, 2004).

Diagnosis: Adjustment Disorder (309.0–309.9)

An adjustment disorder consists of "clinically significant emotional or behavioral symptoms in response to an identifiable psychosocial stressor or stressors" (APA, 2004, p. 623). An adjustment disorder is categorized as with or without depressed mood, anxiety, and/or disturbance of conduct; it can be acute, chronic, recurrent, or continuous (APA, 2004). Stressors may be a single event or multiple events, and examples include the termination of romantic relationship, significant business difficulties, and living in a high crime neighborhood (APA, 2004). (Note: A stress disorder, clinically referred to as an acute stress disorder, is significantly more severe than an adjustment disorder; it is a response to a traumatic event involving death, serious injury, or physical integrity that causes feelings of intense helplessness, fear, or horror; as well as additional symptoms [APA, 2004]).

Condition: Impaired Mental Wellness—Stress/Anxiety

With the condition of impaired mental wellness–stress/anxiety, the individual does not meet the diagnostic criteria for stress disorder, anxiety disorder, or adjustment disorder, but nonetheless has emotional or behavioral symptoms in response to a psychosocial stressor(s).

In addition to its link to the diagnoses of stress disorder, anxiety disorder, and adjustment disorder, a defining component of the condition of impaired mental wellness–stress/anxiety is that it is disproportionate in response to the situation or event and that it is non-constructive (Corsini & Wedding, 2007). The condition also is based upon the concept of state anxiety, where the patient/client perceives tension in response to a specific circumstance (Corsini & Wedding, 2007). For example, a patient walks into the office of a physical therapist who is wearing a white lab coat and a stethoscope, and the patient's blood pressure rises in direct response to seeing the medical professional, lab coat, and stethoscope.

During my career as a physical therapist, many of my patients/clients have presented with impaired mental wellness–stress/anxiety in addition to their physical therapy diagnosis. An example is one of my former home health patients who, during our initial session, refused to ambulate with her walker because she had fallen when first trying to use it in her hospital room (before a physical therapist had been ordered, I might add).

Diagnosis: Major (296) and Minor Depression (311)

A major depressive episode "is a period of at least two weeks during in which there is either a depressed mood or the loss of interest or pleasure in nearly all activities" (APA, 2004, p. 320), which is accompanied by at least four additional symptoms from the following: changes in appetite or weight, psychomotor activity, and sleep; difficulty concentrating, thinking, or making decisions; feelings of guilt or worthlessness; decreased energy; or suicide ideation, plans, or attempts or recurrent thoughts of suicide. Additionally, "the symptoms must persist for most of the day, nearly every day" and must be accompanied by significant impairment or distress in occupational, social, or other important areas of functional (or, if the functioning appears to be normal, markedly increased effort must be required) (APA, 2004, p. 320).

Similar to a major depressive episode, a minor depressive episode is characterized by a depressed mood or the loss of interest, but it is accompanied by two to four additional symptoms and involves less of an impairment (APA, 2007).

Ten percent of Americans suffer from a depressive illness (National Institute of Mental Health [NIMH], 2000). Currently, only 23% of those with depression receive treatment (U.S. DHHS, 2000).

Condition: Impaired Mental Wellness—Depression

While some physical therapy patients/clients have been diagnosed with depression, others present with the condition of impaired mental wellness–depression. With the condition of impaired mental wellness–depression, the individual does not meet the diagnostic criteria for depression but may have a loss of interest, difficulty concentrating, making decisions, and/or decreased energy (e.g., in physical therapy). A former home health patient was not clinically depressed according to the diagnostic criteria, but he had lost interest in some activities that were previously enjoyed, and he had difficulty concentrating and making decisions, including during physical therapy. During the initial examination, he reported that he used to feel more "upbeat," but recently more "blue."

Condition: Impaired Emotional Wellness—Self Esteem

Some physical therapy patients/clients present with a poor self-esteem (i.e., they don't feel good about themselves) (Adams et al., 1997). If a patient/client has a negative or poor self-esteem, it can adversely impact her/his ability to participate in and benefit from physical therapy. For example, a woman having a low self-esteem may not want to exercise in a common area or participate in a group exercise.

Diagnosis: Body Dysmorphic Disorder (300.7)

Body dysmorphic disorder is a type of somatoform disorder in which the patient/client is preoccupied "with an imagined or exaggerated defect in physical appearance" (APA, 2004, p. 445). For this diagnosis to be made, the preoccupation must cause functional impairment or significant emotional distress, must not be restricted to concerns about "fatness," and not better accounted for by another mental disorder, such as anorexia nervosa (APA, 2004). A prime example of a physical therapy patient/client with this diagnosis is a male bodybuilder who is preoccupied with the appearance of certain of his skeletal muscles, and has sought physical therapy because he has sustained an injury secondary to his exercise regimen.

Diagnosis: Anorexia Nervosa (307.1)

According to the APA (2004), the essential characteristics of anorexia nervosa are a refusal to maintain even a minimally low body weight (e.g., a body mass index ≤ 17.5 kg/m^2), an intense fear of gaining weight, and a significant disturbance in the perception of the size (or shape) of her (or his) body. The severely decreased body weight is obtained and preserved through voluntary dieting and fasting as well as compulsive exercise, self-induced vomiting, and/or abuse of laxatives, diuretics, and/or enemas (APA, 2004).

Diagnosis: Bulimia Nervosa (307.51)

According to the APA (2004), the essential characteristics of bulimia nervosa are binge eating and inappropriate compensatory behaviors, on average, at least twice a week for 3 months; additional criteria include a lack of control during the binge-eating episodes and an excessive emphasis on body image; that is, body weight and shape. In these individuals, body image largely determines self-esteem (APA, 2004). Self-induced vomiting occurs in 80% to 90% of the cases; the abuse of laxatives occurs in one-third of the cases; and other common compensatory behaviors include excessive exercise, fasting, the abuse of diuretics, and rarely an enema (APA, 2004). Individuals with bulimia nervosa are not significantly underweight (as are those with anorexia nervosa) but present somewhat underweight, average weight, or overweight/overfat.

Diagnosis: Binge Eating (783.6)

According to the APA (2004), binge-eating disorder is similar to bulimia nervosa, but there is not an inappropriate compensatory behavior and it does not meet the diagnostic criteria to be considered bulimia nervosa. Patients/clients who binge eat typically feel powerless to food and feel emotional distress, guilt, and depression (APA, 2004). In samples drawn from weight-control programs, the prevalence of binge eating averages 30% (APA, 2004). Individuals who binge eat are often overweight/overfat.

Condition: Night-Eating Syndrome

The criteria for night-eating syndrome (NES) are skipping breakfast 4 or more days per week, consuming more than one-half of the total caloric intake after 7:00 PM, difficulty sleeping 4 or more days per week (Gluck, Geliebter, & Satov, 2001). Night-eating syndrome is associated with low self-esteem, depression, and less weight loss in the obese (Gluck et al., 2001). Although night-eating syndrome is not considered a diagnostic eating disorder, it deserves consideration (Gluck et al., 2001).

V-Code: Malingering (V65.2)

According to the APA (2004, p. 683), "The essential characteristic of malingering is the intentional production of false or grossly exaggerated physical or psychological symptoms, motivated by external incentives such as avoiding military duty, avoiding work, obtaining financial compensation, evading criminal prosecution, or obtaining drugs." This source states that malingering should be suspected if there is a medicolegal connection (e.g., the person is referred by an attorney); there is a marked discrepancy between the objective findings and the subjective report; there is a lack of cooperation during the examination or plan of care; or the person has antisocial behavior that is not due to a mental disorder (e.g., professional racketeer or thief).

Diagnosis: Factitious Disorder (300.16; 300.19)

The essential characteristics of a factitious disorder are the intentional production of psychological or physical symptoms or signs and a motivation to assume the sick role without other external incentives (APA, 2004). The patient/client may also alter her/his medical records, inflict self-injury, alter her/his lab results, and so on (APA, 2004). One of my former home health patients developed a factitious disorder. Although she initially had a need for skilled physical therapy, she later began to fake her functional deficits in the hopes that I would continue to see her.

V-Code: Noncompliance with Treatment (V15.81)

While the reasons for "noncompliance with treatment" may include maladaptive coping styles or personality traits (e.g., denial of injury), personal value judgments, cultural or religious beliefs about the disadvantages and advantages of the treatment, or the discomfort or expense of treatment, the V-Code may only be assigned "when the problem is sufficiently severe to warrant independent clinical attention" (APA, 2004, p. 683).

Condition: Impaired Social Wellness

If a patient/client is antisocial but not clinically antisocial, and otherwise is (at least fairly) a functional and productive member of society, she or he may be assigned the condition of impaired social wellness. Those with this condition are less likely to interact appropriately with a physical therapist, other clinical staff, and other patients (e.g., group therapy). (Note: Adult Antisocial Behavior (V71.01) is assigned when the symptoms are not due to a mental disorder, but rather to a choice in social conduct. For example, the actions of a criminal or a dealer of illegal substances.)

During my career as a physical therapist, I have had a few patients/clients who presented with impaired social wellness (in addition to their physical therapy diagnosis). I have found that these patients typically are quick to anger, are controlling, easily frustrated, and/or condescending.

Summary: Mental Diagnoses

While it is outside their scope for physical therapists to assign a mental diagnosis, we should be well versed in the APA's DSM-IV (2004). When indicated, the physical therapist should assign a mental wellness condition. Mental disorders are based upon information obtained in the examination, particularly the information in the mental and social wellness sections. Perhaps the most common mental and social wellness conditions that physical therapists may assign are (1) impaired mental wellness–stress/anxiety, (2) impaired mental wellness–depression, and (3) impaired social wellness.

SECTION 8: MENTAL AND SOCIAL WELLNESS GOALS AND PROGNOSIS

The mental and social wellness goals are a subset within the physical therapy goals. These wellness goals should be based upon the patient's/client's evaluation and the diagnosis and/or condition, and guided by optimal mental and social wellness guidelines as well as the patient's/client's personal goals. Ultimately, the mental and social wellness goals should be based upon realistic expectations and your clinical judgment. Mental and social wellness goals may be broad or specific. Generally, it is more appropriate to indicate specific goals rather then rely upon broad goals. An example of a broad mental wellness goal is to enhance mental wellness. An example of a specific mental wellness goal is to increase compliance to the stress-reduction home program to at least 10 minutes per day at least 3 days per week.

The mental and social wellness prognosis is a subset within the physical therapy prognosis. The prognosis is a qualitative descriptor (excellent, good, fair, or poor) of the likelihood that the patient/client will achieve a specific goal or group of goals. It is helpful to determine the individual prognosis for each goal, including each mental and social wellness goal, rather than assign only a global prognosis. For example, the prognosis to achieve the goal of "increase compliance to a mental wellness home program" might be excellent; but the prognosis to achieve the goal of "increase social wellness when in the physical therapy clinic" might be only fair. In addition to each specific prognosis, the global physical therapy prognosis may also be identified.

Summary: Goals and Prognosis

The mental and social wellness goals are a subset within the global physical therapy goals. Ultimately, these wellness goals should be based upon realistic expectations and your clinical judgment. Generally, it is more appropriate to indicate specific goals rather then rely upon broad goals. The mental and social wellness prognosis is a subset within the global physical therapy prognosis. It is helpful to determine the individual prognosis for each goal, including each mental and social wellness goal rather than assign only a global prognosis.

SECTION 9: MENTAL AND SOCIAL WELLNESS PLAN OF CARE

The mental and social wellness plan of care should fully consider the stages of the wellness model: primordial, pre-contemplation, contemplation, assessment, action, maintenance, and permanent maintenance. Although as part of the examination you would have already assessed the patient's/client's mental and social wellness, the patient/client may be in a lower stage (e.g., primordial or pre-contemplation stage). A goal should be to raise her/his level of consciousness to the contemplation stage. If the patient/client is not in the contemplation stage by the close of the initial session, then the primary mental and social wellness goal should be to achieve the contemplative stage. To raise awareness of the importance of mental and social wellness and her/his current deficits, you may directly educate the patient/client and then indirectly educate her or him by requiring the completion of a homework assignment. Other goals related to mental and social wellness should be deferred until the patient/client achieves the stage of contemplation insofar as mental and social wellness is concerned. Once the patient/client has achieved the contemplation stage, you may advance her or him to the action stage. In terms of mental and social wellness, this might mean that you direct the patient/client to begin to practice the healthier mental and social wellness patterns that you have discussed together. For example, instruct the patient/client to begin a "stress-reduction exercise diary" to record the details of her/his weekly stress-reduction exercise sessions in order to enhance compliance.

Mental Health Models

When devising the mental and social wellness plan of care, it is helpful for the physical therapist to consider mental health models. These could include Freudian therapy, Alderian therapy, analytical therapy, existential therapy, person-centered therapy, behavior therapy, cognitive therapy, brief or rational emotive therapy (RET), reality therapy, and multimodal therapy. Aspects of these models, either alone or in combination with aspects of other mental health models, will prove useful in your approach toward treatment, especially with difficult patients/clients.

Psychoanalytic Theory

Developed and advanced by Sigmund Freud (1856–1939), a distillation of some aspects of psychoanalysis comprises three tenets: (1) causality, or how the unconscious affects actions; (2) the notion that people do anything to get pleasure and avoid pain; and (3) the notion that people are inherently bad and we compete against each other. In the physical therapy realm, examples of these components are (1) an elderly female patient doesn't want to participate in her therapeutic exercise program and says, "I just don't like exercise." She's not sure why she doesn't like to exercise, but upon questioning, it is uncovered that when she was child, she had been repeatedly "rough housed" by older brothers; (2) a physical therapist assumes that her patient isn't really trying and just wants palliative care; and (3) a physical therapy patient considers her fellow patients "meddlesome" and refuses to join the group therapy session.

Adlerian Theory

Individual therapy, developed and advanced by Alfred Adler (1870–1937), considers the external social environment as well as the inner beliefs and feelings of the patient. Five components are (1) a holistic view of the patient; (2) the notion that people are fellow human beings and are neither good nor bad; (3) freedom of choice; (4) social interest; and (5) the goal of therapy is competence. In the physical therapy realm, respective examples of these components are (1) A physical therapist takes into account all aspects of a patient when developing her/his plan of care; (2) a physical therapist encourages and motivates her/his patients; (3) a physical therapist offers her patients treatment alternatives; (4) a physical therapist provides pro bono services to the economically disadvantaged; and (5) a physical therapist appreciates her patient's maximum optimal function when developing long-term goals.

Jungian Psychoanalysis

Analytical therapy was developed and advanced by Dr. Carl Jung (1875–1961), whose theories focused on the collective unconscious, shared archetypes of perceiving and behavior patterns, and the power of symbols that can drive humans toward well-being and vitality or psychiatric pathology. Two components of Jungian analysis are (1) self-knowledge and the potential for self-healing; and (2) symptoms hold the key to a cure. In the physical therapy arena, examples of these components are (1) during the initial session and each subsequent visit, the physical therapy incorporates the self-report of the patient; and (2) during the initial session, the physical therapy critically reflects upon the symptoms of the patients, and integrates these symptoms with the signs to develop an appropriate physical therapy diagnosis.

Person-Centered Therapy

Developed by Carl Rogers (1902–1987) and advanced by Nathaniel J. Raskin, as "nondirective therapy," person-centered therapy emphasizes empathy of the therapist for the patient and the belief that everyone is good and healthy. Three components are (1) trust and unconditional positive regard; (2) the patient is the locus of evaluation and should experience her/his self and the world with flexibility and openness; and (3) the "actualizing tendency," where each person has an internal motivation to develop her/his potential to the fullest possible extent. In the physical therapy realm, these can be exemplified by (1) a physical therapist offers unconditional positive regard for her patient and takes time to bond with the patient to build mutual trust; (2) a physical therapist encourages his patient to take responsibility for his therapy and be open and flexible with his rehabilitation process; and (3) a physical therapist appreciates his patient's drive toward maximum optional function when developing the long-term goals.

Behavior Therapy

Behavior therapy, also known as behavior modification therapy, seeks to exchange maladaptive/undesirable behaviors with healthy behaviors. It can be divided into classical conditioning, operant conditioning, and the social learning theory. *Classical conditioning* is a type of associative learning in which an unconditioned or conditioned stimulus naturally evokes an unconditioned response. For example, a physical therapist walks into a patient's room in the hospital and the patient frowns. The therapist smiles, and the patient smiles in return. This continues for several visits. One session, the therapist walks into the patient's room, and the patient smiles before she sees the therapist's face. *Operant conditioning* relates to the modification of voluntary behavior through the use of consequences, which are positive and negative reinforcement. The *social learning theory*, developed by Dr. Albert Bandura (1925–), involves external stimuli, external reinforcement, and the cognitive mediational process. A scenario to illustrate this theory is when my family was on vacation; my daughter and I saw a rock-climbing wall on a deck of the cruise ship. My daughter wanted to climb the rock wall to the top and ring the bell. External stimuli included the rock wall, the height of the ship in relation to the ocean below us, the other passengers, and so on. The external reinforcement included me cheering her on. She engaged in a cognitive mediational process to first think through the climbing procedures and then advance herself to the top of the rock wall and ring the bell **(Figure 8-4)**.

Cognitive Therapy

Developed by Dr. Aaron Beck (1921–), who studied patients diagnosed with depression, cognitive therapy is rooted in the notion that how one thinks largely determines how one feels. It employs guided discovery, which involves the following processes: (1) determine how the function developed; (2) apply the inductive model; (3) determine a hypothesis; (4) initiate a cognitive shift; (5) conduct verbal discussions and behavioral experiments; (6) examine the alternatives; and (7) perform readjustments as indicated. (Note: The inductive model is the process of using observations to develop general principles about a specific subject.) A relevant scenario to illustrate cognitive therapy is when a physical therapy patient is not compliant with her home program because she doesn't feel motivated. The function (noncompliance) developed secondary to the patient's thoughts that exercise takes too much time. The therapist's use of the inductive model reveals that the patient has poor time-management skills. The hypothesis is that the patient does not prioritize exercise in her hectic schedule. The therapist then initiates a cognitive shift in the

---

Anxiety Scale in Physical Therapy
(To be completed by the patient/client)

Surname: _____   First: _____   Date: ___/___/_____

0 = I'm completely calm and I have absolutely no fear of doing the activity.

1

2

3

4

5

6

7

8

9

10 = I'm completely anxious and afraid. I will *not* do the activity.

(Note: #1 to #9 to be determined during the question-and-answer period between the physical therapist and the patient/client.)

Figure 8-4 Anxiety Scale in Physical Therapy

patient by raising her level of consciousness to the contemplative stage, to value exercise. The therapist then teaches the patient an appropriate home exercise program and helps motivate her to perform it regularly. The therapist will adjust the program as indicated.

Rational Emotive Therapy

Also known as brief therapy, rational emotive therapy was developed by Dr. Albert Ellis (1913–2007). He theorized that our daily "activating events" cause us to think about and interpret what is happening, and our interpretation is what forms our belief about these events. Once a belief is developed, this and similar events cause us to experience a specific emotional consequence that is based only on that belief. It involves the following components: (1) acceptance that the client is fallible; (2) homework and discipline help change beliefs; and (3) different therapies are effective at different times for different patients/clients. Physical therapists should recognize and accept that patients/clients will make mistakes as they learn (e.g., not fully comply with the instructions of the physical therapy, including the home exercise program). To assist the patient/client, the physical therapist must first differentiate between the patient's rational and constructive thoughts and the irrational and nonconstructive thoughts. To facilitate the patient's/client's rehabilitation, the physical therapist then parlays her/his "bag-of-tricks" strategies, which may include but are not limited to role playing, assertion training, desensitization, humor, operant conditioning, and social support.

Reality Therapy

William Glasser (1925–) originated reality therapy on the premise that most human problems are based on unsatisfactory or no relationships with those we need, so the focus is on learning how to make or enhance the connections with others now, rather than dwelling on the past. Two relevant components are (1) the basic psychological needs of a person are belonging, freedom, power, and fun; and (2) therapy should be simple in terminology. In the physical therapy realm, examples are (1) a physical therapist is careful that her patient feels that he is an integral part of the rehab team, does not force him to engage in a treatment or therapy, seeks his input regarding treatment alternatives, and incorporates activities that she thinks will be fun for her patient; and (2) a physical therapist refrains from using technical and medical jargon when discussing issues with his patients.

Multimodal Therapy

According to Dr. Arnold Lazarus (1932–) all humans think, experience, and respond to our environment and other people through our senses. We also react biologically to influences of food, medication, and our environment. These are divided into "modalities" (five senses, imaging, and biochemical reactions) to use to categorize the presenting problem. The modalities incorporate the physical, interpersonal, behavior, affect, sensation, imagery, and cognition domains. For example, the physical modality involves physical activity, such as gait training and therapeutic exercise and the interpersonal modality involves communication. *Bridging* is the act of addressing a patient in her/his preferred (or current) modality as a vehicle to transition to the modality of the therapist's choosing. For example, if a therapist walks into a treatment room and finds her patient crying, she may utilize the affective modality and then move the patient to a physical modality (i.e., manual therapy). In multimodal therapy, it is common to utilize multiple interventions from different theories and treatment strategies rather than just one.

Plan of Care for Specific Conditions or Disorders

If a patient/client presents with mental health symptoms that may be severe enough to warrant a diagnosis of stress, anxiety, or adjustment disorder, the physical therapy plan of care should include notification of the symptoms to the patient's/client's medical doctor, who will thereby be alerted to consider mental health counseling and/or psychotropic medications. If a patient/client presents with the diagnosis of stress, anxiety, adjustment disorder, or impaired mental wellness–stress/anxiety, it is advised that the physical therapist incorporate the bridging component of multimodal therapy into the plan of care.

For the patient/client presenting with impaired mental wellness–stress/anxiety, the physical therapist can employ techniques that have been found to decrease stress. These interventions include but are not limited to coping (Arnett et al., 2008; Devereux, Hastings, Noone, Firth, & Totsika, 2009; Golbasi, Kelleci, & Dogan, 2008); social support (Sinokki et al., 2008; Ye et al., 2008); progressive muscle relaxation (Conrad, Isaac, & Roth, 2008); systematic desensitization through the construction of an anxiety hierarchy (Andrews & Hunt, 1998); guided imagery (Nunes et al., 2007; Toth et al., 2007; Watanabe et al., 2006);

physical exercise (Martinsen, 2008), meditation (Grepmair et al., 2008; Manzoni, Pagnini, Castelnuovo, & Molinari, 2008; Rungreangkulkij & Wongtakee, 2008); and/or hypnosis (Weisberg, 2008). Meditation and hypnosis should only be utilized by those physical therapists who have obtained specialized training. (Note: Physical exercise as an intervention is discussed in Chapter 7; other interventions are discussed in Section 10.)

When developing the plan of care for a patient/client who presents with impaired wellness–stress/anxiety, it is critical the physical therapist appreciate that there is no single method that is effective for reducing stress in all people and in every situation, so several methods should be applied to effectively manage stressful situations (Holahan & Moos, 1986). A physical therapist also should be aware that individuals tend to use the same methods they have used in the past to deal with stress (Stone & Neale, 1984). Thus, if the habitual techniques are helpful, the plan of care might be to increase their frequency and/or duration, and perhaps augment them with additional strategies. If the previous techniques were not helpful, the plan of care might be to teach the patient/client new stress-reduction strategies.

If a patient/client presents with symptoms of depression and the symptoms may be severe enough to warrant a diagnosis of depression, the physical therapy plan of care should include notification of the depressive symptoms to the patient's/client's medical doctor. This communication is critical because mental health counseling and/or medication can help 80% of patients with depression (U.S. DHHS, 2000). If a patient/client presents with the diagnosis of depression or the condition of impaired mental wellness–depression, it is advised the physical therapist incorporate the bridging component of multimodal therapy into the plan of care. Unless otherwise contraindicated, physical exercise is also an appropriate intervention to alleviate depression (Martinsen, 2008) and should be included in the plan of care.

If a patient/client presents as a malingerer, she or he is not appropriate for physical therapy. In such cases, the evaluation should state the examination indicates the patient/client is malingering and the diagnosis is malingerer. The plan of care should be to discontinue the patient/client from physical therapy and, as applicable, notify her/his insurance provider (or applicable agency), medical doctor, and/or a mental health provider of the findings.

If a patient/client presents with a factitious disorder, body dysmorphic disorder, or an eating disorder, the physical therapist must be mindful the disorder is a mental rather than a physical diagnosis and facilitate mental health treatment (if it is not already in place). If the patient/client does not present with a physical comorbidity pertinent to physical therapy, then physical therapy is not warranted. If the patient/client concurrently presents with a physical disorder pertinent to physical therapy, the plan of care will be affected by the mental diagnosis. For example: If a home health patient presents with symptoms of a factitious disorder (e.g., is feigning symptoms to receive social companionship), the plan of care might consist of referrals to social support groups as well as a report to his medical doctor and, if necessary, the recommendation for a referral to a mental health provider. However, physical therapy should be discontinued unless there are additional symptoms that independently warrant skilled physical therapy care. If a private clinic patient seeks treatment from a physical therapist because she has sustained an injury secondary to excessive exercise and it is obvious that the patient is suffering from anorexia nervosa, the plan of care should include a report to her medical doctor detailing her signs (e.g., height, weight, BMI, percent body fat) and symptoms (e.g., mental wellness tests and measures related to self-esteem), and a recommendation for a referral to a mental health professional and a dietician. Additionally, the physical therapy plan of care will need to take into account the physical repercussions of the mental disorder of anorexia nervosa. For example, it may not be appropriate for the patient to engage in therapeutic exercise until her nutritional intake and body weight/muscle mass is enhanced.

If a patient/client presents with noncompliance with treatment, the physical therapy plan of care may include the following interventions: clarification of values, cognitive therapy, cognitive/behavioral therapy, behavioral therapy, and the development of a contract related to the plan of care and noncompliance.

If a patient/client presents with impaired social wellness, the physical therapy plan of care may include role modeling as well as training in assertiveness, differentiation of self, and centering.

Summary: Plan of Care

The mental and social wellness plan of care should fully consider the stages of the wellness model. When devising the mental and social wellness plan of care, it is helpful for the physical therapist to consider the mental health models that may include Freudian therapy, Alderian therapy, analytical therapy, existential therapy, person-centered therapy, behavior therapy, cognitive therapy, brief or rational emotive therapy, reality therapy, and multimodal therapy. Borrowing relevant aspects of these theories and therapeutic strategies, either alone or in combination, will help the physical therapist to effectively tailor a plan of care to meet patient/client needs, which directly impacts the duration and success of the outcomes. In many cases, it is advisable for the physical therapist to incorporate the bridging component of multimodal therapy into the plan of care. The plan of care should specify whether the patient's/client's medical doctor will be notified of the symptoms and whether a mental health (or other) referral will be recommended. It also should specify which interventions will be provided or whether physical therapy is not indicated.

SECTION 10: MENTAL AND SOCIAL WELLNESS INTERVENTIONS AND OUTCOMES

The mental and social wellness interventions are identified in the same section as the other physical therapy interventions. Important interventions related to mental and social wellness are patient/client education and a home program. The education intervention includes teaching the patient/client about aspects of mental and social wellness; a mental and social wellness home program consists of instructing the patient/client to practice (in the patient's/client's home and other environments such as work) certain mental and social wellness activities. For example, a physical therapist might teach a patient/client the theory behind a particular stress-reduction exercise, instruct her or him how to perform the exercise, educate her or him about the importance of regular stress-reduction activities, and then request she or he practice it at least 10 minutes per day, at least 4 days per week. (Note: As you will notice, this intervention satisfies the three aspects of wellness: cognitive, psychomotor, and affective.)

Interventions to Enhance Impaired Mental Wellness–Stress/Anxiety

Interventions that are appropriate for patients/clients with the condition of impaired mental wellness–stress/anxiety include coping strategies, social support, progressive muscle relaxation, systematic desensitization, construction of an anxiety hierarchy, guided imagery, hypnosis, meditation, and medications.

Coping is a technique that can be employed to reduce stress. Lazarus and Launier (1978) defined coping as "Efforts, both action oriented and intrapsychic, to manage (that is, to master, tolerate, reduce, minimize) environmental and internal demands and conflicts among them which tax or exceed a person's resources "(p. 311). Coping strategies may modify the stressor, alter one's own evaluation of the stressor in order to reduce perceptions of threat, and decrease the risk of consequences to one's health (Vogel, 1985).

Social support, which is defined as the perceived comfort, caring, esteem, or direct help a person receives from others (Cobb, 1976), also can be used to decreased stress. A physical therapist can encourage her/his patients/clients to expand the depth and breadth of their social network, which can be comprised of family, friends, and/or peers; neighbors; colleagues at work, school, church; and those in community organizations, such as legal, health, and social welfare services.

In the early 20th century, Jacobson (1938) introduced the idea of using skeletal muscle relaxation to reduce both physical and psychological stress, an easy strategy for physical therapists. To engage in skeletal (i.e., progressive) muscle relaxation, the patient/client is instructed to focus her/his attention on specific skeletal muscle groups, and to alternately tighten and relax these muscles, usually from the head to the toes or the reverse direction.

Systematic desensitization is a technique frequently used in conjunction with relaxation to reduce more complex personal issues surrounding fears and/or anxieties (Lazarus & Rachman, 1957; Sue, 1972), and is based on the idea that fears are learned by classical conditioning. The therapy is believed to reverse this process of association with negative events or feelings by pairing the feared object or situation with neutral feelings (Lazarus & Rachman, 1957). Wolpe (1961) suggested that reversal comes as a result of counterconditioning, whereby the calm response replaces the fear and/or anxiety response. In my practice, I develop an anxiety scale that is an adaptation of the one introduced by Lazarus and Rachman (1957).

When a physical therapist instructs a patient/client in systematic desensitization, a fear with which the patient/client presents is preselected. An example is a patient first learning or relearning how to ambulate without a walker. The physical therapist asks, "What is the specific event related to walking without a walker that you would score your anxiety as 10 on a scale of 0 to 10, with 0 being totally calm and 10 being completely anxious and afraid?" The patient might respond, "I feel terrified of walking all alone without my walker and I won't do it." The therapist and patient make note of that experience and equates it to the score of 10. The therapist next asks, "Now, think of the state of being absolutely calm, and we'll call this zero. On this scale of 0 to 10, how do you rate yourself at this moment?" With additional questioning, the balance of the anxiety hierarchy is clarified.

According to Lazarus and Rachman (1957), two things are accomplished with a hierarchy scale: (1) the beginning and end points of anxiety hierarchy have been established; and (2) the therapist and the patient/client have developed a common understanding of how anxious the patient/client is feeling at any time relating to the preselected event. Following completion of the anxiety hierarchy, the patient/client is asked to sit with eyes closed and visualize an event that is far in the future and will cause distress as it approaches, but is causing little to no stress now. The patient/client is asked to rate the stress level and then to visualize moving closer to the date of the future event. When tension is felt above a predetermined threshold (e.g., 4 on the scale of 10), the patient/client indicates this by raising a hand, for example. If tension were experienced as the patient visualized walking with a walker with the therapist only standing close to the patient, but no longer holding onto the gait belt, the therapist and patient would work together to relax the muscles (e.g., muscle relaxation) while the patient was still thinking of the usually tension-producing scene. Gradually, and with much practice, the patient learns to visualize all the scenes in the anxiety hierarchy while breathing deeply and steadily, and feeling relaxed. Some of the most dramatic demonstrations of systematic desensitization procedures have been with those with snake and spider phobias (McGlynn, 1971; McGlynn & Walls, 1976; Ost, 1978).

The goal of guided imagery is to stop, or at least lessen, worry and distress. To facilitate a guided imagery session, the physical therapist instructs the patient/client to

1. Select an upcoming situation or even about which she or he feel anxious or stressed.
2. Use contract/relax to relax the body.
3. Assume a comfortable position with eyes closed and body relaxed.
4. Imagine her- or himself as the director of a movie that she or he is going to run in her/his "mind's eye."
5. As the director, remind the patient/client that she or he can start or stop the movie at any point that discomfort occurs.
6. Begin with the situation, imagining everything about it (what is said, what is done, etc.)
7. When she or he notices discomfort or distress, stop the movie and use contract/relax to relax.
8. Once relaxed, begin at the point just before anxiety was felt.
9. Continue until successful outcome. (modification of Clark, 1996)

According to the American Psychological Association (2009), hypnosis is the procedure of one person providing suggestions for changes in subjective experience, and alternations in emotion, sensation, perception, thought, and/or behavior to another person. Unlike many of the other techniques a physical therapist may implement to reduce stress in his or her patients, hypnosis requires specialized training and instructors should obtain a certification.

The National Board for Certified Clinical Hypnotherapists is a reputable organization from which a medical professional can find out about training and obtain a certification.

To reduce stress, physical therapists also may instruct their patients/clients to meditate. In meditation, the participant increases her/his ability to elicit the relaxation response at will, which can be especially useful in times of distress. This is achieved by sitting upright in a relaxed position with eyes closed and mentally repeating a word or a sound to prevent distressing thoughts from occurring (Russell, 1972). While a certification to teach others to meditate is more rare than a certification to hypnotize, a physical therapist should obtain specialized training in meditation before incorporating it into her/his practice.

In certain cases, medications such as benzodiazepines (e.g., Alpraxolam and Ativan) prescribed by medical doctors are indicated to reduce stress. Such medications reduce physiological arousal and feelings of anxiety (Hoffman & Mathew, 2008). Unlike nonpharmacological stress-reducing options, however, stress-reducing medication may have adverse side effects.

Interventions for Patients/Clients Who Are Noncompliant with Treatment

Interventions that are appropriate for patients/clients who are noncompliant with their treatment include, but are not limited to, clarification of values, cognitive therapy, cognitive/behavioral therapy, behavioral therapy, the development of a contract related to the plan of care, and noncompliance.

Clarification of values can be employed to enhance compliance. To utilize this intervention, ask your patient/client to

1. Assess one of her/his physical therapy, fitness, health, and/or wellness goals.
2. Consider the alternatives to obtaining the goal and the pros and cons of each alternative (e.g., full vs. partial vs. no compliance).
3. Choose and act freely, but with thoughtfulness.
4. With your facilitation, evaluate the outcome. (adaptation of Clark, 1996)

A cognitive strategy that can be utilized to enhance compliance is self-affirmation, where a positive thought is linked to a positive behavioral goal. Examples are "It's getting easier and easier to exercise," and "I feel better when I exercise." To practice self-affirmation, you can instruct the patient/client to state out loud a positive thought related to a behavioral goal for a specific number of times per day (to her- or himself or to a partner), write the affirmation on paper and look at it a specific number of times per day, or listen to a supportive audio tape.

To employ cognitive/behavioral therapy to enhance compliance, the physical therapist develops realistic and measurable long-term and short-term goals; encourages the patient/client to adopt a positive attitude; develops a contract with the patient/client; provides feedback and revises the plan as needed; educates the patient/client to the importance of social support systems for encouragement; and/or provides or refers the patient/client to another healthcare practitioner for lifestyle counseling (modification of the ACSM, 2006).

To develop a contract related to the plan of care, the physical therapist:

1. Integrates the appropriate goals into the plan of care.
2. Provides a copy of the plan of care with the patient's/client's responsibilities clearly delineated, and explains the rationales for these responsibilities.
3. If the patient/client wants previous treatment (e.g., palliative) that is now inappropriate, explains the rationale of why it is now inappropriate.
4. Provides the rationale for the necessity of compliance; notifies the patient/client of the deadline, and that she or he will discontinue physical therapy if noncompliance is continued past the deadline.
5. Requires the patient/client to sign the plan of care (to continue physical therapy at this point in time).
6. If the patient/client continues noncompliance past the deadline, discontinues the patient/client from physical therapy. (modification of Goude, 2002)

Interventions for Patients/Clients with the Condition of Impaired Social Wellness

Interventions that are appropriate for patients/clients with the condition of impaired social wellness include assertiveness training, role modeling socially appropriate interactions, teaching her or him to differentiate at a higher level, and teaching her or him to center the self.

A cornerstone of healthy socialization is being assertive rather than passive and/or aggressive (Bond, 1988a). Assertive behavior involves honest self-expression regarding (1) positive and negative feelings; (2) self-initiation (e.g., making a request and/or speaking up); and (3) setting limits (e.g., saying "No") (Bond, 1988e). The opposite of assertive behavior is passive–aggressive behavior. The following case illustrates the difference between assertive, passive, and aggressive behaviors: A manager has just told John, a physical therapist, that his performance is not "up to par." John's reaction would be aggressive if his initial reaction was "She's at me again!" His reaction would be passive if it was "She's going to fire me!" and assertive if it was "I wonder what she means specifically?"

Obstacles to assertive behavior include internal discomfort and not wanting to hurt someone's feelings (Bond, 1988b), while the benefits are personal and professional empowerment.

Although the relationship between assertiveness and physical therapists has not been investigated, Kilkus (1993) explored the assertiveness of nurses and found that it was correlated to gender, age, degree, and setting. If physical therapists mirror nurses, men are more assertive than women, those with advanced age and higher degree are more assertive than their peers, and those employed in the independent settings (e.g., academia and home health) are more assertive than those in the traditional settings (e.g., acute and skilled nursing facility). Physical therapists can and should enhance their own assertiveness as well as facilitate the assertiveness in their patients/clients. Strategies to enhance self-assertiveness include formal education using research and textbooks and self-help groups that emphasize self-knowledge, personal experience, and other resources within the group, and emphasize enabling rather than teaching (Slater, 1990). In nurses, Slater found that self-help groups are as effective as traditional pedagogy. It is likely that this is true for physical therapists.

To model assertive behavior to patients/clients, physical therapists should use appropriate body language (Bond, 1988c), demonstrate good posture and direct eye contact (Bond, 1988c), use "I" and avoid "you" in their statements (Slater, 1990). A physical therapist also can instruct a patient/client to practice assertiveness with the use of a mirror, videotape, and/or role play (Clark, 1996). Another assertive behavior is employing the "broken-record response" when a patient/client doesn't accept what the physical therapist says. To use the technique, simply repeat the same response, no matter the number of times a question is asked or how it is phrased (Clark, 1996). This strategy can be used in many situations; for example, in response to a patient/client repeatedly asking if you can provide more palliative treatment. The broken-record response might be "No, and we've already discussed the reasons why."

To help socialize a patient/client, a physical therapist can interact with her or him in a socially appropriate manner. According to Purtilo (1999), guidelines for interacting with a patient/client are to

1. Invite the patient to sit down.
2. Show respect.
3. Maintain eye contact.
4. Listen attentively.
5. Use a calming tone of voice.
6. Do not use derogatory labels.
7. Clarify you will work with the patient/client to identify and address the problem(s).
8. Engage the patient/client to work with you to identify solutions/goals.
9. If there are multiple issues, begin with the most immediate concern and progress.

Differentiation of self is the ability to separate negative emotions from the intellect (Clark, 1996). A lower level of differentiation of self is characterized by a fusion of the emotional and intellectual centers and increases the risk of triangles (i.e., inappropriately involving a third party). A higher level of differentiation of self is characterized by the ability to assess, separate, and control one's emotions. Consider the following case: If a patient/client speaks rudely to a physical therapist and the therapist rushes through the patient's/client's treatment, the therapist is demonstrating a low level of differentiation. A physical therapist can facilitate a higher level of differentiation in a patient/client who is exhibiting a lower level by interacting with her or him in a socially appropriate manner by communicating with her or him in an assertive, rather than a passive or aggressive manner.

Centering is positive self-talk (similar to positive affirmation) to feel objective and stable (Clark, 1996). If one feels centered, one is more likely to be able to differentiate at a high level and more likely to effectively listen to others without becoming defensive, aggressive, or otherwise socially inappropriate. While some people are inherently able to center, others need much practice. A centering exercise takes less than 2 minutes to perform and is easily taught: (1) ask the patient/client to think about a recent negative emotional event for about 15 seconds (use a timer rather than staring at a watch/clock); (2) next, the patient/client lists a few words that captures the mood of the 15-second period; (3) then, utilize self-talk to feel more objective and stable about the event or situation. For example, "Mary is a nice person. Being rude to Mary won't improve the problem. It would be healthy for me to have more patience with others." Continue this for about 30 seconds; (4) next, reconsider the recent negative event for another 15 seconds; (5) finally, take a final 15 seconds to list a few words that capture the patient's/client's (hopefully) improved mood. A modification of this exercise involves two people (Clark, 1996). The first person talks about a negative event twice; the second person identifies how she or he feels after listening to the same story before centering and then after centering. Because most people are not inherently adept at centering in every circumstance, it is helpful for most to practice this invaluable skill.

Mental and Social Wellness Outcomes

Mental and social wellness outcomes are the cumulative effects physical therapy has upon the mental and social wellness of the patient/client. As a goal is achieved, an outcome is realized. Upon discharge from physical therapy, each goal that has been met contributes to the mental wellness outcome and the social wellness outcome of the patient/client.

Summary: Interventions and Outcomes

The mental and social wellness interventions are identified in the same section as the other physical therapy interventions. Important interventions related to mental and social wellness are patient/client education and a home program. Interventions to reduce stress include coping, social support, progressive muscle relaxation, systematic desensitization, construction of an anxiety hierarchy, guided imagery, hypnosis, meditation, and medications. Interventions to enhance compliance include clarification of values, cognitive therapy, cognitive/behavioral therapy, behavioral therapy, the development of a contract related to the plan of care, and noncompliance. Interventions to enhance social wellness include assertiveness training, role modeling socially appropriate interactions, teaching the patient/client to differentiate at a higher level, and teaching her or him to center. Mental and social wellness outcomes are the cumulative effects physical therapy has upon the mental and social wellness of the patient/client.

chapter nine

Wellness Preferred Practice Pattern

*Too many people confine their exercise to jumping to
conclusions, running up bills, stretching the truth,
bending over backward, lying down on the job,
sidestepping responsibility and pushing their luck.*

■ ■ ■ ■ ■

Unknown

OBJECTIVES

Upon completion of this chapter, you should be able to:

1. Explore the components of an examination (history, client report, systems review, and tests and measures) as they relate to (physical, mental, and social) wellness.
2. Explain the evaluation and condition/diagnosis as they relate to wellness.
3. Explore the prognosis, plan of care, and goals as they relate to wellness.
4. Examine the concepts of interventions and outcomes as they relate to wellness.

SECTION 1: SCOPE OF CARE

When a physical therapist initiates an "episode of care" (a duration of time for the patient/client to undergo physical therapy) with an individual, either a restorative patient or wellness client, it is appropriate to apply the elements of client management as described in the *Guide to Physical Therapist Practice* (APTA, 2001b). According to this invaluable resource, there are six elements of client management: (1) the examination, including the history, the systems review, and tests and measures; (2) the evaluation; (3) the diagnosis; (4) the prognosis, including the plan of care and goals; (5) interventions; and (6) outcomes. As with the Preferred Practice Patterns described in the *Guide to Physical Therapist Practice*, the wellness elements of patient/client management should be approached in a comprehensive manner.

When a patient/client (i.e., those presenting with a wellness complaint if not also a restorative complaint) reports for the initial session of physical therapy, the attending physical therapist should obtain the wellness history and screen areas of wellness in the systems review. If the history, systems review, and/or patient/client report suggest that wellness-related tests and measures are indicated, then the physical therapist should perform the appropriate tests and analyze the results. If a wellness test or measure is performed, the physical therapist also must address wellness in the evaluation. As applicable, wellness should be addressed in the condition/diagnosis, prognosis, plan of care, goals, and interventions. If, after completing the wellness tests and measures, the physical therapist concludes that the patient is not appropriate for wellness-related physical therapy, then this should be indicated in the evaluation. In the plan of care, the therapist should inform the patient that there is no wellness condition to be remedied. If there is no additional condition or diagnosis that the physical therapist will treat, then she or he will conduct only the initial session and within that session enact a discontinuance; this procedure is discussed in the *Documentation Guidelines to Physical Therapist Practice* (APTA, 2001b). If the wellness issue is outside the expertise of the physical therapist, he or she should refer the patient/client to an appropriate medical professional(s).

If the physical therapist concludes that the patient/client is appropriate for wellness-related physical therapy, this should be indicated in the evaluation and the wellness condition(s) and, if applicable, the wellness diagnosis/diagnoses should be documented. As appropriate, the physical therapist may provide the indicated wellness interventions directly and/or refer the patient/client to another provider (or providers). This could mean that a patient/client would see the physical therapist to remedy a knee injury, a dietician for dietary counseling for obesity, and a YWCA swimming program to help develop social wellness and physical wellness by participating in a water aerobics exercise class.

Summary: Scope of Care

Physical therapists practicing wellness should understand the elements of patient/client management as described in the *Guide to Physical Therapist Practice* (APTA, 2001b). These wellness elements essentially mirror those of the American Physical Therapy Association's 2004 proposal. As with the Preferred Practice Patterns described in the *Guide*, the wellness elements should be approached in a comprehensive manner. When a patient/client reports for the first session of physical therapy, the physical therapist should endeavor to learn whether the patient/client has a wellness condition. If so, the therapist should address the wellness condition and/or refer the patient/client to another provider, as indicated.

SECTION 2: THE WELLNESS EXAMINATION

The *Guide to Physical Therapist Practice* (APTA, 2001b, p. 43) defines examination as "the process of obtaining a history, performing a systems review, and selecting and administering tests and measures to gather data about the patient/client . . . . The examination process may also identify possible problems that require consultation with or referral to another provider." As it is necessary to comprehensively examine patients/clients who are classified in any of the existing (*Guide*) Preferred Practice Patterns, it is likewise indicated to conduct a thorough examination of wellness. The wellness examination is comprised of the history, client report, systems review, and tests and measures.

Wellness History

The physical therapist should determine pertinent historical data about the patient/client. These data can be obtained through the patient/client's self-report, family report, caregiver report, or the patient's/client's medical record. As with many of the Preferred Practice Patterns in the *Guide to Physical Therapist Practice,* the history should include (1) general demographics, including age, gender, race/ethnicity, primary language, and education; (2) social history, including cultural beliefs, family and caregiver resources, and social interactions, social activities, and support systems; (3) occupation, including current and prior occupation and school and community; (4) growth and development, including hand dominance; (5) living environment, including devices and equipment (e.g., assistive devices, adaptive, orthotic, protective, supportive, prosthetic), living environment and community resources, and projected discharge destination; (6) general health status, including general health perception, physical function (e.g., mobility, sleep patterns, restricted bed days), psychological function (e.g., memory, reasoning ability, depression, anxiety), and role function (e.g., community, leisure, social, work); (7) social function (e.g., social activity, social interactions, social support); (8) social health habits (past and current), including behavioral health risks (e.g., drug abuse), and level of physical fitness; (9) family history, including familial health risks, medical/surgical history, including gastrointestinal, obstetrical, prior hospitalizations, surgeries, and preexisting medical and other health-related problems, and psychological history; (10) current condition(s) and chief complaint(s), including concerns that led the patient/client to seek the services of a physical therapist, concerns or needs of client who requires the service of a physical therapist, current interventions (if any), and previous occurrence of chief or similar complaint; (11) functional status and activity level, including current and prior functional activity status, such as activities of daily living (ADL), instrumental activities of daily living (IADL), leisure activities, and occupation (work/school/play); (12) medications, including medication(s) for the current condition, medications previously taken for the current condition(s), and medications for other conditions; and (13) other clinical tests, including laboratory and diagnostic tests, review of available records (e.g., medical, education, surgical), and review of other clinical findings (e.g., nutrition and hydration).

The history section of a wellness examination also should include (1) the history of weight, obesity, and, if known, body composition; (2) fitness related resources, such as health clubs, in home equipment, appropriate outdoors environment, and weather; (3) body image; (4) behavioral health risks, such as tobacco use and alcohol use; (5) family history of obesity, overfatness, and underfatness; (6) obesity related surgeries, such as gastric bypass surgery, liposuction, and abdominoplasty; (7) mental, psychological, and social disorders, such as the eating disorders of anorexia nervosa and bulimia nervosa, anxiety disorder, dysthymic disorder, or body dysmorphic disorder; (8) data about the current condition(s) and/or chief complaint(s), including the onset of the wellness problem or (9) previous occurrence of chief or similar complaints, such as a history of bulimia nervosa followed by a current complaint of overfatness or obesity; (10) prior fitness levels (e.g., maximal oxygen consumption); (11) data about the past activity level, including formal exercise, informal exercise, leisure activities, and hobbies; (12) data about the current and past medication(s) for the current wellness condition, including details about each medication, such as if it is a prescription, over-the-counter (OTC), or herbal substance, and possible adverse effects; (13) information about the patient's/client's past mental and social wellness; and (14) historical overview of the patient's/client's alimentation.

Wellness Patient/Client Report

In addition to the patient/client making statements and answering questions pertinent to the examination history, other statements and questions will be pertinent to other aspects of the initial and subsequent sessions; these include the examination systems review, examination tests and measures, and the interventions. These patient/client reports should be considered when developing the evaluation, determining the condition, and if applicable, the diagnosis, and developing the prognosis and plan of care.

Wellness Systems Review

The physical therapist should perform a systems review of the wellness of the patient/client. The data should be obtained through direct assessment or a patient/client self-report, family report, caregiver report, or the patient's/client's medical record, as available and applicable. The wellness aspects of a systems review are presented below.

Physical Activity Readiness Questionnaire

The systems review should begin with the "Physical Activity Readiness Questionnaire," which is commonly known as the PAR-Q (© 2007, Canadian Society for Exercise Physiology). The PAR-Q was designed to determine whether an individual (between the ages of 15 and 69) should consult with a physician before beginning an exercise program or increasing her/his level of physical activity. The questions in The Physical Activity Readiness Questionnaire (Par-Q; 2007, p. 1) are

1. Has your physician ever said that you have a heart condition and that you should only do physical activity recommended by a physician?
2. Do you feel pain in your chest when you do physical activity?
3. In the past month, have you had chest pain when you were not doing physical activity?
4. Do you lose your balance because of dizziness or do you ever lose consciousness?
5. Do you have a bone or joint problem that could be made worse by a change in your physical activity?
6. Is your physician currently prescribing drugs (for example, water pills) for your blood pressure or heart condition?
7. Do you know of any other reason why you should not do physical activity?

A PDF version of "The Physical Activity Readiness Questionnaire" is available at http://www.lcsd.gov.hk/en/forms/parq.pdf

It is relevant to note that no deaths have been reported from submaximal tests (up to 79% to 85% of maximum heart rate) in adults aged 18 through 65 who have "passed" the Par-Q (ACSM, 2006). If a patient/client does not pass the questionnaire, the patient/client should be directed to her or his primary care physician (PCP) or her or his cardiologist to obtain medical clearance. This is true even in direct-access states. In these cases, the physical therapist may still conduct the sedentary aspects of the systems review (e.g., the heart rate, blood pressure, respiratory rate, edema) but should not proceed to active aspects of the systems review (e.g., gross range of motion, gross strength) or to the tests and measures. Once the patient/client has obtained clearance to begin an exercise program or increase her or his level of physical activity (as applicable, assuming such clearance is provided), the physical therapist may complete the systems review and, if indicated, proceed to the tests and measures.

Cardiovascular/Pulmonary and Cardiac Risks

As per the *Guide to Physical Therapist Practice* (APTA, 2001b), the cardiovascular and pulmonary aspect of the systems review should include heart rate, blood pressure, respiratory rate, and edema. In addition to these items, the patient's/client's cardiac risk should be identified. According to the American College of Sport Medicine (ACSM, 2006), there are three categories of cardiac risk: (1) low risk, younger individuals (males less than age 45; females less than age 55) who are asymptomatic and do not have more than one risk factor; (2) moderate risk, older individuals (males age 45 or older, females age 55 or older) or those who have two or more risk factors; and (3) high risk, anyone (an individual of any age) who has one or more signs or symptoms of a cardiovascular, pulmonary, or metabolic disease.

Cardiac risk factors include a myocardial infarction, coronary revascularization, sudden death in a first-degree relative less than age 55 (if male) or less than age 65 (if female), cigarette smoking (or quit within the past 6 months), systolic blood pressure equal to or greater than 140 mm Hg or diastolic blood pressure equal to or greater than 90 mm Hg or antihypertensive medication, hypercholesterolemia (total cholesterol above 200 mg/dL, low-density lipoprotein [LDL] greater than 130 mg/dL, high-density lipoprotein [HDL] less than 35 mg/dL, or on lipid-lowering medication), impaired fasting glucose (110 mg/dL or greater), obesity (body mass index [BMI] equal to or greater than 30 kg/mg (or waist girth greater than 100 cm), and a sedentary lifestyle (ACSM, 2006). (Note: The superiority of body composition to BMI is discussed in Chapter 7.) Signs and symptoms of a cardiovascular, pulmonary, or metabolic disease include pain or discomfort in the chest, neck, jaw, arms, and so on (i.e., ischemia); shortness of breath (SOB) at rest or with mild exertion; syncope (transient loss of consciousness) or dizziness; orthopenea (inability to breathe unless standing or sitting in an erect, upright position)/paroxysmal nocturnal dyspnea (cardiac asthma); ankle edema; palpitations or tachycardia (irregular heart beat); intermittent claudication (temporary arterial blockage in the leg[s], causing pain after walking or other exercise); heart murmur; and unusual fatigue or shortness of breath with usual activities (ACSM, 2006).

Similar to the course of action that a physical therapist should take if a patient/client does not pass the Par-Q, those who present with risk factors that contraindicate the beginning or the advancement of an exercise program must obtain medical clearance before the physical therapist proceeds to the active sections of the examination. In these instances, the physical therapist may complete sedentary aspects of the systems review such as the heart rate, blood pressure, respiratory rate, and edema. Once the patient/client has obtained medical clearance to begin an exercise program or increase her or his level of physical activity (as applicable, assuming such clearance is provided), the physical therapist may complete the systems review and proceed to the tests and measures.

Basal Metabolism

The wellness systems review should consist of a basal metabolic rate (BMR) screen. This screen is not a test or measure of basal metabolism but a gross estimate based upon oral and/or written comments of the patient/client to the physical therapist. (The BMR screen is discussed in Chapter 7.)

Body Composition

The wellness systems review should include a body composition screen. This screen should succinctly address body composition and body composition wellness. A screen for body composition and body composition wellness is in Chapter 7.

Integumentary

Similar to the Preferred Practice Patterns in the *Guide to Physical Therapist Practice* (APTA, 2001b), the wellness systems review should include an integumentary screen. This should include the presence of scar formation, skin color, and skin integrity.

Mental Status

The wellness systems review should include a mental status screen. Similar to the Preferred Practice Patterns (APTA, 2001b); orientation (to person, place, and time), communication, affect, cognition, language, and learning style should be screened.

Mental and Social Wellness

The wellness systems review should include a mental and social wellness screen. This screen should succinctly address each major aspect of mental and social wellness. A screen for mental and social wellness is included in Chapter 8.

Musculoskeletal

Similar to the Preferred Practice Patterns (APTA, 2001b), the wellness systems review should include a musculoskeletal screen. The musculoskeletal aspect of the systems review should include gross range of motion, gross strength, and gross symmetry. (Note: Height and weight are not included in the musculoskeletal aspect of the systems review because they are key components of body composition. Hence, they are screened in the body composition and body composition wellness component of systems review.

Neuromuscular

Similar to the Preferred Practice Patterns in the *Guide to Physical Therapist Practice* (APTA, 2001b), the wellness systems review should include a neuromuscular screen. The neuromuscular aspect of the systems review should include gross coordination such as balance, transfers, and locomotion.

Nutritional Wellness and Nutrition

The wellness systems review should include a nutritional wellness screen. This screen should succinctly address each major aspect of nutritional health and wellness. A screen for nutritional wellness is included in Chapter 5.

Wellness Changes

The final component of the systems review should be a screen of the patient's/client's stage of wellness (i.e., primordial, pre-contemplation, contemplation, preparation, action, maintenance, permanent maintenance). The stage of wellness screen is the final screen because you will have already examined other aspects of the patient's/client's health and wellness (e.g., Par-Q, nutritional wellness) and will have a notion of whether she or he has a wellness-related problem. If the patient/client has at least one wellness-related problem; for example, an issue related to fitness wellness, begin the screen with a question related to the primordial and pre-contemplation stages. For example, you could ask her or him "Do you believe that you have a problem or might have a problem related to how much you exercise?" If the patient/client denies that she or he has a wellness problem, then she might be in the primordial or pre-contemplative stage of wellness. However, if the patient's/client's reply suggests that she or he is aware that she or he has a wellness-related problem, then progress to a question related to the contemplation and preparation stages. For example, you could ask her or him "What do you think you might want to do about your lack of exercise?" If the patient/client replies "I don't know," then she or he might be in the contemplation or preparation stage. If the patient/client verbalizes that she or he is already exercising a little, then she or he may be in the action or maintenance stage. (Note: During the systems review, it is not appropriate to screen for the permanent maintenance phase.)

Examination: Tests and Measures

Guided by the patient/client history, self-report, and systems review, the physical therapist should perform indicated tests and measures. These tests and measures can be performed through a psychomotor test or through a comprehensive interview. When a patient/client is asked to write and/or verbalize responses to a comprehensive written and/or verbal examination, the responses are regarded as results. The tests and measures of a physical therapy examination that are typically most pertinent to wellness are aerobic capacity, aerobic capacity wellness, BMR, body composition, body composition wellness, flexibility, flexibility wellness, muscular fitness, muscular fitness wellness, mental wellness, nutritional wellness, social wellness, and the stage of wellness.

Tests and measures related to wellness are discussed within the corresponding chapters of this book. For example, nutritional wellness tests and measures are provided in Chapter 5. Tests and measures that are considered more traditional (e.g., those related to the integumentary, musculoskeletal, and neuromuscular systems) are not discussed in this book because they are extensively detailed in traditional physical therapy textbooks (e.g., Kendall et al., 2005).

Although the stages of wellness were introduced in Chapter 1, tests and measures related to these stages were not. To examine the stages of wellness, the physical therapist must first consider the results of the stages of the wellness screen. If this screen suggests that a patient/client is in the primordial or the pre-contemplative stage, the physical therapist begins the tests and measures of the stages of wellness by asking the patient/client more detailed questions about her/his awareness of the wellness-related problem(s) that were suggested during the analysis of the systems review. For example, if the systems review suggested the patient/client has a problem related to fitness wellness and also suggested she or he is in the primordial or pre-contemplative stage, then the physical therapist might ask the patient/client why she or he doesn't exercise. A response that would indicate that the patient/client is in the primordial stage is "I don't exercise because I'm fine just the way I am." A reply that would indicate that she or he is in the pre-contemplation stage is "Well, I've heard that people are supposed to exercise; but I don't think I need to until I'm older." If the systems review suggests the patient/client's body composition and body composition wellness are poor and she or he is in the contemplation or preparation stage, then the physical therapist might ask the patient/client what she or he is doing to address her/his wellness problem. A response that would indicate that the patient/client is in the contemplation stage is "I know that I eat too much junk food and never exercise and I've read some magazine articles about how to lose weight, but I just don't feel I'm ready to make any changes right now." A reply that would indicate that she or he is in the preparation stage is "I know that I'm too fat and I really do want to lose weight. This is why I came here to see you for help." If the systems review suggested that the patient/client might have a problem related to flexibility wellness and also suggested she or he is in the action stage of flexibility wellness, then the therapist could ask the patient/client detailed questions about her or his new flexibility program to confirm that she or he has indeed entered the action stage. To determine whether a patient/client is in the maintenance or permanent maintenance stage of an aspect of wellness, the physical therapist must evaluate the results of the corresponding tests and measures and ask the patient/client questions that will help to distinguish whether she or he simply regularly practices the wellness behavior or whether she or he has been faithfully engaging in the regimen for a long period of time and considers it an integral part of her/his life.

Summary: Wellness Examination

The wellness-related history, systems review, patient/client report, and tests and measures are components within the physical therapy history, systems review, patient/client report, and tests and measures, respectively. Except those precluded by not passing the PAR-Q and not subsequently permitted by a physician, the systems review of each physical therapy patient/client should screen body composition and body composition wellness, fitness and fitness wellness, nutritional wellness, mental wellness, social wellness, and the stages of wellness. Guided by the patient/client history, self-report, and systems review, indicated tests and measures related to wellness should be performed. In all cases, the physical therapist should test and measure the stage of wellness.

SECTION 3: WELLNESS EVALUATION AND CONDITION/DIAGNOSIS

The *Guide to Physical Therapist Practice* (APTA, 2001b, p. 43) defines the evaluation as "A dynamic process in which the physical therapist makes clinical judgments based on the data gathered during the examination. This process also may identify possible problems that require consultation with or referral to another provider." It defines diagnosis as "both the process and the end results of the evaluating examination data, which the physical therapist organizes into clusters, syndromes, or categories to help determine the prognosis (including the plan of care) and the most appropriate treatment strategies."

If the examination identifies problems related to wellness, the evaluation must include a section related to the applicable areas and the diagnosis section should include the applicable conditions and/or diagnoses. The wellness conditions and diagnoses serve as one-word summations of the evaluation, are used to help guide the prognosis, plan of care, and goals, and impact the interventions and outcomes.

Wellness conditions include impaired aerobic capacity, impaired aerobic capacity wellness, impaired muscular fitness, impaired muscular fitness wellness, impaired mental and/or social wellness, impaired body composition, and so on. These conditions do not meet a threshold to be labeled or referred to as a diagnosis—as yet. Obesity was only recognized as a diagnosis (with the ICD-9-CM code 278.00; ICD, International Classification of Disease) in 2004; before then it was categorized as a condition and had no ICD-9-CM code.

In restorative therapy, physical therapists must assign (e.g., establish or borrow from the referral source) a diagnosis that is listed in an ICD-9-CM resource. In contrast, it may or may not be appropriate for a physical therapist to assign a diagnosis to a wellness-related problem. If the therapist will directly treat a wellness-related problem, it is appropriate to label it a primary diagnosis or condition, as applicable. However, if the therapist will not treat the problem directly, then it is appropriate to label it as a secondary diagnosis or condition, as applicable. Whether the assignment of a diagnosis (and ICD-9-CM) is warranted, the physical therapist must designate a condition if the patient/client presents with a wellness-related problem.

To appreciate the difference between what I label a condition versus a diagnosis, compare the diagnoses listed in an Impaired Preferred Practice Pattern of the *Guide to Physical Therapist Practice* (APTA, 2001b). For instance, the "Impaired Muscle Performance Preferred Practice Pattern" (in the Musculoskeletal section) includes the diagnosis "782.2 Muscular wasting and disuse atrophy, not elsewhere specified," which is more severe than the condition of "impaired muscular strength." Other diagnoses are associated with impaired muscle performance but are distinct from it. For example, the diagnosis "733.0 Osteoporosis" can lead to or exacerbate impaired muscle performance and/or be partially caused or exacerbated by osteoporosis. Additional examples are found in other sections, such as the Neuromuscular section. An example in this section involves the Impaired Neuromotor Development Preferred Practice Pattern, which includes the diagnoses of "315.4 Coordination disorder" and "741 Spina bifida." Examples in the Impaired Aerobic Conditioning Practice Pattern in the Cardiovascular/Pulmonary section include the diagnoses "492 Emphysema" and "493 Asthma."

Summary: Wellness Condition/Diagnosis

In restorative therapy, the physical therapist must assign (e.g., establish or borrow from a referral source) to each patient/client at least one diagnosis that is listed in an ICD-9-CM resource. In contrast, it may or may not be appropriate for the physical therapist to assign a wellness-related diagnosis to a patient/client. (Note: Perhaps the most common wellness-related diagnosis is obesity.) As indicated, the physical therapist should assign applicable wellness-related conditions (e.g., impaired nutritional wellness, impaired aerobic capacity, impaired aerobic capacity wellness, impaired muscular fitness, impaired muscular fitness wellness, impaired body composition, impaired body composition wellness, and numerous types of impaired mental or social wellness). Although conditions do not meet the threshold level to be labeled or referred to as a diagnosis, they impact physical therapy outcomes and should help guide the physical therapy prognosis, plan of care, and goals.

SECTION 4: WELLNESS PROGNOSIS, PLAN OF CARE, GOALS, INTERVENTION, AND OUTCOMES

Prognosis

The *Guide to Physical Therapist Practice* (APTA, 2001b, p. 43) defines the prognosis (including plan of care) as "The determination of the level of optimal improvement that may be attained through intervention and the amount of time required to reach that level." According to the APTA (2001b), the patient/client and/or family members and significant others as applicable and appropriate are involved in establishing the prognosis, plan of care, goals, and outcomes.

The wellness prognosis is influenced by the results of the examination, the analysis contained in the evaluation, and the condition(s) and/or diagnosis(es). The prognosis for patients/clients should be rated as excellent, very good, good, average, or poor. If the prognosis is poor, the physical therapist should consider whether it is possible to amend the goals so that they are more modest so that the prognosis level can be increased.

Plan of Care and Goals

According to the APTA (2001b, p. 43), the plan of care "Is based on the examination, evaluation, diagnosis, and prognosis . . . . Identifies goals and outcomes of all proposed interventions . . . . [Takes] into consideration the expectations of the patient . . . and others as appropriate . . . . Includes the frequency and duration of all proposed interventions . . . . Involves appropriate coordination and communication of care with other professionals/ services . . . [and] includes plan for discharge."

As it is necessary to develop a comprehensive plan of care for patients/clients that can be classified in any of the existing *Guidelines to Physical Therapist Practice,* (APTA, 2001b) Preferred Practice Patterns, it is likewise necessary, if indicated, to develop a thorough wellness-related plan of care. The wellness plan of care includes the goals, objectives, and interventions to reach these goals and objectives, the frequency schedule, and a tentative discharge date. The wellness plan of care is determined by the results of the examination, the analysis contained in the evaluation, and the condition(s) and/or diagnosis.

The goals and objectives must be objective, realistic, and target a dimension of wellness, such as aerobic capacity wellness, nutritional wellness, mental wellness, or social wellness. Some goals may involve the expertise of another provider, such as a psychologist or dietician.

Interventions may be directly provided by the physical therapist, such as teaching, or activities that the patient/client performs either under the supervision of the physical therapist or alone (e.g., home program).

The frequency is the number of sessions each week until the tentative discharge date. For example, five times per week for 1 week, then twice per week for 1 week, and then one time per week for 4 weeks. Unlike restorative therapy, wellness therapy need not be concerned with a low frequency that could be viewed as maintenance therapy. In fact, it is typical for wellness therapy to begin with a higher frequency and then taper off as the patient/ client is educated and able to independently practice what she or he has been taught.

The tentative discharge date from wellness-related physical therapy is just that: tentative. As indicated, the wellness patient/client should be reexamined. If in the reevaluation it is determined that the discharge date should be modified, this should be documented in a revised plan of care.

Wellness Intervention

The *Guide to Physical Therapist Practice* (APTA, 2001b, p. 43) defines intervention as "The purposeful and skilled interaction of the physical therapist and, if appropriate, with other individuals involved in the care of the client, using various physical therapy methods and techniques to produce changes in the condition that consistent with the [evaluation], diagnosis and prognosis . . . ." I propose that the wellness interventions mirror the description of the "global" interventions identified by the APTA.

Wellness Outcomes

The *Guide to Physical Therapist Practice* (APTA, 2001b, p. 43) defines outcomes as "results of client management, which include the impact of physical therapy interventions in the following domains: pathology/pathophysiology (disease, disorder, or condition); impairments, functional limitations, and disabilities; risk reduction/prevention; health, wellness, and fitness; societal resources; and client satisfaction." I propose that wellness outcomes focus on the health and wellness aspect of these global outcomes.

Summary: Prognosis, Plan of Care, Goals, Intervention, and Outcomes

The wellness plan of care, prognosis, intervention, and outcomes are similar to what is presented in the Preferred Practice Patterns in the *Guide to Physical Therapist Practice* (APTA, 2001b) but are individualized according to the field of wellness. The wellness plan of care includes the goals and objectives, the interventions to reach the goals and objectives, the frequency schedule, and the tentative discharge date. The goals and objectives must be objective, realistic, and pertain to one or more wellness conditions. The wellness interventions are to be tailored to the wellness plan of care and goals to ensure successful completion of the outcomes.

chapter ten

Wellness and Physical Therapy Case Scenario

Knowing is not enough; we must apply.
Willing is not enough; we must do.

▪ ▪ ▪ ▪ ▪ ▪ ▪ ▪ ▪ ▪ ▪ ▪ ▪ ▪ ▪ ▪ ▪ ▪

Johann Wolfgang von Goethe (1749–1842)

OBJECTIVES

Upon successful completion of this chapter, you should be able to:

1. Examine a case scenario of a patient/client who presents with impaired wellness and explore her or his examination, evaluation, prognosis, plan of care, goals, and interventions.
2. Create and present a case scenario of a real or fictional patient/client who has a diagnosis and/or condition related to fitness wellness, body composition wellness, nutritional wellness, and mental/social wellness, as well as other diagnoses and/or conditions.
3. Apply the theoretical knowledge acquired.

SECTION 1: CASE SCENARIO

In this chapter, a case scenario that incorporates information from Chapters 4 through 8 (i.e., physical wellness and its subdimensions of nutrition, fitness, and body composition, as well as mental and social wellness) is presented. This case scenario has been designed to apply a patient/client with wellness-related problems to the Wellness Preferred Practice Pattern presented in Chapter 9. This case illustrates how you, in your role as a physical therapist, can integrate wellness as you examine a patient/client; evaluate your findings; assign one or more conditions and, if appropriate, one or more diagnoses; develop an appropriate prognosis, plan of care, and goals; and provide appropriate therapeutic interventions, which may or may not include one or more referrals.

Patient/Client History

General Demographics

Carol Smith is a 48-year-old Caucasian female. Her date of birth is May 6, 1960. Her primary language is English; she possesses a bachelor of arts in education and teaches high school English. She is married (James, age 50), and she and her husband have one daughter (Rachel, age 15).

Current Conditions/Chief Complaints

The concerns that led Carol to a physical therapist is that she has "gained some weight" and is now "way too fat." The proposed condition is overfatness. The date of onset of the condition is unknown, but Carol reports that she started gaining weight about 5 years ago. There are no current or past therapeutic interventions, but she reports she's tried over-the-counter (OTC) diets and diet pills. Carol's goal is to reduce her body fat. Carol's perception of her emotional response to the current clinical situation is distressed.

Medical/Surgical History

Carol's medical and surgical history is unremarkable in the following systems: cardiovascular, endocrine, gastrointestinal, genitourinary, gynecological, integumentary, musculoskeletal, neuromuscular, and pulmonary. Regarding her obstetrical history, Carol had a cesarean section 15 years ago.

Mental/Psychological History

Carol denies a history of mental or psychological disorders, but reports that she felt depressed for a few months following the premature death of her brother 25 years ago.

General Health Status

Carol perceives her general health status to be good but not excellent. She reports having difficulty going to sleep and/or staying asleep one or two nights per week. Carol denies anxiety and depression.

Health/Social Habits

Carol reports that she does not smoke and is a "light" social drinker (i.e., one glass of wine per week). She denies street drug use or abuse of medications.

Growth and Development

Carol is right handed. Her developmental history is unremarkable.

Medications

Carol does not take any medications for her current condition of overfatness, but 2 years ago she used OTC diet pills for about a week when "I was on one of my diets." As needed, she takes Advil or Motrin for headaches and menstrual cramps.

Family History

Carol reports that her paternal grandmother was diagnosed with arthritis at about age 70, and with diabetes and coronary artery disease at about age 75; she passed away at age 88. Her paternal grandfather was diagnosed with glaucoma and arthritis at age 80 and with coronary artery disease at the age of 90; he died at the age of 92. Her maternal grandmother was diagnosed with multiple strokes between the ages of 80 and 88 and died at age 88. Her paternal grandfather was diagnosed with coronary artery disease at about age 65 and died at age 78. Carol reports that her mother, currently age 74, was diagnosed with cervical cancer at about age 35 and with colon cancer at about age 65, but that her mother is now in full remission. Carol reports that her father, currently age 76, is in excellent health.

Functional Status and Activity Level

Carol is independent in all self-care and home management functional activities, including activities of daily living and instrumental activities of daily living. She is also independent in all functional tasks related to her employment.

Mental and Social Wellness

The "Mental and Social Wellness History" survey was utilized (see **Figure 10-1**). The results suggest that, historically, Carol has had an unsatisfactory level of emotional, antistress, and environmental wellness; she had a satisfactory level of mental and social wellness.

Body Composition Wellness History

The "Body Composition History" survey was utilized (see **Figure 10-2**). Carol reports that she weighed about 125 lbs 5 years ago and weighs about 160 lbs now. She reports that during the course of her life, she would describe herself as being "not too fat or too thin." She reports that during the past 5 years, she would describe herself as being "somewhat overfat." She denies ever having a body composition test.

Fitness Wellness History

The "Fitness Wellness History" survey was utilized (see **Figure 10-3**). Carol reports that she would describe herself as an "occasional exerciser" over the course of her life and as a "couch potato" during the past year. Carol reports that during the course of her life she occasionally engaged in aerobic capacity and strengthening activities and rarely engaged in flexibility activities. She reports that during the past year she has not engaged in any activities related to aerobic capacity, strengthening, or flexibility. (She has recently begun to exercise; refer to the tests and measures.) Carol denies ever having her maximal oxygen consumption tested.

Nutritional Wellness History

The "Nutritional Wellness History" survey was utilized (see **Figure 10-4**). Carol perceives that her nutritional intake has been "unhealthy" during the last year and "somewhat healthy, somewhat unhealthy" over the course of her life. She reports that she's been on a low-calorie diet about 10 times in her life. Regarding her low-calorie diets, Carol estimates

---

Mental and Social Wellness History

(To be completed by the patient/client)

Surname: _Smith_ First: _Carol_ Date: _4_/_20_/_09_

Please answer each of the questions honestly. Your honesty will help us to better assist you to meet any goals you may have related to your wellness.

1. During the **past 5 years,** have you been confident that **"things would work out"** as well as they reasonably could (i.e., have you been optimistic)?
   ☑ Yes   ❏ Somewhat   ❏ No

2. During the **past 5 years,** have you had a **strong self-esteem** (i.e., have you felt good about yourself)?
   ❏ Yes   ❏ Somewhat   ☑ No

3. During the **past 5 years,** have you **avoided activities that cause you stress?**
   ❏ Yes   ❏ Somewhat   ☑ No

4. During the **past 5 years,** has the **social support available to you been adequate?**
   ☑ Yes   ❏ Somewhat   ❏ No

5. During the **past 5 years,** have you **contributed to your community?**
   ☑ Yes   ❏ Somewhat   ❏ No

6. During the **past 5 years,** have you **taken time to enjoy nature?**
   ❏ Yes   ❏ Somewhat   ☑ No

7. During the **past 5 years,** have you helped to **conserve the environment?**
   ❏ Yes   ❏ Somewhat   ☑ No

Figure 10-1 History of Mental and Social Wellness

the average duration was 2 weeks and the longest duration was 2 months. Carol perceives that during the course of her life, she has eaten a low amount of dark green and orange vegetables, healthy oils and fats, whole grains, "alternative" proteins, a medium amount of fruits, fish, poultry, egg whites, egg yolks, and salt; and a high amount of red meat, butter, refined grains, and sweets.

Body Composition History
(To be completed by the patient/client)

Surname: *Smith*   First: *Carol*   Date: *4* / *20* / *09*

1. About how much did you weigh **5 years ago**? ___*125*___ lbs _____ I don't know
2. About how much do you weigh **now**? ___*160*___ lbs _____ I don't know
3. During the **course of your life**, how would you describe yourself? (check one)
   - ❑ morbidly obese
   - ❑ very fat/obese
   - ❑ somewhat overfat
   - ☑ not too fat or too thin
   - ❑ somewhat underfat/thin but with good muscle mass
   - ❑ somewhat underfat/thin with average muscle mass
   - ❑ very underweight/thin with poor muscle mass (i.e., frail)

4. During the **past 5 years**, how would you describe yourself?
   - ❑ morbidly obese
   - ❑ very fat/obese
   - ☑ somewhat overfat
   - ❑ not too fat or too thin
   - ❑ somewhat underfat/thin but with good muscle mass
   - ❑ somewhat underfat/thin with average muscle mass
   - ❑ very underweight/thin with poor muscle mass (i.e., frail)

5. Have you ever had a test to measure your percent of body fat?
   - ❑ Yes ☑ No ❑ I don't know

6. If you have had a body fat test, provide as much information about it as you can about the following:
   - Approximate date of the test: _____
   - The result of the test: _____% body fat
   - Your approximate body weight on the date of the test: _____ lbs
   - The type of test: ❑ underwater weighing ❑ skinfold calipers ❑ BOD POD
     ❑ handheld device or scale ❑ other: _____

NOTE: As part of this "Body Composition History" survey, you also should complete the "Fitness History" survey and the "Nutrition History" survey.

Figure 10-2 History of Body Composition Wellness

Fitness Wellness History
(To be completed by the patient/client)

Surname: *Smith*   First: *Carol*   Date: *4* / *20* / *09*

1. If you consider yourself throughout the **course of your life**, how would you best describe yourself?
   ❏ a "couch potato"   ☑ an occasional exerciser   ❏ a regular exerciser   ❏ an "athlete"

2. Over the **course of your life**, how often have you done physical activities (such as jogging or carrying boxes at least 12 minutes) that increase your **endurance**?
   ❏ regularly   ☑ occasionally   ❏ rarely   ❏ never   ❏ I don't know

3. Over the **course of your life**, how often have you done physical activities (such as weight lifting or strengthening calisthenics) that increase your **strength**?
   ❏ regularly   ☑ occasionally   ❏ rarely   ❏ never   ❏ I don't know

4. Over the **course of your life**, how often have you done activities (such as stretching or yoga) that increase your **flexibility**?
   ❏ regularly   ❏ occasionally   ☑ rarely   ❏ never   ❏ I don't know

5. If you consider yourself throughout the course of the **past year**, how would you best describe yourself?
   ☑ a "couch potato"   ❏ an occasional exerciser   ❏ a regular exerciser   ❏ an "athlete"

6. During the **past year**, how often have you done physical activities (such as jogging or carrying boxes at least 12 minutes) that increase your **endurance**?
   ❏ regularly   ❏ occasionally   ❏ rarely   ☑ never   ❏ I don't know

7. During the **past year**, how often have you done physical activities (such as weight lifting or strengthening calisthenics) that increase your **strength**?
   ❏ regularly   ❏ occasionally   ❏ rarely   ☑ never   ❏ I don't know

8. During the **past year**, how often have you done activities (such as stretching or yoga) that increase your **flexibility**?
   ❏ regularly   ❏ occasionally   ❏ rarely   ☑ never   ❏ I don't know

9. Tests to measure endurance (or, technically, maximal oxygen consumption) include walking on a treadmill, walking and then jogging on a treadmill, riding a stationary bike, and walking or jogging on a track. Have you ever had any of these tests?
   ❏ yes   ☑ no

If you have had an endurance test (i.e., to measure maximal oxygen consumption), provide as much information about the test as you can:

- Approximate date and year of the test: _____
- The result of the test: ❏ excellent   ❏ good   ❏ okay   ❏ poor
- Your maximum oxygen consumption: _____ mL/kg·min
- Did you wear an air mask?   ❏ yes   ❏ no

Figure 10-3 History of Fitness Wellness

Nutritional Wellness History

(To be completed by the patient/client)

Surname: _Smith_ First: _Carol_ Date: _4_/_20_/_09_

Please answer each of the questions honestly. Your honesty will help us to better assist you meet any goals you may have related to your nutrition, body composition (i.e., fat weight versus muscle weight), and/or level of fitness.

1. During the *course of your life*, how healthy (or unhealthy) do you think your nutritional intake has been? (check only one)
   ❑ healthy ☑ somewhat healthy, somewhat unhealthy ❑ unhealthy ❑ I don't know

2. During the *past year*, how healthy (or unhealthy) do you think your nutritional intake has been? (check only one)
   ❑ healthy ❑ somewhat healthy, somewhat unhealthy ☑ unhealthy ❑ I don't know

3. Of the following, which describes your **low-calorie "dieting"**? (check all that apply)
   ❑ I've never been on a low-calorie diet
   ❑ I've been on a low-calorie diet once in my life and it lasted about _____ weeks / months / years
   ☑ I've been on a low-calorie diet about __10?__ times in my life, the average one lasted about __2__ (weeks)/ months / years, and the longest lasted about __2__ weeks /(months)/ years
   ❑ I've been on a low-calorie diet so many times in my life I can't count them

4. During the *course of your life*, has your diet been high, medium, or low in **dark green and orange vegetables**, such as broccoli, green beans, spinach, squash, and carrots?
   ❑ high ❑ medium ☑ low ❑ I don't know

5. During the *course of your life*, has your diet been high, medium, or low in **fruits**?
   ❑ high ☑ medium ❑ low ❑ I don't know

6. During the *course of your life*, has your diet been high, medium, or low in **whole grains** (e.g., whole-grain bread, pasta, rice)?
   ❑ high ❑ medium ☑ low ❑ I don't know

7. During the *course of your life*, has your diet been high, medium, or low in **healthy oils and fats**?
   ❑ high ❑ medium ☑ low ❑ I don't know

8. During the *course of your life*, has your diet been high, medium, or low in **nuts, seeds, beans, and tofu**?
   ❑ high ❑ medium ☑ low ❑ I don't know

9. During the *course of your life*, has your diet been high, medium, or low in **fish, poultry, and egg whites**?
   ❑ high ☑ medium ❑ low ❑ I don't know

10. During the *course of your life*, has your diet been high, medium, or low in **egg yolks**?
    ❑ high ☑ medium ❑ low ❑ I don't know

11. During the *course of your life*, has your diet been high, medium, or low in **red meat and butter**?
    ☑ high ❑ medium ❑ low ❑ I don't know

12. During the *course of your life*, has your diet been high, medium, or low in **refined grains** (e.g., white bread, white pasta, white rice)?
    ☑ high ❑ medium ❑ low ❑ I don't know

13. During the *course of your life*, has your diet been high, medium, or low in **sweets** (e.g., cookies, cake, candy) and **sugary drinks**?
    ☑ high ❑ medium ❑ low ❑ I don't know

14. During the *course of your life*, has your diet been high, medium, or low in **salt**?
    ❑ high ☑ medium ❑ low ❑ I don't know

15. During the *course of your life*, has your **alcohol** intake been high, medium, or low?
    ❑ high ❑ medium ☑ low ❑ I don't know

Figure 10-4 History of Nutritional Wellness

Living Environment

Carol lives in a ranch-style home (single level) with a large yard in Jupiter, Florida. Jupiter is a mid-sized community on the eastern seaboard.

Social History

Carol is spiritual, but not religious. Her family and caregiver resources are her husband and her daughter. Carol's social interactions include her nuclear and extended family, colleagues at work, and a small network of friends. Carol is an active member of her daughter's parent–teacher association (PTA).

Occupation (Job/School/Play)

Carol teaches English in a local private high school. Carol's leisure activities include watching television, dining out, playing board games, ceramics, and participating in her daughter's school activities, such as helping her daughter with her school work and socializing with the other moms of her daughter's swim team.

Systems Review

Mental Status, Cognition, Affect, Communication, Language, Learning Style

Carol is alert and oriented to person, place, and time. Her affect is attentive, cooperative, and pleasant. She is articulate with no speech or hearing deficits. Her primary language is English. A verbal screen of Carol's learning style suggests a preference for sequential and practical learning.

Pain

Carol reported that she hasn't had pain since her last menses. In addition to pain with her menstrual cycle, she has an occasional headache (i.e., less than once per week).

Cardiovascular/Pulmonary

Carol's resting heart rate is 72 beats per minute; her resting blood pressure is 120/70 mm Hg; and her resting respiratory rate is 14 breaths per minute. No edema is observed. Carol completed and passed the Physical Activity Readiness Questionnaire (Par-Q).

Integumentary

Carol's skin color and integrity are unremarkable.

Neuromuscular

Carol's gross coordinated movements (including mobility, transfers, and balance) are within normal limits.

Musculoskeletal

Carol's gross range of motion is limited in bilateral calves and bilateral hamstrings but is otherwise within functional limits. Carol's gross strength is within functional limits. She presents with bilateral pes planus. Otherwise, her posture is unremarkable. Carol wears custom shoe inserts for bilateral pes planus.

Basal Metabolic Rate/Resting Metabolic Rate

Carol's basal/resting metabolic rate (BMR/RMR) may be impaired because she is overfat and/or because she has a history of low-calorie dieting. It is therefore indicated to examine Carol's BMR/RMR in the tests and measures.

Body Composition and Body Composition Wellness

The "Body Composition Screen" was utilized (see **Figure 10-5**). Carol's height is 5′6″, weight is 163 lbs, and her BMI is 26.3. My visual estimate is that her fat mass category is moderately overfat and she has little muscle mass. Carol denies being on a diet to lose fat or gain muscle. Items #1 and #2 of the "Fitness Wellness Screen" (**Figure 10-6**) and items #1 and #2 of the "Nutritional Wellness Screen" (**Figure 10-7**) suggest that Carol's diet is poor and that she does not exercise. (Note: The results of this screen indicate that body composition should be examined in the tests and measures.)

Body Composition Screen
(To be completed by the patient/client)

Surname: _Smith_   First: _Carol_   Date: _4_/_20_/_09_
Name of the Physical Therapist (PT): _Sharon Fair, PT_

1. Height: __5__ feet __6__ inches
2. Weight: __163__ lbs
3. Body Mass Index (BMI): _26.3_ (m²/kg) (e.g., per http://www.bmi-calculator.net/)
4. The physical therapist's visual estimate of patient's/client's fat mass category:
   - ❑ Extremely underfat (i.e., less than 18% body fat for female; less than 5% body fat for male)
     Note: This person may appear healthy or frail, depending on her/his muscle mass.
   - ❑ Moderately underfat (i.e., about 18% to 21% fat for female; about 5% to 9% for male)
   - ❑ Average body fat level (i.e., about 22% to 29% fat for female; about 10% to 19% for male)
   - ☑ Moderately overfat (i.e., about 30% to 39% fat for female; about 20% to 29% body fat for male)
   - ❑ Obese (i.e., greater than 40% fat for female, greater than 30% for male)
   - ❑ Morbidly obese (i.e., greater than 50% fat for female, greater than 40% fat for male)
5. The physical therapist's visual estimate of the patient's/client's muscle mass category:
   - ☑ Little muscle mass. *Note: This person may appear frail, average, or overfat depending upon her/his amount of body fat mass.*
   - ❑ Adequate muscle mass
   - ❑ Significant muscle mass (e.g., she or he appears as though she or he regularly strength trains)
   - ❑ Extremely significant muscle mass (e.g., she or he resembles or almost resembles a bodybuilder)
6. Ask the patient/client: Are you on a diet to lose fat mass (fat weight)?   ❑ Yes ☑ No
7. Ask the patient/client: Are you on a specific diet to gain muscle?   ❑ Yes ☑ No

Figure 10-5 Systems Review of Body Composition

Fitness Wellness Screen

(To be completed by the patient/client)

Surname: _Smith_____   First: _Carol_____   Date: _4_ / _20_ / _09___

Please answer each of the questions honestly. Your honesty will help us to better assist you meet any goals you may have related to your fitness and/or body composition (e.g., fat weight versus muscle weight).

1. If you consider yourself throughout the **past month**, how would you best describe yourself?

   ☑ a "couch potato"   ❑ an occasional exerciser   ❑ a regular exerciser   ❑ an "athlete"

2. If you consider yourself throughout the **past week**, how would you best describe yourself?

   ☑ a "couch potato"   ❑ an occasional exerciser   ❑ a regular exerciser   ❑ an "athlete"

3. Over the **past month**, how often have you done physical activities (such as jogging or carrying boxes at least 12 minutes) that increase your **endurance**?

   ❑ regularly   ❑ occasionally   ❑ rarely   ☑ never   ❑ I don't know

4. Over the **past week**, how often have you done physical activities (such as jogging or carrying boxes for at least 12 minutes) that increase your **endurance**?

   ❑ regularly   ❑ occasionally   ☑ rarely   ❑ never   ❑ I don't know

5. Over the **past week**, for about how many hours did you do physical activities that increase your endurance?

   _1/2_ hours

6. Over the **past month**, how often have you done physical activities (such as weight lifting or strengthening calisthenics) that increase your **strength**?

   ❑ regularly   ❑ occasionally   ❑ rarely   ☑ never   ❑ I don't know

7. Over the **past week**, how often have you done physical activities (such as weight lifting or strengthening calisthenics) that increase your **strength**?

   ❑ regularly   ❑ occasionally   ❑ rarely   ☑ never   ❑ I don't know

8. Over the **past month**, how often have you done activities (such as stretching or yoga) that increase your **flexibility**?

   ❑ regularly   ❑ occasionally   ❑ rarely   ☑ never   ❑ I don't know

9. During the **past week**, how often have you done activities (such as stretching or yoga) that increase your **flexibility**?

   ❑ regularly   ❑ occasionally   ❑ rarely   ☑ never   ❑ I don't know

10. Do you ever use anabolic steroids?   ❑ yes   ☑ no

Figure 10-6 Fitness and Fitness Wellness Systems Review

Nutritional Wellness Screen

(Note: To be completed by the patient/client)

Surname: *Smith*_____   First: *Carol*_____   Date: _4_/_20_/_09_

Please answer each of the questions honestly. Your honesty will help us to better assist you meet any goals you may have related to your nutrition, body composition (i.e., fat weight versus muscle weight), and/or level of fitness.

1. During the *past month*, how healthy (or unhealthy) do you think your nutritional intake has been? (check only one)
   ❏ healthy   ❏ somewhat healthy, somewhat unhealthy   ☑ unhealthy   ❏ I don't know

2. During the *past week*, how healthy (or unhealthy) do think your nutritional intake has been? (check only one)
   ❏ healthy   ❏ somewhat healthy, somewhat unhealthy   ☑ unhealthy   ❏ I don't know

3. Are you on a special diet (such as low-calorie or weight-loss diet or any type of diet prescribed by a physician or a dietician) at this time?   ❏ yes   ☑ no

4. Is your diet high, medium, or low in **dark green and orange vegetables**, such as broccoli, green beans, spinach, squash, and carrots?
   ❏ high   ❏ medium   ☑ low   ❏ I don't know

5. Is your diet high, medium, or low in **fruits**?
   ❏ high   ☑ medium   ❏ low   ❏ I don't know

6. Is your diet high, medium, or low in **whole grains** (e.g., whole-grain bread, pasta, rice)?
   ❏ high   ❏ medium   ☑ low   ❏ I don't know

7. Is your diet high, medium, or low in **healthy oils and fats**?
   ❏ high   ❏ medium   ☑ low   ❏ I don't know

8. Is your diet high, medium, or low in **nuts, seeds, beans, and tofu**?
   ❏ high   ❏ medium   ☑ low   ❏ I don't know

9. Is your diet high, medium, or low in **fish, poultry, and egg whites**?
   ❏ high   ☑ medium   ❏ low   ❏ I don't know

10. Is your diet high, medium, or low in **egg yolks**?
    ❏ high   ☑ medium   ❏ low   ❏ I don't know

11. Is your diet high, medium, or low in **red meat and butter**?
    ❏ high   ❏ medium   ☑ low   ❏ I don't know

12. Is your diet high, medium, or low in **refined grains** (e.g., white bread, white pasta, white rice)?
    ☑ high   ❏ medium   ❏ low   ❏ I don't know

13. Is your diet high, medium, or low in **sweets** (e.g., cookies, cake, candy) and **sugary drinks**?
    ☑ high   ❏ medium   ❏ low   ❏ I don't know

14. Is your diet high, medium, or low in **salt**?
    ❏ high   ☑ medium   ❏ low   ❏ I don't know

15. Is your **alcohol** intake high, medium, or low?
    ❏ high   ❏ medium   ☑ low   ❏ I don't know

Figure 10-7 Nutritional Wellness Systems Review

Fitness and Fitness Wellness

The "Fitness Wellness Screen" was utilized (see Figure 10-6). Carol reports that she considers herself to be a "couch potato" during the past month and the last week. She reports that during the past week she has engaged in endurance exercise for one-half hour, but did not participate in any other exercise. She denies the use of anabolic steroids. (Note: The results of this screen indicate that fitness wellness should be examined in the tests and measures.)

Nutritional Wellness

The "Nutritional Wellness Screen" was utilized (see Figure 10-7). Carol reports that during the past month and the last week, her nutritional intake has been unhealthy. She denies that she is on a special diet as this time. Carol reports that her current diet is low in dark green and orange vegetables, healthy oils and fats, whole grains, "alternative" proteins, and alcohol; medium in fruits, fish, poultry, egg whites, egg yolks and salt; and high in red meat, butter, refined grains, and sweets and sugary drinks. (Note: The results of this screen indicate that nutritional wellness should be examined in the tests and measures.)

Mental and Social Wellness

The "Mental and Social Wellness Screen" was utilized (see **Figure 10-8**). The results of the screen suggest that Carol's "pure" mental wellness (i.e., confidence) and social wellness are satisfactory; and her emotional wellness (i.e., low self-esteem), antistress wellness, and environmental wellness are unsatisfactory. (Note: The results of this screen indicate that mental wellness should be examined in the tests and measures, especially as they impact her presenting condition of overfatness.)

Tests and Measures

Basal Metabolic Rate and Caloric Balance

As measured with a BodyGem, Carol's basal metabolic rate (BMR) is 1150 calories per day. Based upon her gender, age, height, and weight (and as determined by the "BMR Calculator," available at http://www.bmi-calculator.net/bmr-calculator/), her estimated basal metabolic rate is 1436 calories per day.

Carol filled out a food journal (see Figure 10-12), which was utilized to assess caloric intake. Raw data are itemized in the food journal. Carol reports that the results of the journal are representative of her food intake.

Flexibility/Range of Motion

Bilateral ankle dorsiflexion is from neutral to 5 degrees. Straight leg raise is 65 degrees on the right and 60 degrees on the left.

Muscular Fitness/Muscle Performance

Carol's five repetition maximum of various muscle groups was tested using Cybex® plate-loaded equipment and dumbbells. The results are bench press, 50 lbs (Cybex); bicep curl, 15 lbs (dumbbells); latissimus pull-down, 40 lbs (Cybex); tricep extension,

---

Mental and Social Wellness Screen

(To be completed by the patient/client)

Surname: _Smith_____ First: _Carol_____ Date: _4_/_20_/_09_

Please answer each of the questions honestly. Your honesty will help us to better assist you to meet any goals you may have related to your wellness.

1. Do you believe **"things will work out"** as well as they reasonably can (i.e., are you optimistic)?
   ☑ Yes ☐ Somewhat ☐ No

2. Do you have a strong **self-esteem** (i.e., do you feel good about yourself)?
   ☐ Yes ☐ Somewhat ☑ No

3. Do you tend to **minimize (or avoid) activities that cause you stress?**
   ☐ Yes ☐ Somewhat ☑ No

4. Do you feel **"burned out"**?
   ☐ Yes ☑ Somewhat ☐ No

5. Do you feel you have **enough social support?**
   ☑ Yes ☐ Somewhat ☐ No

6. Do you adequately **contribute to your community?**
   ☑ Yes ☐ Somewhat ☐ No

7. Do you take time to **enjoy nature?**
   ☐ Yes ☐ Somewhat ☑ No

8. Do you **conserve the environment?**
   ☐ Yes ☐ Somewhat ☑ No

Figure 10-8 Mental and Social Wellness Screen

15 lbs (dumbbells); knee extension, 50 lbs (Cybex); hip abduction, 70 lbs (Cybex); hip adduction, 60 lbs (Cybex); and hip extension, 40 lbs (Cybex). Maximum calisthenics: crunches = 15; non-military push-ups = 5. Using a Cybex lumbar extension stand, the maximum number of pain-free lumbar extensions is 5.

Aerobic Capacity

As tested with the Rockport walk test, Carol's maximal oxygen consumption is 25 mL/kg·min.

Fitness and Fitness Wellness

The "Fitness and Fitness Wellness Survey" was utilized. The results are provided in **Figure 10-9**.

Fitness and Fitness Wellness Survey

(PT to examine patient/client and fill in this survey)

Surname: _Smith_____   First: _Carol_____   Date: _4_/_20_/_09_

Name of the Physical Therapist (PT): _Sharon Fair, PT_____

Note to the PT: Dialog with the patient/client to complete these tests and measures. Utilize lay terminology unless there is direct evidence that more clinical terminology is indicated.

For the PT to state to the patient/client: I will be asking you numerous questions to obtain information about your exercise and fitness habits. Please answer as honestly, accurately, and completely as possible. This will enable me to help you meet any goals you may have related to your fitness and/or body composition (e.g., fat weight versus muscle weight). At the end of this survey, you will have the opportunity to ask me questions. Are you ready to start?

Section A: Cognitive Aspects of Fitness Wellness

1. Please rate the amount of cardiovascular/endurance/aerobic capacity exercise in which you've engaged during the past month:

   ☑ much too little   ❑ too little   ❑ just right   ❑ too much   ❑ I don't know

2. Please rate the amount of strength training/muscular fitness exercise in which you've engaged during the past month:

   ❑ much too little   ☑ too little   ❑ just right   ❑ too much   ❑ I don't know

3. Please rate the amount of stretching/flexibility exercise in which you've engaged during the past month:

   ❑ much too little   ❑ too little   ❑ just right   ❑ too much   ☑ I don't know

4. Tell me what you know about what a person should do in terms of cardiovascular/endurance/aerobic capacity exercise:
   It needs to be done at a moderate pace—not too fast, not too slow. You should do it about 2 to 3 times/week.

5. Tell me what you know about what a person should do in terms of strength training/muscular fitness exercise:
   Strength training causes you to add muscle. Women need to be careful not to strength train too hard so they don't get bulky.

6. Tell me what you know about what a person should do in terms of stretching/flexibility exercises:
   Stretching isn't as important as "real exercise." You don't have to practice them unless you feel really tight somewhere.

7. Under what circumstances can leisure activities (such as cleaning the house, playing basketball, and shoveling snow) "count" as cardiovascular/endurance/aerobic capacity exercise?
   Certain grueling sports can count as exercise, but I can't do any of them.

Figure 10-9 Fitness Wellness Tests and Measures

8. Under what circumstances can leisure activities (such as cleaning the house, playing basketball, and shoveling snow) "count" as strengthening/muscular fitness exercise?
   I'm really not sure. I suppose the example you just said could help.

9. What is the purpose of a warm-up?
   You do a warm-up before you exercise so you can exercise harder without getting tired.

10. What is the purpose of a cool-down?
    This isn't necessary.

11. Tell me what you know about exercise and dehydration:
    You only have to drink something if you exercise for hours and hours.

12. Tell me what you know about anabolic steroids:
    I don't know anything about them except some men use them to bulk up and that they aren't healthy.

13. Do you believe it can be safe to use anabolic steroids?   ❑ yes   ☑ no   ❑ I don't know

14. Tell me what you know about the **risks** of anabolic steroids:
    I don't know.

Section B-1: Psychomotor Aspects of Aerobic Capacity Wellness

1. Have you engaged in cardiovascular (aerobic capacity) exercise during the past week?
   ☑ yes   ❑ no

If yes: Please describe your cardiovascular (aerobic capacity) routine during the past week by telling me what type of exercise you did and on what day.

If no, but usually does: Complete this section and indicate when this aerobic capacity program was last performed. *If no, and does not usually:* Skip to the next section (Muscular Fitness Wellness).

DESCRIPTION OF EXERCISE	Monday	Tuesday	Wednesday	Thursday	Friday	Saturday	Sunday
Duration (in minutes)			*30*				
Mode of exercise (e.g., bike, swim, aerobic dance)			*brisk walk*				
Intensity of exercise utilizing the Perceived Activity Scale or terms *light, moderate,* or *heavy*			*moderate*				

Figure 10-9 Fitness Wellness Tests and Measures (continued)

2. If what you've just told me about your cardiovascular program is not typical behavior, tell me what you usually do and why it was different last week. (*Note to PT*: Specify what is typically performed in previous table and provide additional data below.)

   This is the first time I've exercised in I can't remember how long. I did it because I knew I'd be coming here today.

Section B-2: Psychomotor Aspects of Muscular Fitness Wellness

1. Have you engaged in strengthening exercises during the past week?

   ❑ yes ☑ no

If yes: Please describe your strengthening routine during the past week by telling me what type of exercise you did and on what day.

If no, but usually does: Complete this section and indicate when this strengthening program was last performed. *If no, and does not usually:* Skip to the next section (Flexibility Wellness).

Muscle–Strengthened	# of days	# of repetitions	# of sets	Mode (e.g., calisthenics, free)
Back of arms				
Front of arms				
Shoulder				
Chest				
Upper Back				
Lower Back				
Abdomen				
Front of thighs				
Back of thighs				
Outer thighs				
Inner thighs				
Calves				

2. If what you've just told me about your strength training program is not typical behavior, tell me what you usually do and why it was different last week. (*Note to PT*: Specify what is typically performed in previous table and provide additional data below.)

_____

_____

_____

Figure 10-9 Fitness Wellness Tests and Measures (continued)

Section B-3: Psychomotor Aspects of Flexibility Wellness

1. Have you engaged in a flexibility program during the past week, such as stretching, yoga, or tai chi?

   ❑ yes ☑ no

If yes: Please describe your stretching routine during the past week by telling me what type of exercise you did and on what day.

If no, but usually does: Complete this section and indicate when this flexibility program was last performed. *If no, and does not usually:* Skip to the next section (Leisure Wellness).

Muscle Group	# of days	Duration (in seconds)	Intensity (*no, mild,* or *severe* discomfort)	Mode (e.g., stretch on own, yoga position)
Chest	_____	_____	_____	_____
Shoulders	_____	_____	_____	_____
Back of upper arms	_____	_____	_____	_____
Back	_____	_____	_____	_____
Hips	_____	_____	_____	_____
Front of thighs	_____	_____	_____	_____
Back of thighs	_____	_____	_____	_____
Calves	_____	_____	_____	_____
Other:	_____	_____	_____	_____

2. If what you've just told me about your stretching (flexibility) program is not typical behavior, tell me what you usually do and why it was different last week. (*Note to PT*: Specify what is typically performed in previous table and provide additional data below.)

_____

_____

_____

Section B-4: Psychomotor Aspects of Leisure Wellness

Note to the PT: Based upon what the patient/client reports, select the most appropriate section of this survey in which to record each activity. Do **not** record an item in this section as well as in either of the Exercise sections. For example, if a patient/client plays 1 hour of basketball per day, do not include it in this section *and* in the Aerobic Capacity Wellness section.

1. During the past week, what was the average number of hours per day during which you engaged in a **sedentary activity** (e.g., sleeping, reading, being on the Internet/computer, watching TV/playing video games)? *Note*: Because the total includes sleep, the minimum hours recorded should typically be 7 or 8.

   ___*18*___ hours

Figure 10-9 Fitness Wellness Tests and Measures (continued)

2. During the past week, what was the average number of hours per day during which you engaged in an **activity of light intensity** (e.g., cleaning windows, raking leaves, weeding, painting, lawn mowing with a power mower, slowly waxing floor, playing doubles tennis)?
   ___2___ hours

3. During the past week, what was the average number of hours per day during which you engaged in an activity of **moderate intensity** (e.g., easy digging in a garden, pushing a lawn mower, light backpacking, house cleaning, skating, moderate-intensity basketball)?
   ___4___ hours

4. During the past week, what was the average number of hours per day during which you engaged in an activity of **heavy intensity** (e.g., sawing wood, heavy shoveling, carrying a heavy weight, digging a ditch, canoeing without rests, mountain climbing, high-intensity basketball)?
   ___0___ hours

5. During the past week, what was the average number of hours per day during which you engaged in an activity of **very heavy intensity** (e.g., carrying a very heavy weight or a load up steps, shoveling heavy snow, or playing paddleball, touch football, handball, or vigorous basketball)?
   ___0___ hours

6. If what you have just told me about your household activities is not typical behavior, tell me what you usually do and why it was different last week:
   ___N/A___
   _____
   _____

Section B-5: Other Dimensions of Fitness Wellness

1. Do you warm-up before you exercise?   ☑ yes   ☐ no
   If yes, what do you do?
   ___I walked somewhat faster than my usual pace for about 5 minutes.___

2. Do you cool-down after you exercise?   ☐ yes   ☑ no
   If yes, what do you do?
   _____

3. If you warm-up before you exercise, about how often do you do it (e.g., 100% of the time, once per week)?
   ___I usually never exercise, but when I did this week I did warm up.___

4. If you cool-down after you exercise, about how often do you do it (e.g., 100% of the time, once per week)?
   ___N/A___
   _____

Figure 10-9 Fitness Wellness Tests and Measures (continued)

5. Do you drink water or another beverage before, during, or after you exercise? ☑ yes ☐ no

    If yes, what, when, and how much do you drink?

    A half cup of juice after I finished walking.

6. Have you used a tobacco product within the past month? ☐ yes ☑ no

    If yes, tell me about your usage.

    Smoking is disgusting!

Specific directions to the physical therapist for items 7 and 8: *If the patient/client talks positively and openly about anabolic steroids, it is important the physical therapist not speak to him or her in a judgmental tone. In an open atmosphere, the patient/client may more readily admit that she or he uses steroids.*

7. Have you ever used anabolic steroids? ☐ yes ☑ no

    If yes, tell me about it.

8. Do you currently use anabolic steroids? ☐ yes ☑ no

    If yes, tell me about it.

    N/A

Section C: Affective Aspects of Fitness Wellness

On a scale of 1 to 10, with 1 being no commitment and 10 being total commitment,

1. How committed are you to engaging in cardiovascular (aerobic capacity) exercise?

    2 times/wk? __*10*__ ; 3 times/wk? __*9*__; 4 times/wk? __*8*__; 5 times/wk? __*7*__;
    6 times/wk? __*1*__; every day? __*0*__

2. How committed are you to engaging in strengthening exercises 2 times/wk? __*8*__;
    3 times/wk? __*7*__

3. How committed are you to engaging in flexibility exercises 2 times/wk? __*3*__,
    3 times/wk? __*2*__

4. How committed are you to performing leisure activities that promote cardiovascular (aerobic capacity), e.g., tennis and other sports, laser tag, sand or snow art/play, gardening? __*7*__

5. How committed are you to performing leisure activities that promote strength (muscular fitness), e.g., heavy yard work or house cleaning, carrying items that are heavy for you? *4* _____

6. What kinds (modes) of exercise do you like and what kinds (modes) of exercise do you not like? (For example, one person might really like to swim, "kind of" like to strength train, and hate to use the treadmill.) *Carol would like to start to garden.*

    Walking outside. I don't like any other kind of exercise—walking on a treadmill,
    strength training, stretching or anything else. I know some people are into this
    yoga or kickboxing craze, but I wouldn't do it. I might like swimming.

Figure 10-9 Fitness Wellness Tests and Measures (continued)

Section D: Athleticism
Note to the PT: There is no need to assess athleticism in both this exam and in the Tests & Measures related to Nutrition; you can just transfer the results.

1. Over the past year, have you engaged in a "grueling" exercise program (i.e., at least 2 to 3 hours per day on at least 5 or 6 days per week)?

   ❏ yes   ☑ no   ❏ I don't know

2. Over the past month, have you engaged in a "grueling" exercise program (i.e., at least 2 to 3 hours per day on at least 5 or 6 days per week)?

   ❏ yes   ☑ no   ❏ I don't know

3. In the foreseeable future, do you intend to engage in a "grueling" exercise program, (i.e., at least 2 to 3 hours per day on at least 5 or 6 days per week)?

   ❏ yes   ☑ no   ❏ I don't know

Section E: Fitness Wellness Goal(s)
What is/are your fitness goal(s)?

To have more endurance and increase my walking to help me lose weight.

Figure 10-9 Fitness Wellness Tests and Measures (continued)

Nutritional Wellness

The "Nutritional Wellness Survey" was utilized. The results are provided in Figure **10-10**.

Body Composition

Carol's body fat is 34.1% as measured with a Bod Pod®. Her deposits of fat are primarily in her abdominal region as opposed to in her hip and thigh regions. Her appearance is muscular.

Body Composition Wellness

The "Body Composition Wellness Survey" was utilized. The results are provided in **Figure 10-11**.

The results of Sections A, B-1, B-2, B-3, B-4, B-5, C, and E of the "Fitness and Fitness Wellness Survey" (Figure 10-9) are components of the "Body Composition Wellness Survey." These results are provided in the respective sections of Figure 10-9.

The results of Sections A, C, D, E, F, and G of the "Nutritional Wellness Survey" (Figure 10-10) are components of the "Body Composition Wellness Survey." These results are provided in the respective sections of Figure 10-10.

As of today's session, Carol has completed one day of her "Food Journal." These results are provided in **Figure 10-12**. Carol reports the results are largely representative of her lifestyle in terms of the where, with whom, and state of mind. She reports the food choices vary day to day, but what she's written is typical in terms of the "healthiness of food." She reports she'll try to complete additional days of her journal within the next week.

Nutrition and Nutritional Wellness Survey

(Note: To be completed by the patient/client)

Surname: _Smith_____ First: _Carol_____ Date: _4_/_20_/_09__

Name of the Physical Therapist (PT): _Sharon Fair, PT_____

Note to the PT: Dialog with the patient/client to complete these tests and measures. Utilize lay terminology unless there is direct evidence that more clinical terminology is indicated.

For the PT to state to the patient/client: I will be asking you numerous questions to obtain information about your nutritional habits. Please answer as honestly, accurately, and as completely as possible. This will enable me to help you meet any goals you may have related to your nutrition, body composition (i.e., fat weight versus muscle weight), and/or level of fitness. At the end of this survey, you will have the opportunity to ask me questions. Are you ready to start?

Section A: Vegetarianism (Nutritional Status)

- Do you consider yourself to be a vegetarian?   ❑ Yes   ☑ No   ❑ I don't know
- Do you consider yourself to be a vegan?   ❑ Yes   ❑ No   ☑ I don't know
- Do you always avoid meat products?   ❑ Yes   ☑ No   ❑ I don't know
- Do you always avoid eggs and egg products?   ❑ Yes   ☑ No   ❑ I don't know
- Do you always avoid milk and milk products?   ❑ Yes   ☑ No   ❑ I don't know

Section B: Athleticism *Previously tested*

Note to the PT: There is no need to assess athleticism in both this exam and in the Tests and Measures related to fitness—just transfer the results.

1. During the past year, have you engaged in a "grueling" exercise program (i.e., at least 2 to 3 hours per day on at least 5 or 6 days per week)?   ❑ Yes   ❑ No   ❑ I don't know

2. During the past month, have you engaged in a "grueling" exercise program (i.e., at least 2 to 3 hours per day on at least 5 or 6 days per week)?   ❑ Yes   ❑ No   ❑ I don't know

3. In the foreseeable future, do you intend to engage in a "grueling" exercise program (i.e., at least 2 to 3 hours per day on at least 5 or 6 days per week)?   ❑ Yes   ❑ No   ❑ I don't know

Section C: Cognitive Aspect of Nutritional Wellness

1. Tell me what you know about fiber:
   To get enough fiber, you have to eat a lot of breads and starchy foods, which
   isn't always healthy
   _____

2. What do vegetables contain? For example, do they contain fat?
   No, they don't have fat. They don't have any protein either. They have lots of
   vitamins, but I'm not sure about minerals

3. About how many cups of water should a person drink each day? _2_

4. During the past week, how healthy (or unhealthy) do you think your nutritional intake has been?
   _Very unhealthy_____
   _____
   _____
   _____

Figure 10-10 Nutritional Wellness Tests and Measures

Section D: Psychomotor (Behavioral) Aspect of Nutritional Wellness

1. Think about how many **refined grains** (e.g., white rice, white bread, white pasta, only the white part of a potato without the skin) you ate *during the past 3 days*. Did you eat:
   - ☑ a lot almost every day or every day?
   - ❏ some almost every day or every day?
   - ❏ a lot on most days and none on other days?
   - ❏ some on some days and none on other days?
   - ❏ very little or none?

2. Think about how many **refined grains** you ate *during the past week*. Did you eat:
   - ☑ a lot almost every day or every day?
   - ❏ some almost every day or every day?
   - ❏ a lot on most days and none on other days?
   - ❏ some on some days and none on other days?
   - ❏ very little or none?

3. Think about how many **whole grains** (e.g., whole grain bread, whole wheat pasta, brown rice, oats) you ate *during the past 3 days.* Did you eat:
   - ❏ a lot almost every day or every day?
   - ❏ some almost every day or every day?
   - ❏ a lot on most days and none on other days?
   - ❏ some on some days and none on other days?
   - ☑ very little or none?

4. Think about how many **whole grains** you ate *during the past week*. Did you eat:
   - ❏ a lot almost every day or every day?
   - ❏ some almost every day or every day?
   - ❏ a lot on most days and none on other days?
   - ❏ some on some days and none on other days?
   - ☑ very little or none?

5. Think about how many **dark green and orange vegetables** (e.g., broccoli, green beans, spinach, carrots, squash, sweet potatoes) you ate *during the past 3 days*. Did you eat:
   - ❏ a lot almost every day or every day?
   - ❏ some almost every day or every day?
   - ❏ a lot on most days and none on other days?
   - ❏ some on some days and none on other days?
   - ☑ very little or none?

6. Think about how many **dark green and orange vegetables** you ate *during the past week*. Did you eat:
   - ❏ a lot almost every day or every day?
   - ❏ some almost every day or every day?
   - ❏ a lot on most days and none on other days?
   - ❏ some on some days and none on other days?
   - ☑ very little or none?

Figure 10-10 Nutritional Wellness Tests and Measures (continued)

7. Think about how many **"starchy" vegetables** (e.g., corn, peas) you ate *during the past 3 days.* Did you eat:
   - ❏ a lot almost every day or every day?
   - ❏ some almost every day or every day?
   - ❏ a lot on most days and none on other days?
   - ❏ some on some days and none on other days?
   - ☑ very little or none?

8. Think about how many **"starchy" vegetables** you ate *during the past week.* Did you eat:
   - ❏ a lot almost every day or every day?
   - ❏ some almost every day or every day?
   - ❏ a lot on most days and none on other days?
   - ☑ some on some days and none on other days?
   - ❏ very little or none?

9. Think about how many dairy products you consumed *during the past 3 days.*
   - About how many cups of _____ skim, _____ 1%, _____ 2%, __1__ whole milk did you drink each day?
   - About how many cups of other high-calcium foods did you eat per day? __0__

10. Think about how many dairy products you consumed *during the past week.*
    - About how many cups of _____ skim, _____ 1%, _____ 2%, __3__ whole milk did you drink each day?
    - About how many cups of other high-calcium foods did you eat per day? __0__

11. Think about how much **red meat** you ate *during the past 3 days.* Did you eat:
    - ☑ a lot almost every day or every day?
    - ❏ some almost every day or every day?
    - ❏ a lot on most days and none on other days?
    - ❏ some on some days and none on other days?
    - ❏ very little or none?

12. Think about how much **red meat** you ate *during the past week.* Did you eat:
    - ☑ a lot almost every day or every day?
    - ❏ some almost every day or every day?
    - ❏ a lot on most days and none on other days?
    - ❏ some on some days and none on other days?
    - ❏ very little or none?

13. Think about how many **nuts, seeds, beans, and tofu** fats you consumed *during the past 3 days.* Did you eat:
    - ❏ a lot almost every day or every day?
    - ❏ some almost every day or every day?
    - ❏ a lot on most days and none on other days?
    - ❏ some on some days and none on other days?
    - ☑ very little or none?

Figure 10-10 Nutritional Wellness Tests and Measures (continued)

14. Think about how many **nuts, seeds, beans, and tofu** fats you consumed *during the past week.*
    Did you eat:
    ❑ a lot almost every day or every day?
    ❑ some almost every day or every day?
    ❑ a lot on most days and none on other days?
    ❑ some on some days and none on other days?
    ☑ very little or none?

15. Think about how much **fish, poultry, and egg whites** you consumed *during the past 3 days.*
    Did you eat:
    ❑ a lot almost every day or every day?
    ❑ some almost every day or every day?
    ❑ a lot on most days and none on other days?
    ❑ some on some days and none on other days?
    ☑ very little or none?

16. Think about how much **fish, poultry, and egg whites** you consumed *during the past week.*
    Did you eat:
    ❑ a lot almost every day or every day?
    ❑ some almost every day or every day?
    ❑ a lot on most days and none on other days?
    ☑ some on some days and none on other days?
    ❑ very little or none?

17. Think about how many **egg yolks** you consumed *during the past week.* Did you eat:
    ❑ 15 or more   ❑ 8 to 14   ☑ 5 to 7   ❑ 1 to 4 or   ❑ none?

18. Think about how much **healthy oils and fats** (e.g., olive, canola, soy, corn, sunflower, peanut, other vegetable oils) you ate *during the past 3 days.* Did you eat:
    ❑ a lot almost every day or every day?
    ❑ some almost every day or every day?
    ❑ a lot on most days and none on other days?
    ❑ some on some days and none on other days?
    ☑ very little or none?

19. Think about how much **healthy oils and fats** (e.g., olive, canola, soy, corn, sunflower, peanut, other vegetable oils) you ate *during the past week.* Did you eat:
    ❑ a lot almost every day or every day?
    ❑ some almost every day or every day?
    ❑ a lot on most days and none on other days?
    ❑ some on some days and none on other days?
    ☑ very little or none?

20. Think about how much **fried food** you ate *during the past 3 days.* Did you eat:
    ☑ a lot almost every day or every day?
    ❑ some almost every day or every day?
    ❑ a lot on most days and none on other days?
    ❑ some on some days and none on other days?
    ❑ very little or none?

Figure 10-10 Nutritional Wellness Tests and Measures (continued)

21. Think about how much **fried food** you ate *during the past week*. Did you eat:
    - ☑ a lot almost every day or every day?
    - ❑ some almost every day or every day?
    - ❑ a lot on most days and none on other days?
    - ❑ some on some days and none on other days?
    - ❑ very little or none?

22. Think about how much **butter** you ate *during the past 3 days*. Did you eat:
    - ☑ a lot almost every day or every day?
    - ❑ some almost every day or every day?
    - ❑ a lot on most days and none on other days?
    - ❑ some on some days and none on other days?
    - ❑ very little or none?

23. Think about how much **butter** you ate *during the past week*. Did you eat:
    - ☑ a lot almost every day or every day?
    - ❑ some almost every day or every day?
    - ❑ a lot on most days and none on other days?
    - ❑ some on some days and none on other days?
    - ❑ very little or none?

24. Think about how many **sweets** (e.g., cookies, cake, candy) and sugary drinks you consumed *during the past 3 days*. Did you eat:
    - ☑ a lot almost every day or every day?
    - ❑ some almost every day or every day?
    - ❑ a lot on most days and none on other days?
    - ❑ some on some days and none on other days?
    - ❑ very little or none?

25. Think about how many **sweets** (e.g., cookies, cake, candy) and sugary drinks you consumed *during the past week*. Did you eat:
    - ☑ a lot almost every day or every day?
    - ❑ some almost every day or every day?
    - ❑ a lot on most days and none on other days?
    - ❑ some on some days and none on other days?
    - ❑ very little or none?

26. Think about how much **fruit** you ate *during the past 3 days*. Did you eat:
    - ❑ a lot almost every day or every day?
    - ❑ some almost every day or every day?
    - ❑ a lot on most days and none on other days?
    - ❑ some on some days and none on other days?
    - ☑ very little or none?

27. Think about how much **fruit** you ate *during the past week*. Did you eat:
    - ❑ a lot almost every day or every day?
    - ❑ some almost every day or every day?
    - ❑ a lot on most days and none on other days?
    - ☑ some on some days and none on other days?
    - ❑ very little or none?

Figure 10-10 Nutritional Wellness Tests and Measures (continued)

28. Think about how much **salt** you consumed *during the past 3 days*. Did you eat:
    - ☑ a lot of foods high in salt?
    - ❑ just a few salty foods?
    - ❑ very few or no salty foods?

29. Think about how much **salt** you consumed *during the past week*. Did you eat:
    - ☑ a lot of foods high in salt?
    - ❑ just a few salty foods?
    - ❑ very few or no salty foods?

30. Think about if you added **salt** to your food (at the table) *during the past week?* Did you:
    - ☑ often or always add salt?
    - ❑ sometimes add salt?
    - ❑ never add salt?

31. Think about how much **alcohol** (e.g., beer, wine, liquor) you consumed *during the past 3 days.* About how many drinks did you drink each day? __0__
    About how many total drinks did you drink total (during the past 3 days)? __0__

32. Think about how much **alcohol** you consumed *during the past week.* About how many drinks did you drink each day? __< 1__
    About how many drinks did you drink total (during the whole week)? __1__

33. Think about how much **alcohol** you consumed *during the past month.* About how many drinks did you drink each day? __4__

34. Do you regularly take a multivitamin? ❑ Yes ☑ No

35. Do you regularly take a supplement with calcium and vitamin D? (This may be as part of a multivitamin.) ❑ Yes ☑ No

36. If you are following any special diet (such as a low-calorie or weight-loss diet or any type of diet prescribed by a physician or dietician), please tell me about it:
    _____N/A_____
    _____
    _____
    _____

37. Please tell me anything else that you believe is important about your current eating habits.
    _____N/A_____
    _____
    _____
    _____

Section E: Affective Aspect of Nutritional Wellness
On a scale of 1 to 10, with 1 being no commitment and 10 being total commitment, how committed are you to

1. Eating *some* dark green or orange vegetables (almost or) every day? __8__
2. Eating *a lot* of dark green or orange vegetables (almost or) every day? __2__
3. Eating other kinds of vegetables (almost or) every day? __8__

Figure 10-10 Nutritional Wellness Tests and Measures (continued)

4. Eating some fruits (almost or) every day? __8__

5. Choosing whole grains (e.g., whole grain bread, whole grain pasta, brown rice) rather than refined grains (e.g., white bread, white pasta, white rice) *some* of the time? __4__

6. Choosing whole grains rather than refined grains *most or all* of the time? __2__

7. Consuming some healthy oils (e.g., olive, canola and vegetable oils)? __8__

8. Choosing fish, poultry, eggs, nuts, seeds, beans, and tofu rather than red meat *some* of the time? __8__

9. Choosing fish, poultry, eggs, nuts, seeds, beans, and tofu rather than red meat *most or all* of the time? __2__

10. Eating some fish, poultry, eggs, nuts, seeds, beans, and tofu? __8__

11. Consuming two servings of milk or the equivalent of other high-calcium foods or taking a calcium/vitamin D supplement (almost or) every day? __8__

12. Rarely or never eating red meat? __5__

13. Rarely or never eating butter? __7__

14. Rarely or never eating refined grains (e.g., white bread, pasta, rice)? __6__

15. Rarely consuming sugary drinks (e.g., sodas)? __2__

16. Rarely consuming sugary foods (e.g., cake, cookies)? __8__

17. Limiting your salt intake? __8__

18. If a woman: Drinking less than one alcoholic drink per day? If a man: Drinking less than one to two alcoholic drinks per day? __10__

Section F: Food Preferences

1. What "healthy foods" do you like? Please be certain to list the kinds of vegetables you like.
   salad with low-calorie thousand island dressing, squash, corn, green beans, asparagus, broccoli with cheese, whole-grain pasta and bread and rice, leaner hamburger, beans, low-fat milk

2. What are your one or two favorite "unhealthy foods"?
   ice cream and sugary cereals

Section G: Nutritional Wellness Goal(s)

What is/are your goal(s) related to eating/nutrition?
Eat a healthier diet. Not eating the unhealthy foods my husband eats, but eating healthy food like my daughter

Figure 10-10 Nutritional Wellness Tests and Measures (continued)

Body Composition Wellness Survey

(PT to examine patient/client and fill in this survey)

Surname: _Smith_ First: _Carol_ Date: _4_ / _20_ / _09_
Name of the Physical Therapist (PT): _Sharon Fair, PT_

Note to the PT: Dialog with the patient/client to complete these tests and measures. Utilize lay terminology unless there is direct evidence that more clinical terminology is indicated.

For the PT to state to the patient/client: I will be asking you numerous questions to obtain information about your habits that affect body composition (i.e., body fat and muscle.) Please answer as honestly, accurately, and completely as possible. This will enable me to help you meet any goals you may have related to your body composition. At the end of this survey, you will have the opportunity to ask me questions. Are you ready to start?

Section A: Cognitive Aspect of Body Composition Wellness

1. What is a good diet for a person who wants to lose weight/body fat?
   Eat some whole grain foods, but not too much because they're starchy. Eat a lot of vegetables and fruits and drink a lot of fruit juices

2. What exercises should a person do to lose body fat?
   Do a lot of hard exercise like running. I've heard that if you go into a sauna with a sweatsuit you'll lose even more weight

3. What exercises should a person do to gain muscle?
   Lift a lot of heavy weights at a gym, "no pain, no gain"

4. Can leisure activities (such as cleaning the house, playing basketball, and shoveling snow) help you to lose body fat and gain muscle? ❏ Yes ☑ No ❏ I don't know

If the patient/client replies yes, ask him or her how.

Section B: Psychomotor Aspect of Body Composition Wellness

1. Weight, Clothing Sizes, and Percent Body Fat

	Current	1 month ago	3 months ago	6 months ago	1 year ago
Weight in lbs.	160	159	157	154	148
Dress (if woman) Shirt (if man)	16	14	14	14	12-14
Pants Size	14	12	12	12	10-12
% Body Fat (if known)	—	—	—	—	—

Figure 10-11 Body Composition Wellness Tests and Measures

2. Tell me about how your clothes have fit you over the past year.
   My clothes were very tight a month ago, that's why I had to go up in size. Over the past year, they've been getting tighter and tighter.

3. Self-Weighing Habits:
   - About how often do you weigh yourself on a scale? _____*every day*_____

   If the patient/client weighs her/himself **at least once a month**, ask her/him the following questions:
   - What time of the day do you typically weigh yourself? _____*in the morning*_____
   - Do you typically weigh yourself before or after your first meal of the day (e.g., breakfast)?
     ☑ before ☐ after ☐ varies ☐ I don't know
   - Typically, do you weigh yourself before or after a bowel movement?
     ☑ before ☐ after ☐ varies ☐ I don't know
   - Do you typically use the same scale every time that you weigh yourself?
     ☑ yes ☐ no ☐ varies ☐ I don't know
   - Do you typically you use a medical or calibrated scale?
     ☑ yes ☐ no ☐ varies ☐ I don't know

4. If the Systems Review revealed the patient/client is on a diet to lose fat and/or gain muscle, ask her/him to describe the diet.
   N/A

Section C: Affective Aspect of Body Composition Wellness

Note to the PT: Rephrase these questions as appropriate to the specific patient/client. For example, if the patient/client is a young man and the goal is to gain muscle, substitute "gain muscle mass" for "lose fat and/or gain muscle mass." If the patient/client understands the phrase "improved body composition," you may use that as the substitute at the end of each question.

On a scale of 1 to 10, with 1 being no commitment and 10 being total commitment, how committed are you to:

1. Participating in cardiovascular (endurance/aerobic capacity) exercise to lose fat and/or gain muscle mass? ___8___
2. Participating in strength training (muscular fitness) exercise to maintain or increase your muscle mass? _____ 7
3. Participating in leisure activities (such as taking stairs instead of elevators, washing your own car instead of going to a car wash) that will help you to lose fat and/or maintain or increase your muscle mass? ___7___
4. Eating (consuming) the types of foods (e.g., vegetables; foods high in fiber, low in sugar, or low in fat) that will help you to lose fat and/or gain muscle mass? ___8___
5. Practicing mental and/or social activities to help you to lose fat and/or gain muscle mass? ___7___

Figure 10-11 Body Composition Wellness Tests and Measures (continued)

Section D: Body Composition and Body Composition Wellness Goal(s)
What is/are your body composition (fat/muscle) goal(s)?

Get back to a size 6 pants!

This Body Composition Wellness Survey includes the tests in Sections A, C, D, E, F, and G of the Nutritional Wellness Survey and the tests in Sections A, B-1, B-2, B-3, B-4, B-5, C, and E of the Fitness and Fitness Wellness Survey. If these tests have not already been completed, complete them now. The Food Journal is a part of this Body Composition Survey.

- *If the patient/client has not completed at least 1 day of the Food Journal:* Provide the Food Journal to her/him and instruct her/him to record the items she or he has eaten so far that day and take the journal home and complete the remainder of it at the end of the day. Also instruct the patient/client to complete the rest of the Food Journal over the next 2 days.

- *If the patient/client has completed only 1 or 2 days of the Food Journal:* Collect what has been completed and instruct her/him to complete the remainder.

- *If the patient/client has completed 3 days of the Food Journal by the first PT session:* Collect it.

Figure 10-11 Body Composition Wellness Tests and Measures (continued)

Mental and Social Wellness

The "Mental and Social Wellness Survey" was utilized. The results are provided in **Figure 10-13**.

Resources/Support and Barriers

Carol's resources and barriers relevant to a therapeutic program to address her body composition and related conditions were examined through questioning.

Community resources include a fitness facility that offers group instruction in aerobic dance, spinning (i.e., stationary cycling), step aerobic, and kickboxing. Available equipment includes treadmills, ellipticals, stairmasters, stationary bicycles, free weights, strength training machines, and supplies for calisthenics. There is also a heated swimming pool and racquetball. An asset is the distance from her job (5 miles). The barriers are the monthly membership fee of $45.00 and the distance from her home (15 miles). Additional community support systems include a network of close friends, some of whom are health conscious and a few who exercise on a regular basis and/or consume a healthy diet, and overeating support groups.

Resources in Carol's home include a treadmill and an exercise-friendly community (e.g., safe neighborhood, walking path). Family support includes her daughter, who eats

FOOD JOURNAL

** Please try to record information after each meal, or at the end of each day **

Date: 4 / 19 / 2009   Day (circle one):   Mon   Tue   Wed   Thur   Fri   Sat   (Sun)

Last Name: _Smith_   First: _Carol_

Time	Describe each food/drink you ate/drank	Where?	With Whom?	State of Mind?	calories
Examples: 2 PM	Examples: McDonald's double cheeseburger, large fries, large diet Coke	Examples: driving in car, on way to pick up son	Examples: alone	Examples: hungry, in a hurry	15
9 PM	2 PBJ sandwiches (white bread, ~ 2 T peanut butter each, ~ 2 T jelly each), can diet Sprite	in bed	with husband	bored— watching tv show	65 30 160
9:45 PM	3 scoops chocolate ice cream	➤	➤	➤	100 150
8 AM	coffee with 1 t sugar	driving to work	alone	hurried/ stressed	415 210
12 PM	Egg sandwich - 1 egg cooked with butter (a little less than a t.) 2 slices white bread	at desk	alone	grading papers	150
	mayonnaise 1 tablespoon 1 orange soda				
6 PM	McDonald's quarter lb burger small fries	coffee table in living room	with husband	talking about our days at	270
	Coke			work - stressed	
10 PM	Snickers bar	in bed	with husband	watching tv news bored	290 80
10:45 PM	4 peanut butter cookies 1/2 cup milk	in bed	with husband		——— 1935

Figure 10-12 Nutritional Wellness and Mental and Social Wellness Tests and Measures—Food Journal

Mental and Social Wellness Survey

(PT to examine patient/client and fill in this survey)

Surname: _Smith_ First: _Carol_ Date: _4_/_20_/_09_

Name of the Physical Therapist (PT): _Sharon Fair_

Note to the PT: Dialog with the patient/client to complete these tests and measures. Utilize lay terminology unless there is direct evidence that more clinical terminology is indicated.

For the PT to state to the patient/client: I will be asking you numerous questions to obtain information about your nutritional habits. Please answer me as honestly, accurately, and as completely as possible. This will enable me to help you meet any goals you may have related to your mental wellness, social wellness, and other areas—such as body composition. At the end of this survey, you will have the opportunity to ask me questions. Are you ready to start?

Section A: Cognitive Aspect of Mental and Social Wellness

1. Tell me what you know about mental and emotional wellness:
   To be happy with your life

2. Tell me what you know about stress and burn out:
   Stress is inevitable. Too much stress causes the body to burn out and breakdown

3. Tell me what you know about social wellness:
   It's important to have strong relations with your family members and some good friends

4. Tell me what you know about environmental wellness:
   People should conserve the environment, but it's difficult to find the time

Section B: Psychomotor Aspect of Mental and Social Wellness

Part 1: Mental Wellness (Define/discuss each term that is unfamiliar to the patient/client.)

1. As much as it is reasonably possible, are you confident that things will work out as well as they reasonably can?
   ☑ Yes ☐ Somewhat ☐ No

2. Do you believe that everything will probably work out the best that it can?
   ☑ Yes ☐ Somewhat ☐ No

3. Do you live your life as though everything will probably work out the best that it can?
   ☑ Yes ☐ Somewhat ☐ No

4. Do you believe that you tend to influence the events in your life?
   ☐ Yes ☑ To a certain extent ☐ No

Figure 10-13 Mental and Social Wellness Tests and Measures

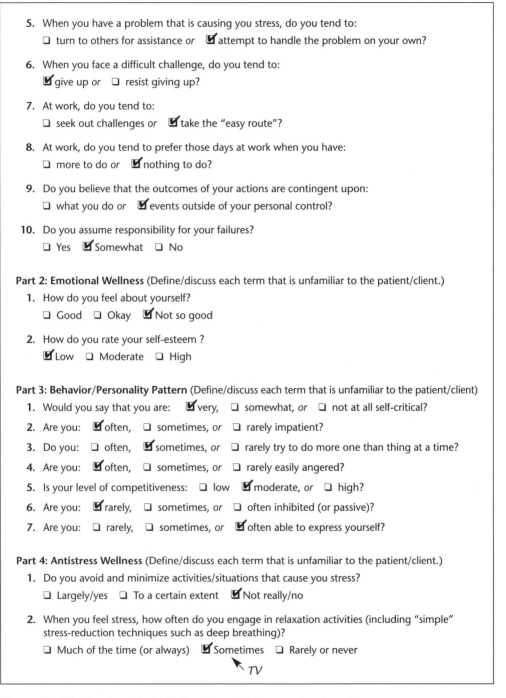

5. When you have a problem that is causing you stress, do you tend to:
   ❑ turn to others for assistance *or*   ☑ attempt to handle the problem on your own?

6. When you face a difficult challenge, do you tend to:
   ☑ give up *or*   ❑ resist giving up?

7. At work, do you tend to:
   ❑ seek out challenges *or*   ☑ take the "easy route"?

8. At work, do you tend to prefer those days at work when you have:
   ❑ more to do *or*   ☑ nothing to do?

9. Do you believe that the outcomes of your actions are contingent upon:
   ❑ what you do *or*   ☑ events outside of your personal control?

10. Do you assume responsibility for your failures?
    ❑ Yes   ☑ Somewhat   ❑ No

Part 2: Emotional Wellness (Define/discuss each term that is unfamiliar to the patient/client.)

1. How do you feel about yourself?
   ❑ Good   ❑ Okay   ☑ Not so good

2. How do you rate your self-esteem ?
   ☑ Low   ❑ Moderate   ❑ High

Part 3: Behavior/Personality Pattern (Define/discuss each term that is unfamiliar to the patient/client)

1. Would you say that you are: ☑ very,   ❑ somewhat, *or*   ❑ not at all self-critical?
2. Are you: ☑ often,   ❑ sometimes, *or*   ❑ rarely impatient?
3. Do you: ❑ often,   ☑ sometimes, *or*   ❑ rarely try to do more one than thing at a time?
4. Are you: ☑ often,   ❑ sometimes, *or*   ❑ rarely easily angered?
5. Is your level of competitiveness: ❑ low   ☑ moderate, *or*   ❑ high?
6. Are you: ☑ rarely,   ❑ sometimes, *or*   ❑ often inhibited (or passive)?
7. Are you: ❑ rarely,   ❑ sometimes, *or*   ☑ often able to express yourself?

Part 4: Antistress Wellness (Define/discuss each term that is unfamiliar to the patient/client.)

1. Do you avoid and minimize activities/situations that cause you stress?
   ❑ Largely/yes   ❑ To a certain extent   ☑ Not really/no

2. When you feel stress, how often do you engage in relaxation activities (including "simple" stress-reduction techniques such as deep breathing)?
   ❑ Much of the time (or always)   ☑ Sometimes   ❑ Rarely or never

   ↖ *TV*

Figure 10-13 Mental and Social Wellness Tests and Measures (continued)

Part 5: Burn Out Secondary to Stress (Define/discuss each term that is unfamiliar to the patient/client. Check all symptoms that apply. Ensure the patient/client understands that the symptoms/signs must be linked to/caused from stress {rather than independent of stress}. If a patient/client acknowledges a symptom in #1, she or he may acknowledge a higher level of that symptom in #2 or #3. For example, she or he may report "headache" in #1 and then report "chronic headaches" in 3-A).

1. Stress in your life causes you to have which of the following, if any?

   ❑ Irritability/anxiety ❑ Decreased ability to concentrate/forgetfulness ☑ Headaches
   ❑ Insomnia/trouble sleeping ❑ Bruxism/grinding your teeth
   ❑ Heart palpitations/arrhythmia/transient hypertension ❑ None   *occasional*

2. Stress in your life causes you to have which of the following, if any? (Check all that apply.)

   ❑ Cynical attitude/resentful ❑ Persistent tiredness in the morning
   ❑ Lateness for work or school ❑ Procrastination/turn in work late
   ❑ "I don't care" attitude; frequently skipping work or school; social withdrawal
   ❑ Increased alcohol, coffee, tea, or cola ❑ Decreased sexual desire ❑ None

3-A. Stress in your life causes you to have which of the following, if any?

   ❑ Chronic sadness or depression ❑ Chronic stomach or bowel problems
   ❑ Chronic mental fatigue ❑ Chronic physical fatigue ❑ Chronic headaches ❑ None

3-B. Which of the following, if any, are you considering?

   ❑ Moving away from friends and/or family ❑ Quitting your job or dropping out of school
   ❑ Harming yourself ❑ None

Part 6: Intellectual Wellness (Define/discuss each term that is unfamiliar to the patient/client.)

1. Is the amount of stimulating intellectual activity you have in your life:

   ❑ Too much ☑ Too little, *or* ❑ Just about right?

2. Does the amount of intellectual activity in your life cause you to be: ❑ Overwhelmed
   ☑ Bored, or ❑ Appropriately engaged/challenged (i.e., neither overwhelmed nor bored)?

Part 7: Occupational Wellness (Define/discuss each term that is unfamiliar to the patient/client.)

1. Do you maintain a balance between your job and family time?
   ☑ Yes ❑ Somewhat ❑ No

2. Do you maintain a balance between your job and personal time?
   ☑ Yes ❑ Somewhat ❑ No

Part 8: Social Wellness (Define/discuss each term that is unfamiliar to the patient/client)

1. Is the social support available to you adequate?
   ☑ Yes ❑ Somewhat ❑ No

2. Do you adequately contribute to your community?
   ☑ Yes ❑ Somewhat ❑ No

Figure 10-13 Mental and Social Wellness Tests and Measures (continued)

Part 9: Family Wellness (Define/discuss each term that is unfamiliar to the patient/client.)

Preface: Whom do you consider to be your immediate family members?

_____*husband*_____

1. How well does your family work together to solve its problems?

   ❏ Very well ☑ Moderately well ❏ Poorly

2. How would you describe the direction of your family?

   ☑ Forward/upward ❏ Static ❏ Backwards/downward

3. Is your family held together by positive emotions (such as caring) rather than convenience?

   ❏ Yes ❏ To a certain extent ☑ No

Part 10: Environmental Wellness (Define/discuss each term that is unfamiliar to the patient/client.)

1. How often do you take the time to enjoy nature?
   ❏ I enjoy nature on a regular basis.
   ❏ I occasionally take the time to enjoy nature.
   ☑ I (rarely) or never take the time to enjoy nature.

2. How well do you conserve the environment? (Consider if you stop junk mail; recycle, conserve water; conserve electricity; use paper shopping bags; use a fuel-efficient vehicle, car pool, or use mass transportation, etc.)
   ❏ I do a lot to conserve the environment.
   ❏ I do some things to conserve the environment.
   ☑ I do very (little) or nothing to conserve the environment.

Section C: Affective Aspects of Mental and Social Wellness

On a scale of 1 to 10, with 1 being no commitment and 10 being total commitment, how committed are you to:

1. telling yourself that "things will work out"? ___8___
2. accepting responsibility for your failures? ___8___
3. living a life that promotes your self-esteem? ___8___
4. avoiding or minimizing events that cause you stress? ___10___
5. choosing intellectual activities that do not cause you to be bored, but are not overwhelming either? ___7___
6. making sure that you have social support when you need it? ___7___
7. working with your family to solve problems and helping your family to move forward? ___9___
8. keeping a balance between your work and family/personal time? ___7___
9. enjoying nature? ___7___
10. preserving the environment? ___3___

Section D: Mental/Social Wellness Goal(s)

What is/are your mental and/or social wellness goal(s)?

*Improve self-esteem and possibly spend more time with daughter*
_____
_____
_____
_____
_____

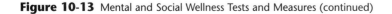

Figure 10-13 Mental and Social Wellness Tests and Measures (continued)

nutritiously, exercises regularly, and encourages Carol to do the same. An obstacle is her husband, who overeats, doesn't exercise, and doesn't consider Carol "that overweight." (Carol reports that her husband is about 6 feet tall, weighs about 240 pounds, and is "rather fat.") An additional barrier within the home is an excess amount of unhealthy foods (e.g., sweets and snacks).

Occupational barriers include a lack of exercise facilities except the school gymnasium (which Carol does not feel comfortable using) and a lack of healthy food choices in the school cafeteria.

Evaluation

Fitness

Carol is sedentary and her overall level of fitness is poor. She is not an athlete.

Aerobic Capacity and Aerobic Capacity Wellness

Carol's maximal oxygen consumption of 25 mL/kg·min is in the lower end of the "average" category for her gender and age.

While Carol understands certain aspects of aerobic capacity exercise (e.g., moderate pace), her understanding of other aspects is flawed (e.g., the optimal frequency is two to three times per week). Because Carol's aerobic capacity wellness is unsatisfactory in terms of the cognitive domain and such knowledge is related to her primary goal of losing body fat, education in this topic is indicated. Carol's affective commitment to engage in aerobic capacity exercise up to five times per week is satisfactory. The psychomotor aspect of Carol's aerobic capacity wellness is unsatisfactory because she admits that she has recently engaged in only one 30-minute bout of aerobic capacity exercise.

Carol's knowledge of, behaviors related to, commitment to, and attitudes about aerobic capacity and aerobic capacity wellness suggest that she is in the contemplation stage in terms of aerobic capacity wellness. Because her aerobic capacity wellness has now been examined, it is indicated to develop an aerobic capacity wellness plan of care and advance her to the action stage.

As more than one domain of her aerobic capacity wellness is unsatisfactory, Carol's overall aerobic capacity wellness is unsatisfactory. Carol's aerobic capacity wellness goal to increase her walking complements her body composition goal to reduce body fat.

Flexibility/Range of Motion and Flexibility Wellness

Carol's bilateral range of motion in her calves and hamstrings are moderately limited.

The cognitive, psychomotor, and affective domains of her flexibility wellness are unsatisfactory. For example, she is unaware that stretches should be held static for at least 30 seconds, she does not participate in a stretching program, and her commitment to engage in a flexibility program at least twice weekly is a 3 on a scale of 10. Because Carol's flexibility wellness is unsatisfactory in terms of the cognitive domain, education in this topic is indicated.

Carol's knowledge of, behaviors related to, commitment to, and attitudes about flexibility and flexibility wellness suggest that she is in the primordial stage in terms of flexibility wellness. Because she has not yet achieved the contemplation stage in flexibility wellness, it is important to address her lack of commitment to flexibility wellness rather than prematurely advance her into the action stage.

As Carol is unsatisfactory in at least one domain of flexibility wellness, her overall flexibility wellness is unsatisfactory. She does not have a goal related to flexibility or flexibility wellness.

Muscular Fitness/Muscle Performance and Muscular Fitness Wellness

As assessed in the systems review, Carol's muscle performance is within functional limits. However, her muscular fitness—as measured with fitness equipment and calisthenics—is unsatisfactory. For example, she can complete only 15 crunches and only 5 non-military push-ups.

Because Carol's muscular fitness wellness is unsatisfactory in the cognitive domain and such knowledge is related to her primary goal of reducing body fat, education in this topic is indicated. The affective domain of Carol's muscular fitness wellness is satisfactory because her commitment to engaging in strengthening exercise three times per week is a 7 on a scale of 1 to 10. Carol's psychomotor aspect of muscular fitness wellness is unsatisfactory because she doesn't engage in any type of strength training and does not engage in any heavy or very heavy-intensity activities (which may translate to strengthening activity).

Because Carol's knowledge of, behaviors related to, commitment to, and attitudes about muscular fitness and muscular fitness wellness suggest that she is in the contemplation stage in terms of muscular fitness wellness and her muscular fitness has now been examined, it is indicated to develop a muscular fitness plan of care and advance her to the action stage.

As more than one domain of her muscular fitness wellness is unsatisfactory, Carol's overall muscular fitness wellness is unsatisfactory. Carol does not have a goal related to muscular fitness or muscular fitness wellness.

Leisure Activity Wellness

Because Carol's leisure wellness is unsatisfactory in the cognitive domain and such knowledge is related to her primary goal of reducing body fat, education in this topic is indicated. Although the affective domain of Carol's muscular fitness wellness is satisfactory in terms of increasing leisure activities that promote muscular fitness, it is unsatisfactory in terms of leisure activities that promote aerobic capacity. Her psychomotor aspect of leisure wellness is unsatisfactory.

Because Carol's knowledge of, behaviors related to, commitment to, and attitudes about leisure wellness suggest that she is in the contemplation stage in terms of aerobic capacity leisure wellness and in the pre-contemplation stage in terms of muscular fitness leisure wellness, it is indicated to develop a muscular fitness plan of care and advance her to the contemplation stage.

As more than one domain of her leisure wellness is unsatisfactory, Carol's overall leisure wellness is unsatisfactory.

Fitness Wellness: Other Dimensions

In conjunction with the one time she recently exercised, Carol did an appropriate warm-up but did not cool-down, her intake of appropriate and adequate fluid intakes before and during the exercise bout was deficient, and her intake of fluids following the exercise was inadequate. Education related to hydration and cooling-down after exercise is indicated.

Carol does not use tobacco products or anabolic steroids. There is no indication that education in either of these areas is needed.

Nutrition and Nutritional Wellness

The cognitive domain of Carol's nutritional wellness is unsatisfactory. For example, she thinks that the daily requirement of water is only 1 or 2 cups per day and consuming starchy foods is unhealthy. Because a sound knowledge of nutrition can enhance fat loss, Carol's primary goal, nutritional education is indicated.

The psychomotor domain of Carol's nutritional wellness also is unsatisfactory. For example, her intake of refined grains, red meat, fried foods, butter, sweets, and salt is excessive. In contrast, her intake of whole grains, dark green and orange vegetables, beans (or nuts or seeds or tofu), healthy oils, starchy vegetables, fruit, high-calcium foods and the fish, poultry, and egg white food groups is inadequate. Carol's intake of alcoholic beverages is modest. Because Carol's typical food choices are unhealthy and she does not take a multivitamin, her intake of vitamins and minerals is likely also deficient.

Carol's affective domain of nutritional wellness is largely satisfactory. Although her commitment to eating the recommended amount of dark green and orange vegetables is not satisfactory, her commitment to eating an improved amount is satisfactory. Her commitment to eating the recommended amount of fruits, other vegetables, healthy oils, high-calcium items, butter, and sugary foods is satisfactory. Her commitment to choosing whole grains rather than refined grains and alternative protein foods rather than red meat is unsatisfactory, but her commitment to eating some alternative protein foods is satisfactory. Her commitment to rarely or never eating red meat or refined grains is unsatisfactory, rarely consuming sugary drinks is unsatisfactory, limiting her salt intake is satisfactory and consuming no more than the recommended amount of alcohol is satisfactory.

Carol's knowledge of, behaviors related to, commitment to, and attitudes about nutrition and nutritional wellness suggest that she is in the pre-contemplation stage in terms of nutrition. Because she has not yet achieved the contemplation stage in nutritional wellness, it is important to address her lack of knowledge in this area rather than prematurely advance her to the action stage.

As more than one domain of her nutritional wellness is unsatisfactory, Carol's overall muscular fitness wellness is unsatisfactory. Her nutritional goal to consume a healthier diet is appropriate, but vague. Also, her stipulation of not having to eat healthy foods that she doesn't like is inappropriate because the variety of healthy foods she likes is rather limited. Carol's goals confirm that she needs to be educated in nutritional wellness.

Mental and Social Wellness

Because a comprehensive examination and evaluation of mental and social wellness is beyond the scope of physical therapy, this evaluation of Carol's mental and social wellness is an educated rather than definitive evaluation.

The analysis of the mental and social wellness examination suggests that Carol has a Type A behavior/personality pattern, an external locus of control, and impaired hardiness. It suggests also that her emotional wellness (self-esteem), antistress wellness, intellectual wellness, and environmental wellness (enjoyment and conservation of nature) are unsatisfactory. For example, the only stress-reduction strategy she reports is watching television and she rarely or never takes time to enjoy nature. With one sign/symptom of stress, she may be categorized in the lowest end of stage one of burnout. The aspects of mental and social wellness that appear to be satisfactory are mental wellness (optimism), occupational wellness, social wellness (social support and contributions to community), and family wellness.

Carol's cognitive knowledge of various aspects of mental and social wellness appears satisfactory. For example, she recognizes that mental and emotional knowledge is associated with happiness, stress can cause burnout, it is important to have a strong social network, and it is worthwhile to conserve the environment.

Carol's commitments toward her mental wellness (optimism), promoting an internal locus of control (accepting responsibility), emotional wellness (self-esteem), antisocial wellness, intellectual wellness, social wellness, family wellness, occupational wellness, and the enjoying nature aspect of environmental wellness are satisfactory. Her commitment conservation aspect of environmental wellness is unsatisfactory.

Carol's knowledge of, behaviors related to, commitment to, and attitudes related to the components of mental and social wellness are mixed. The results of her tests and measures suggest that she is in the maintenance stage of mental wellness (optimism), antistress wellness, social wellness, family wellness, and occupational wellness; the contemplation stage of emotional wellness (self-esteem); and the pre-contemplation or primordial stage of intellectual wellness and environmental wellness.

Because her current emotional wellness may be unsatisfactory, her goal of a higher self-esteem is appropriate. Carol's social wellness goal of spending more time walking with her daughter will be an asset in achieving her body composition goal. Carol has no other goals related to mental or social wellness. During the development of the prognosis and plan of care, each strength and weakness of Carol's mental and social wellness should be considered in relation to her primary goal of losing fat.

Basal Metabolic Rate and Caloric Balance

Carols' resting metabolic rate (of 1150 calories per day) is less than what is expected for a woman of her gender, weight, and age (i.e., 1436 calories per day). However, this is logically because of her decreased muscle mass in comparison to her total body weight. Her history of low-calorie diets may have also adversely affected her basal metabolism.

As assessed by her food journal, Carol's input is 1935 calories per day. Because her intake has been slightly exceeding her caloric output, her current caloric expenditure is somewhat less than 1935 calories per day. (Carol's caloric imbalance is evidenced by her recent weight gain and her probable fat mass gain, i.e., her clothes fitting more tightly.) A reasonable estimate for Carol's output is 1820 calories per day. (Note: The 1820 caloric output was estimated as follows: (1) Carol gained 12 pounds within the past year, which equates to 42,000 calories; (3) 42,000 calories divided by 365 days equals an excess of about 115 calories per day; (4) Carol's caloric input of 1935 minus an excess of 115 calories equals a caloric output of 1820.)

Body Composition and Body Composition Wellness

Carol's report of weighing 160 pounds this morning versus her measured 163-pound weight at this session is expected because she is now clothed and has since eaten. Because Carol weighs herself under more reliable conditions at her home in the morning than what is possible in the clinic, and self-monitoring weight positively impacts long-term maintenance of weight loss, her self-reported weight will be utilized throughout the episode of care.

As measured with a BOD POD, Carol's body fat is 34.1%, which classifies her as overfat but not obese. Because her total body weight is 160 pounds, her lean body weight is 105.5 pounds, and her fat weight is 54.5 pounds. In addition to being classified as over-fat, Carol can be classified as being overweight as her BMI is 25.82. Carol's body type is android and her body classification is mesomorph.

The cognitive dimension of Carol's body composition wellness is unsatisfactory. For example, while she recognizes that it is important to eat a lot of vegetables if trying to lose (fat) weight, her understanding of the impact of excessive sweating upon fat loss, dehydration, and potential health consequences are impaired.

Carol weighs herself regularly and under standardized conditions (e.g., upon awakening), so the calculated recent changes in her weight (i.e., 1-pound gain in the last month; 3-pound gain in the last 3 months; 6-pound gain in the last 6 months; and 12 pounds in the last year) are likely accurate. Her increasing clothing size and tightness of her clothes also indicate that most of the weight she has been gaining has been fat.

The analysis of the cognitive aspects of Carol's body composition, nutritional, and fitness wellness examinations indicate that her cognitive knowledge of body composition wellness is unsatisfactory. Because her primary goal is to lose body fat, extensive education in body composition and body composition wellness and education in fitness, fitness wellness, and nutritional wellness is indicated.

The analysis of the psychomotor aspects of Carol's body composition, nutritional, and fitness wellness examinations indicate that her fitness and nutritional behaviors are unsatisfactory in terms of how they affect her body composition and body composition wellness. However, although the results of the body composition wellness examination indicate that she has been steadily gaining weight in the form of body fat during the past year, they also indicate that self-weighing is an appropriate method to assess changes in her body weight because she routinely weighs herself under standardized conditions.

The Food Journal was utilized to test Carol's body composition wellness as it relates to her food intake, the time of day she eats, the environment in which she eats, and her state of mind when she eats. Although she only completed 1 day of her journal, an evaluation of the results is useful. In terms of food choices, the evaluation of what she ate on the 1 day she recorded mirror the results of her nutritional wellness survey. Specifically, her food journal suggests that she does not consume enough calories during the morning hours, consumes too many sugary drinks, eats unhealthy lunches and dinners, and eats too much junk food, especially in the late evening hours. Further evaluation of Carol's food journal suggests that she eats a high percentage of meals in a nontraditional setting, such as in her car or in her bed. She also eats when she feels stressed or bored. Carol's poor eating habits might be linked to her unsatisfactory cognitive nutritional wellness and/or her impaired self-esteem. She might be characterized as an "emotional eater."

Carol's affective commitment to enhance her body composition wellness through aerobic capacity exercise, muscular fitness exercise, leisure activities (in terms of promoting aerobic capacity), healthy eating, and mental and social activities are each satisfactory. Although an evaluation of her reported levels of commitment to activities that impact body composition wellness sometimes conflict (e.g., she reports that her commitment to performing leisure activities to promote her muscular fitness is a 4 on a scale of 1 to 10, yet she reports that her commitment to performing leisure activities to help her lose body fat is a 7 on a scale of 10), this may be due to her lack of body composition wellness knowledge.

Carol's knowledge of, behaviors related to, commitment to, and attitudes about body composition wellness suggest that she is in the contemplation stage. Because her body composition wellness has now been examined, it is indicated to develop a body composition wellness plan of care and advance her to the action stage.

Carol's goal related to body composition is to be able to wear a size 6 pants, just like she did 5 years ago. She emphasizes that this is her primary goal and the reason she has come in for help. As she wore size 6 pants 5 years ago and an obstacle that would necessarily preclude her from achieving this goal has not been identified, her goal is realistic.

Resources/Support and Barriers

Although Carol has some barriers relevant to therapeutic program to address her overfatness and related conditions, she has many resources.

Community resources include a fitness facility that offers group instruction in aerobic dance, spinning (i.e., stationary cycling), step aerobic, and kickboxing. Available equipment includes treadmills, ellipticals, stairmasters, stationary bicycles, free weights, strength-training machines, and supplies for calisthenics. There is also a heated swimming pool and racquetball. An asset is the distance from her job (5 miles). The barriers are the monthly membership fee of $45.00 and the distance from her home (15 miles). Additional community support systems include a network of close friends, some of whom are health conscious and a few of whom exercise on a regular basis and/or consume a healthy diet. Overeating support groups are in her area also.

Resources in Carol's home include a treadmill and an exercise-friendly community (e.g., safe neighborhood, walking path). Family support includes her daughter, who eats nutritiously, exercises regularly, and encourages Carol to do the same. An obstacle is her husband, who overeats, doesn't exercise, and doesn't consider Carol "that overweight." (Carol reports that her husband weighs about 260 pounds.) An additional barrier within the home is an excess amount of unhealthy foods; for example, sweets and snacks.

Occupational barriers include a lack of exercise facilities except the school gymnasium (which Carol does not feel comfortable using), a lack of employee-sponsored fitness activities, and a lack of healthy food choices in the school cafeteria.

Diagnosis/Condition

Carol presents with two primary conditions: impaired body composition wellness and impaired body composition. Her secondary conditions that directly impact her primary conditions are impaired nutritional wellness, impaired aerobic capacity wellness and impaired muscular fitness wellness, impaired mental wellness–stress/anxiety, impaired leisure activity wellness, and impaired emotional wellness–self-esteem. (Note: Although Carol also presents with numerous tertiary conditions [e.g., impaired aerobic capacity, impaired muscular fitness, impaired flexibility, and impaired flexibility wellness], it will be inappropriate to attempt to immediately address these tertiary conditions because doing so would likely overwhelm her and may cause her to discontinue therapy.

Prognosis

Over the course of 1 year, Carol will demonstrate optimal body composition wellness that will enhance her functioning in her home, leisure, occupation, and community environments. During her episode of care, Carol will achieve the goals described in the plan of care.

Plan of Care and Goals

Goals

The primary conditions are impaired body composition and body composition wellness, so the goals relate to these areas. Hence, the broad long-term goals (LTGs) are to improve body composition (i.e., reduce body fat) and enhance body composition wellness. The subsidiary broad LTG is to enhance those aspects of health and wellness that improve body composition and body composition wellness (e.g., enhance nutritional wellness, aerobic capacity wellness, muscular fitness wellness, mental wellness–stress/anxiety, and emotional wellness–self-esteem.)

Carol's specific body composition goal—her reason for seeking help—is to return to her former clothing size. The corresponding body fat goal is 25%.

There are four specific LTGs: (1) engage in 30 minutes of moderate intensity aerobic capacity exercise four or five times per week; (2) engage in 20 minutes of strength-training exercise two or three times per week; (3) adopt healthier eating habits, including food choices, times of day foods are eaten, and environments in which foods are eaten; and (4) seek out and engage in activities to enhance leisure wellness and self-esteem and to decrease stress. These four goals will enable Carol to achieve her body composition goal; the physical therapist should emphasize these goals to help Carol more fully embrace them as goals that directly impact her stated goal of wearing size 6 pants. Moreover, these four wellness goals are healthy and realistic and are independently worthy of pursuit.

While additional LTGs could be initially established to address Carol's other problems (e.g., impaired flexibility and impaired flexibility wellness), it is critical that she does not feel inundated with a plethora of goals. Overloading her with LTGs, which necessarily require the assignment of related short-term goals (STGs), could easily overwhelm her and cause her to discontinue physical therapy. Carol is at risk of overload because she presents with impaired stress wellness and low self-esteem and has a history of inactivity and unhealthy eating patterns. Moreover, the secondary goals of enhancing her aerobic capacity wellness and muscular fitness wellness will necessarily enhance her aerobic capacity and muscular fitness, respectively.

There is one primary STG related to Carol's broad LTGs and that STG is to enhance body composition wellness. Because enhancing body composition wellness is a complex goal that necessarily involves diet and exercise and likely involves mental and/or social activities, it is the secondary STGs that should be specifically itemized and pursued.

Initially, there are seven appropriate STGs for Carol: (1) advance Carol's cognitive understanding of body composition, nutrition, fitness, antistress, and emotional wellness (Note: This goal is appropriate because her cognitive knowledge of these subjects is limited and an enhanced understanding of them will help her to achieve the LTGs); (2) advance Carol from the pre-contemplation to the contemplation stage of nutritional wellness (Note: This STG is appropriate because her current nutritional intake is unhealthy and her commitment to change is overall satisfactory.); (3) advance Carol from the contemplation to the action stage of aerobic capacity wellness; (4) advance Carol from the contemplation to the action stage of muscular fitness wellness (Note: STGs #3 and #4 are appropriate because she does not currently exercise and her commitment to improve it is high); (5) advance Carol from the contemplation to the action stage of antistress wellness (Note: This STG is appropriate because her current antistress wellness is unsatisfactory and her commitment to improve it is high); (6) advance Carol from the contemplation stage to the action stage of leisure wellness that promotes aerobic capacity (Note: This STG is appropriate because she is currently sedentary and her commitment to increase her activities that promote her aerobic capacity is adequate); and (7) Advance Carol from the contemplation to the action stage of emotional wellness (Note: This STG is appropriate because her self-esteem is low and her commitment to improve it is high.)

Depending upon Carol's reaction during the first session, it might be prudent to initially pursue no more than two or three of the STGs and then add on additional STGs as she becomes accustomed to her new lifestyle. The first priority, and that which should be addressed during the initial treatment session, should be to progress her to the contemplation stage of nutritional wellness so that you can then advance her to the action stage. During the initial treatment session, it is also a priority to advance her to the action stage of aerobic capacity wellness and begin to advance her knowledge of body composition, nutrition, fitness, antistress, and emotional wellness. For example, contemporaneously with beginning an exercise program is knowing how to warm-up and cool-down. Advancing her to the action stage of aerobic capacity wellness is a higher priority than advancing her to the action stage of muscular fitness wellness because she has a history of participating in at least some aerobic capacity exercise.

Prognosis of Goals

The prognosis of Carol to achieve the broad LTGs (i.e., to wear size 6 pants and to reduce her body fat to 25% and enhance her body composition wellness) and the primary STG (i.e., enhance her body composition wellness) is good. There are many reasons why the prognosis is realistic: (1) she wore this size 5 years ago; (2) she is committed to adhering to a healthy diet; (3) she is committed to enhancing her aerobic capacity wellness to reduce her body fat; (4) she is committed to enhancing her muscular fitness wellness to reduce her body fat; (5) she is committed to engaging in mental and social activities to enhance her ability to manage her body composition; (6) she is internally motivated to lose fat; (7) she is optimistic (i.e., strong mental wellness); (8) she has social support (e.g., her daughter); and (9) she self-monitors her weight.

Expected Duration to Achieve the Goals

Utilizing the 25% body fat goal as a means to calculate the projected time line to achieve the body composition goal of wearing size 6 pants yields a projection of 7 months. The 7-month estimate is based upon the following: (1) the daily deficit will be 645 calories and will be achieved through reducing Carol's intake to 1420 calories per day (i.e., 400 calories below her estimated caloric output of 1820) and increasing her output by 245 calories per day through formal exercise; (2) the weekly deficit will be at least 4515 calories (i.e., 645 calories per day multiplied by seven plus an additional deficit caused by the increased metabolism secondary to the exercise); (3) the theoretical weight loss will be 1.3 lbs per week and 5.5 lbs per month. Carol's theoretical measurements at the end of each of the 7 months, which will be utilized as the body composition and pant size STGs are in **Table 10-1.**

Because the second global goal and the four specific goals are related to wellness (i.e., activities and behaviors, rather than a static status), target dates need not be mandated. Instead, a gradual increase in wellness that is determined by shorter term gains in wellness should be facilitated.

Anticipated Frequency

While the total number of visits will be dependent upon Carol's progress and needs for continuing reassessments and interventions, a reasonable estimate is 19 sessions: four during the week 1, two during week 2, one during weeks 3 and 4, and one during months 2 through 12.

Table 10-1 Short-Term Goals

Theoretical Goals	Percent Body Fat	Body Weight	Fat Weight	Lean Body Weight	Pants Size
			lbs		
Baseline	34%	160	54.5	105.5	12/14
End of month 1	~32.5%	~154.5	~50.2	~104.3	12
End of month 2	~31%	~149	~46.2	~102.8	10/12
End of month 3	~29.5%	~143.5	~42.3	~101.2	10
End of month 4	~28%	~138	~38.6	~99.4	8/10
End of month 5	~26.5%	~132.5	~35.1	~97.4	8
End of month 6	~25%	~127	~31.75	~95.25	6/8
End of month 7	~24%	~125	~30	~95	6

Note: The composition of weight loss will be of high quality: 75% will be in the form of fat (i.e., 4.1 lbs) and 25% will be in the form of muscle mass (i.e., 1.4 lbs).

Interventions

The primary interventions are patient/client education and a home program. The patient/client education interventions are discussed in the following subsections. The home program consists of instructing the patient/client to practice certain interventions that she or he has been taught.

Educational Instruction Related to Body Composition

Given Carol's baseline body composition wellness and the corresponding goals, the areas of instruction include, but are not limited to (1) water loss (diuresis) during the initial phase of her low-calorie diet secondary to glycogen breakdown rather than fat loss; (2) the likelihood of weight plateaus later in the diet secondary to the body's resistance to significantly change its set point; (3) the long-term value of body composition wellness (e.g., consistently exercising vs. no exercise); (4) the effects and risks of wearing a sweat suit in a sauna; and (5) the value of leisure activities in caloric output and fat loss.

Educational Instruction Related to Fitness Wellness

Given Carol's baseline fitness wellness level and the corresponding goals, the areas of instruction include, but are not limited to (1) the purpose of a warm-up; (2) how to estimate the intensity of the exercise session through palpation of heart rate and rating of perceived exertion; (3) why and how much water to drink before, during, and after an exercise session; (4) why and what she should do to "cool down" following her exercise; and (5) the frequency of the aerobic capacity exercise sessions and the frequency of the muscular fitness exercise sessions during each successive week (**Table 10-2**).

Table 10-2 Frequency of Carol's Exercise Program

Week Number	Aerobic Exercise	Muscular Exercise	Total Number of Sessions
Week 1	2×/week	1×/week	3×/week
Week 2	2×/week	2×/week	4×/week
Week 3	3×/week	2×/week	5×/week
Week 4	4×/week	2×/week	6×/week
Week 5	4×/week	3×/week	7×/week
Week 6+	4× or 5×/week	3×/week if aerobic is 4×/week; 2×/week if aerobic is 5×/week	7×/week

Educational Instruction Related to Aerobic Capacity Exercise

Given Carol's baseline aerobic capacity wellness and the goal to engage in 30 minutes of moderate intensity aerobic capacity exercise four or five times per week, the areas of instruction include, but are not limited to (1) confirmation that Carol's warm-up of a brisk walk is appropriate; (2) how to estimate the intensity of the exercise session through palpation of heart or the perceived activity scale; (3) confirming that her duration of 30 minutes is appropriate; (4) why she should aerobically exercise twice per week for the first 2 weeks, aerobically exercise three times per week for the next week, aerobically exercise four times per week for the next week, and then enter into a maintenance phase of exercising each day through a combination of aerobic exercise 4 or 5 days per week and strength training 2 or 3 days per week (Table 10-2); and (5) confirming that her mode of exercise, brisk walking, is an excellent choice, especially when she can involve her daughter and/or walk outdoors and enjoy nature but discussing alternatives (e.g., swimming and her other resources as she reported in the tests and measures).

Educational Instruction Related to Muscular Fitness Exercise

Given Carol's baseline muscular fitness wellness and the goal to engage in 20 minutes of strength-training exercise two or three times per week, education related to muscular fitness and muscular fitness include but are not limited to (1) providing examples of warm-ups for strength training; (2) proper body mechanics while weight lifting; (3) the benefits of aerobic strength training, especially in terms of fat loss; (4) how to engage in aerobic strength training, including which muscle groups to include; (5) the myth of spot reduction; (6) muscular hypertrophy in men versus women in response to strength training; and (7) why she should strength train once per week for the first week, twice per week for 3 weeks, three times per week for 1 week, and then enter into a maintenance phase of exercising each day through a combination of aerobic exercise 4 or 5 days per week and strength training 2 or 3 days per week (Table 10-2).

Educational Instruction Related to Nutritional Wellness

Given Carol's baseline nutritional wellness as it relates to body composition and the goal to adopt healthier eating habits, the areas of instruction include but are not limited to (1) the role of nutritional intake in caloric balance and fat loss; (2) the healthful aspects of healthful "starchy" foods; (3) importance of drinking clean water and how much to drink each day; (4) fiber intake when trying to lose fat weight and the types of foods that are high in fiber; (5) limit intake to about 1420 calories per day (to ensure the correct caloric intake, utilize the *Nutritive Values of Foods* [U.S. DOA, 2002], a free Internet Web site such as iGoogle calorie calculator [available at http://www.google.com/ig? hl=en&referrer=ign], or other reputable software program [e.g., NutriBase Junior Edition at http://www.dietsoftware.com/pricing.shtml]; (6) eat 2.5 cups or more of vegetables per day; (7) eat 1.5 cups of fruits per day; (8) eat 6 ounces of grains per day, with at least three of these as whole grain; (9) eat 5 ounces of meat and beans per day; (10) drink 3 cups of low-fat or preferably skim milk per day; (11) limit sugars found in cookies and other junk foods; (12) limit fats found in fried foods, mayonnaise, egg yolks, butter, and fatty meats; (13) eat a healthy breakfast (e.g., a high-fiber cereal with low-fat or skim milk); (14) eat a healthy lunch (e.g., a dark green leafy salad with low-calorie dressing); (15) spread her food and calories out over the whole day and do not consume most of them in the evening or night time; (16) eat in environments designated for meals (i.e., at the dining room table rather than in the car); and (17) do not consume a large proportion of "liquid meals"; that is, substitute real food with liquid meals and substitute some of the juice with eating a piece of fruit with the skin.

Given Carol's baseline antistress wellness and the goal to enhance it as it relates to body composition wellness, educate Carol about the stress-reducing benefits of exercise and introduce her to self-help materials.

Education Related to Interventions to Enhance Self-Esteem

Two resources are Mayo Clinic's *Self-Esteem: Boost Your Self-Image with These 5 Steps* (available at http://www.mayoclinic.com/health/self-esteem/MH00129) and *Building Self-Esteem: A Self-Help Guide* (available at http://mentalhealth.samhsa.gov/publications/allpubs/sma-3715/activities.asp).

Referrals

If Carol is unable to comprehend how to adhere to a nutritional program that is lower in calories and/or emphasizes healthy food choices, then it is indicated to refer her to a dietician.

It is indicated to refer Carol to a mental health practitioner if her symptoms of emotional eating continue or worsen.

Outcomes

The cumulative effect of the wellness-related physical therapy on Carol will be positive and significant. She will reverse her 5-year pattern of gaining (fat) weight, reduce her amount of body fat to a healthy level and to one with which she is happy, considerably improve her diet and exercise habits, and enhance her antistress wellness and self-esteem. Her health status—including but not limited to her maximal oxygen consumption, muscular strength, body composition, and risks for health-related disorders—will be reduced. Her exercise habits alone will reduce her risk of developing diabetes, hypertension, colon cancer, depression, and anxiety as well as her risk of dying from heart disease or prematurely (National Center for Chronic Disease Prevention and Health Promotion, 1999, supported in 2008). Secondary to these improvements in health and wellness, her quality of life will be enhanced.

chapter eleven

Community Wellness

If I have one hour to save the world
I would spend fifty-five minutes defining the problem
and only five minutes finding the solution.

■ ■ ■ ■ ■ ■ ■ ■ ■ ■ ■ ■ ■ ■ ■

Albert Einstein (1879–1955)

OBJECTIVES

Upon successful completion of this chapter, you should be able to:

1. Examine the Health Belief Model and discuss how it can be applied to wellness initiatives facilitated by physical therapists.
2. Discuss a variety of wellness and prevention programs identified by the American Physical Therapy Association.
3. List and discuss the phases of a community wellness project, examine the application of these phases to a scenario, and be able apply the process to a wellness initiative.
4. Discuss corporate fitness (community wellness) in the workplace.

SECTION 1: THE HEALTH BELIEF MODEL

The Health Belief Model is one of the oldest and most widely used health models (Ogden, 2007). It is a psychological model that attempts to explain and predict health behaviors of communities by focusing on the attitudes and beliefs of the individuals within those communities. The Health Belief Model was developed in the 1950s by social psychologists (Hochbaum, Rosenstock, & Kegels) working in the U.S. Public Health Services in response to the failure of a free tuberculosis health screening program (Glanz & Rimer, 2005). Since then, it has been adapted to explore a variety of long- and short-term health behaviors, most notably sexual risk behaviors and the transmission of the human immunodeficiency virus (HIV) and acquired immune deficiency syndrome (AIDS). It also can be successfully adapted to explore health behaviors specific to physical therapy and wellness.

The Health Belief Model consists of five constructs: (1) perceived susceptibility, (2) perceived severity, (3) perceived benefits, (4) perceived barriers, (5) cues to action, and (6) self-efficacy (Ogden, 2007). Ogden's description of each of these constructs follow: (1) perceived susceptibility is the individual's opinion about the chances of getting a condition (e.g., the risk of obesity); (2) perceived severity is the seriousness and consequences of a condition (e.g., comorbidities and premature death); (3) perceived benefits is the individual's belief in the efficacy of the advised intervention (e.g., the positive impact that exercise has upon decreasing the risk of obesity); (4) perceived barriers are the opinions about the psychological and tangible costs of the recommended action (e.g., the time, cost, and discomfort related to exercise); (5) cues to action are the strategies to activate readiness (e.g., a person consults with a physical therapist); and (6) self-efficacy is one's confidence in the ability to successfully perform the desired action (e.g., the person is certain he or she can start and adhere to an exercise program).

Summary: The Health Belief Model

The Health Belief Model consists of perceived susceptibility, perceived severity, perceived benefits, perceived barriers, cues to action, and self-efficacy (Ogden, 2007) and can be utilized by physical therapists to enhance community wellness.

SECTION 2: WELLNESS AND PREVENTION PROGRAMS SUGGESTED BY THE AMERICAN PHYSICAL THERAPY ASSOCIATION

According to the American Physical Therapy Association (APTA, 2001b), wellness and prevention programs can be administered at the individual level, the group level, the organization level, and the governmental-policy level.

Individual Interventions

These include (1) pre-performance testing of individuals who are active in sports, and (2) identification of lifestyle factors (e.g., amount of exercise, stress, weight) that may lead to increased risk for serious health problems (APTA, 2001b, p. 41).

Group-Level Interventions

The APTA (2001b, p. 41) has many suggestions of types of group-level interventions.

1. "Healthy Back" programs (e.g., how to prevent and manage back pain).
2. Pregnancy wellness programs
3. Promoting the use of cycling helmets to prevent head injury
4. Smoking cessation to reduce risk for cardiopulmonary disease
5. Workplace ergonomic redesign
6. Postural training to prevent job-related disabilities trauma and repetitive stress injuries
7. Exercise programs that include weight bearing and weight training to increase bone mass and bone density (especially in older adults with osteoporosis)
8. Exercise programs, gait training, and balance and coordination activities to reduce the risk of falls and fractures from falls in older adults
9. Exercise programs and instruction in activities of daily living (ADL) and instrumental (IADLs) for individuals diagnosed with cardiovascular/pulmonary disorders to decrease utilization of healthcare services and enhance function and/or prevent disability and dysfunction
10. Exercise programs to prevent or reduce the development of sequelae in individuals with life-long conditions
11. Identification of lifestyle factors (e.g., amount of exercise, stress, weight) that may lead to increased risk for serious health problems

Group and organization interventions (APTA, 2001b, p. 41) include: (1) Screening and exercise programs to increase bone density (to reduce risk/severity of osteoporosis), (2) Cardiopulmonary Wellness Program to enhance ADLs and IADLs, (3) Work-Place Intervention, (4) Conduct pre-work screenings, (5) Identification of risk factors for neuromusculoskeletal injuries in the workplace, (6) Identification of elderly individuals in a community center or nursing home who are high risk for falls, (7) Identification of children who may need an examination for idiopathic scoliosis, (8) Identification of children who are sedentary and who could benefit from extra-curricular physical activity.

Policy-Level Interventions

The APTA (2001b, p. 41) defines policy-level interventions as "broad-based consumer education and advocacy programs to prevent problems such as head injury by promoting the use of helmets and pulmonary disease by encouraging smoking cessation."

Summary: Examples from the American Physical Therapy Association

The APTA (2001b) provides numerous examples of wellness and prevention interventions.

SECTION 3: COMMUNITY WELLNESS PROJECTS

Phases of a Community Wellness Project

To provide community wellness, and enhance the likelihood that the services are of maximum benefit, the initiative should be well designed before being enacted. My proposal for a community wellness project model consists of eight phases and is based upon an application of the APTA's (2001b) Preferred Practice Pattern. The phases are

1. Select the target population and wellness problem, tentative goal, and tentative intervention(s).
2. Perform an abbreviated meta-analysis of the issue that explores the problem itself, potential interventions, and their potential outcomes.
3. Survey and screen the target population and, as applicable, select groups that can provide pertinent information about the target population.
4. Examine or pretest the target population and evaluate the results (Note: If the problem is related to wellness, use a survey; if the problem is related to health, do not).
5. Identify the prognosis, including a description of the plan of care, goals, and intervention(s).
6. Provide the intervention(s).
7. Perform a reexamination (posttest), and determine the results.
8. Compare the results of the pretest and the posttest or otherwise analyze the outcomes.

Abbreviated Scenario of a Community Wellness Project

An abbreviated example of a physical therapist utilizing the eight-phase model to facilitate community wellness is as follows.

Phase 1: Select the Target Population and Wellness Problem, Tentative Goal, and Tentative Intervention(s)

The physical therapist, Dr. Embury, selects the residents at a local assisted living facility (ALF) as her target population and decides to focus on their apparent problem of inactivity. Dr. Embury selects a tentative goal of increased activity and tentatively believes that the intervention will be some form a group exercise class. Because the target population consists of assisted living residents, Dr. Embury obtains permission from the prospective participants and the assisted living facility, and also ensures that each participant has received the appropriate medical clearance to participate in an exercise program.

Phase 2: Perform an Abbreviated Meta-Analysis of the Issue That Explores the Problems Itself, Potential Interventions, and Their Potential Outcomes

Dr. Embury reviews the empirical evidence related to the efficacy of various exercise programs in the elderly, including traditional modes of exercise such as walking and other modes of exercise such as tai chi. (1) Ourania, Yvoni, Christas, and Ionannis (2003) concluded that the physical abilities of previously sedentary women who exercise as little as once per week for 10 weeks improve significantly. (2) Chen et al. (2008) found that a simplified tai chi exercise program decreased systolic and diastolic blood pressure, increased bilateral hand-grip strength, and increased lower body flexibility in geriatric residents living in long-term care facilities.

Phase 3: Survey and Screen the Target Population and, as Applicable, Select Groups That Can Provide Pertinent Information About the Target Population

Through surveys and discussions with the facility's nursing staff, Dr. Embury screens various aspects related to the residents' proposed problem of inactivity. These are as follows: demographics and other basic information about the population, including the total number of residents, the percent of each gender, and the median age and the age range; their most prevalent diseases and conditions; the mobility and ambulatory levels of the population; exercise preferences of the residents; facility's staffing, financial, and related contributions to the wellness program as well as ability of the residents to self-pay for all or part of the wellness services.

Dr. Embury learns that there are 90 residents of whom 36 (90%) are women and four (10%) are male. Their average age is 82 with a range from age 65 through 92. Their most prevalent diseases and conditions are impaired fitness wellness, impaired mental wellness, impaired social wellness, arthritis (that does not interfere with activity on a daily basis), impaired balance (that necessitates the use of an assistive device to safely ambulate), hypertension (controlled with antihypertensive medication), depression (largely alleviated with antidepressant medication), high cholesterol (largely addressed with medication), and hypothyroidism and anemia (both addressed with medication). All residents are independent in their mobility, but 10% require a standard cane, 10% require a rolling walker (a few of these a regular walker), and 5% need a wheelchair. The most popular exercise choices are any kind of activity involving a ball, dancing, and walking outside. The facility administration is willing to allocate four full-time equivalent (FTE) staff (e.g., one activities/marketing coordinator and three aides) for a total of 3 hours per week to sponsor a wellness program.) A total of 80% of the residents responded that they do not have the financial resources to self-pay for exercise classes; 20% of the residents responded that they could pay about $6.00 to $10.00 to participate in two to three exercise classes per week, and 80% of these were among the 25% who do not require an assistive device to independently ambulate.

Phase 4: Examine or Pretest the Target Population and Evaluate the Results

Because wellness (i.e., habitual practices) is to be measured, Dr. Embury examines the fitness wellness of the residents with a survey. The results of the cognitive component are that 10% are able to name one benefit of regular exercise and 90% of the residents are able to list two or more of the benefits of regular exercise. The results of the psychomotor component are that 80% of the residents do not exercise at all, 10% exercise once per week, 5% exercise twice per week, and 5% exercise three times per week (thus, 20% of the residents exercise at least once per week). In all cases, the mode of exercise is walking and the average duration is 30 minutes. The results of the affective component are that 80% are committed to exercise and 20% are not; specifically, 80% state that, if offered, they agree to join an exercise class at least once per week and 20% state that they will not join a group exercise class. The evaluation of the tests and measures and the information obtained from the screens are that the cognitive and psychomotor aspects of residents' fitness wellness are unsatisfactory/poor, but their affective fitness wellness is satisfactory/good. There are sufficient resources to provide group exercise classes that will enhance the residents' overall wellness, including their fitness wellness, and satisfy their activity preferences. The conditions/diagnoses and mobility levels with which the residents present require consideration when developing and implementing the plan of care, but are manageable. An option for the posttest is the 6-month mark.

Phase 5: Identify the Prognosis, Including a Description of the Plan of Care, Goals, and Intervention(s)

Dr. Embury stipulates that the prognosis of the wellness program is to enhance the physical, mental, and social wellness of the residents of the assisted living facility.

The plan of care of the wellness program is to offer group exercise classes and to train the activities coordinator to facilitate the group classes. The group classes are held three times per week on Mondays, Wednesdays, and Fridays. Each session is 30 minutes in duration. The activity classes are free to the residents. The administration of the assisted living facility will be fully apprised of the wellness plan and the outcomes to ensure their continued support.

The broad goal of the wellness program is to enhance the fitness wellness of the participants. The broad secondary, yet unmeasured, goal is to enhance mental and social wellness. Three specific goals are to (1) enhance the cognitive component of fitness wellness such that 60% of the residents are able to list two or more of the benefits of regular exercise and an additional 20% are able to name one benefit of regular exercise; (2) enhance the psychomotor component of fitness wellness such that 40% of the residents exercise once per week, 25% exercise twice per week, and 25% exercise three times per week (i.e., 60% of the residents exercise at least once per week); and (3) enhance the affective component of fitness wellness such that 90% of the residents are committed to exercise (i.e., 90% state that, if offered, they agree to participate in an exercise class at least once per week).

The Monday and Friday classes consist of activities with a ball (e.g., kicking or throwing a ball to one another while standing or, if required for safety, guarding by an aide or sitting in a chair or wheelchair). Each Monday's class also includes a very brief review of the benefits of regular exercise. The exercise class on Wednesdays consists of one-on-one dancing with another resident or, if required for safety, with an aide or the activities coordinator. It is anticipated that the "dance class" will be primarily attended by those residents with a higher level of mobility; that is, those who do not require an assistive device or only require a cane to ambulate. The duration of each exercise session is 30 minutes. Each exercise session also includes a light warm-up before the exercise session and a light cool-down following the exercise session. The residents also are encouraged to begin or continue an independent walking program. Educational guidance is provided to those who need it.

Phase 6: Provide the Intervention(s)

The activities coordinator leads the group exercise classes as described in Phase 5. Dr. Embury occasionally visits part of a group exercise session and otherwise makes herself available to answer questions the activities coordinator may have.

Phase 7: Perform a Reexamination or Posttest and Determine the Results

Dr. Embury reexamines the residents' cognitive, psychomotor, and affective fitness wellness 6 months following the initiation of the group classes. The same survey instrument from the initial survey is used for the reexamination except for a slight modification of the affective questions. The results are (1) 50% of the residents are able to list two or more of the benefits of regular exercise and an additional 10% are able to name one benefit of regular exercise; (2) half (50%) of the residents exercise once per week, 10% exercise twice per week, and 10% exercise three times per week (i.e., 70% of the residents exercise at least once per week); and (3) 50% of the residents agree to participate in an exercise class once per week as long as it continues to be offered, 10% agree to participate in two exercise classes per week, and 10% participate in three exercise classes per week.

Phase 8: Compare the Results of the Pretest and the Posttest and Otherwise Analyze the Outcomes

Initially, 10% of the residents were able to name one benefit of regular exercise and another 10% were able to list two or more benefits. Following the wellness intervention, 50% of the residents were able to name one benefit of regular exercise and another 10% were able to list two or more benefits. Thus, as measured by the survey, the wellness intervention significantly increased the cognitive aspect of residents' fitness wellness.

Initially, only 5% of the residents exercised three times per week, 5% exercised twice per week, 10% exercised once per week, and 80% did not exercise at all (i.e., 20% exercised at least once per week). Following the wellness intervention, 10% exercised three times per week, 10% exercised twice per week, and 50% did so once per week (i.e., 70% of the residents exercised at least once per week). The duration of the exercise sessions was 30 minutes. Thus, the wellness intervention significantly increased the psychomotor aspect of residents' fitness wellness. Initially, 80% of the residents were committed to fitness wellness. Following the intervention, this dropped to 70%. While it appears that the wellness intervention adversely influenced the affective component of the residents' fitness wellness, it is more likely that the 70% is simply a more realistic percentage of assisted living residents that can be facilitated to be motivated to exercise on a regular basis. The global outcomes are increased fitness wellness.

Summary: One Community Wellness Project

A model for community wellness projects based upon the APTA's (2001b) Preferred Practice Patterns consists of eight phases that can be summarized as tentative selections; an abbreviated meta-analysis; survey and screens; an examination/pretest and evaluation of the results; prognosis, plan of care, goal(s), and intervention(s); provision of the intervention(s); a reexamination/posttest and description of results; and an analysis of the outcomes.

SECTION 4: CORPORATE FITNESS

While community wellness is a humanitarian initiative that promotes the physical, mental, and/or social wellness of its constituents, a corporation sponsoring an in-house wellness program to its employees also enjoys significant financial gains.

MetLife converted a recreational gymnasium into a wellness facility that initiated fitness assessments, customized workouts, and offered exercise classes to enhance cardiovascular health (Corry, 1990). Six months of exercise treatment produced favorable cardiovascular trends with decreases of 3.6% in resting heart rate, 6.4% in total cholesterol, 3.5% in systolic blood pressure, 2.8% in diastolic blood pressure and an increase of 2.7% in HDL cholesterol (Corry, 1990). Such health benefits can translate into reduced absenteeism as well as decreased hospital admissions and lengths of stay (Bly, Jones, & Richardson, 1986; Breuleux, Heck, Hollenback, & Kinzer, 1993).

Johnson and Johnson's "Live for Life" corporate fitness program resulted in an 18% reduction in absenteeism by the third year of the program (Bly et al., 1986). Mean annual inpatient cost increases were $43 and $42 for two Live for Life groups, while it rose $76 for the non-Live for Life group. Live for Life groups also had lower rates of increase in hospital days and admissions. Similarly, Breuleux et al. (1993) concluded that the medical costs of corporate employees that regularly utilized in-house fitness centers were less than the medical costs of those that did not.

Corporate fitness initiatives also result in fewer and less serious workplace injuries. For example, in one corporation, the introduction of an in-house fitness program caused a reduction in workmen's compensation claims from 8.9% to 5.6% and the cost of the average injury from $9,482 to $6,506 (Associated Press, as cited in *Physical Therapy Bulletin Online*, 2002).

There is also a positive correlation between exercise adherence in a corporate fitness program and above average job performance; however, there is a lack of evidence that the relationship is causal (Bernacki & Baun, 1984).

The benefits of corporate fitness are difficult to dispute. In fact, there is an increased cost to companies that do not integrate wellness initiatives (Anderson, Brink, & Courtney, 1995). For instance, claims related to hypertension increased 7%, physician use related to hypertension increased 11%, inpatient hospital stays related to hypertension increased 24%, inpatient hospital stays related to obesity increased 143%, smoking claims increased 31%, claims related to poor eating habits increased 41%, inpatient hospital stays related to stress increased 13%, and physician use related to stress increased 26% (Anderson et al., 1995).

However, while many corporations provide employees the option of participating in on-site fitness centers, utilization rates are low (Schwetschenau, O'Brian, Cunningham, &

Jey, 2008). The perceived barriers for nonparticipation in corporate fitness are external and internal. External environmental barriers, such as inadequate exercise facilities, have been found to significantly account for employees not joining a corporate fitness center and for decreased duration of visits to the facility among members. Internal barriers, such as feeling embarrassed to exercise around coworkers, significantly accounts for the frequency of fitness center visits among members (Schwetschenau et al., 2008). To increase the use of on-site fitness centers, Schwetschenau et al. (2008) recommends that corporations address the perceived barriers of their employees. One option is to allow employees the time and flexibility to integrate wellness activities into their normal work day (for example, walking or cycling to and from work). According to Shepard (1992), this option of daily integration may prove more acceptable and more cost-effective than having to rely upon formal work-site classes.

Summary: Corporate Fitness

While community wellness is considered a humanitarian initiative, there is evidence that it reduces costs in the workplace, including increased efficiency and productivity, increased health, decreased work injuries, decreased absenteeism, decreased employee turnover, and increased labor relations. There is an increased cost to companies that do not integrate wellness (Anderson et al., 1995). Corporations need to address their employees' perceived barriers to participating in the in-house fitness program (Schwetschenau et al., 2008) as well as encourage the integration of wellness activities into their daily lives (Shepard, 1992).

References

Adams, E. J., Grummer-Strawn, L. M., & Chavez, G. (2003). Food insecurity is associated with increased risk of obesity among California women. *Journal of Nutrition, 133,* 1070-1074.

Adams, S. A., Der Ananian, C. A., DuBose, K. D., Kirtland, K. A., & Ainsworth, B. E. (2003). Physical activity levels among overweight and obese adults in South Carolina. *Southern Medical Journal, 96*(6), 141-145.

Adams, T. B., Bezner, J. R., Drabbs, M. E., Zambarano, R. J., & Steinhardt, M. A. (2000). Conceptualization and measurement of the spiritual and psychological dimensions of wellness in a college population. *Journal of American College of Health, 48*(4), 165-173.

Adams, T. B., Bezner, J. R., Gamer, L., & Woodruff, S. (1998). Construct validation of the perceived wellness survey. *American Journal of Health Studies, 14*(4), 212-220.

Adams, T. B., Bezner, J. R., & Steinhardt, M. (1997). The conceptualization and measurement of perceived wellness: Integrating balance across and within dimensions. *American Journal of Health Promotion, 12,* 380-388.

Agatston, A. (2005). *The South Beach diet quick and easy cookbook.* Emmaus, PA: Rodale.

Ainsworth, B. E., Montoye, H. J., & Leon, A. S. (1994). Methods of assessing physical activity during leisure and work. In C. Bouchard, R. J. Shephard, & T. Stephens (Eds.), *Physical activity, fitness, and health: International proceedings and consensus statement* (pp. 146-159). Champaign, IL: Human Kinetics.

Aizen, I., & Fishbein, M. (1980). *Understanding attitudes and predicting social behavior.* Englewood Cliffs, NJ: Prentice-Hall.

Akers, R., & Buskirk, E. R. (1969). An underwater weighing system utilizing "force cube" transducers. *Journal of Applied Physiology, 26,* 649-652.

Akinci, F., Healey, B. J., & Coyne, J. S. (2003). Improving health status of U.S. working adults with type 2 diabetes. *Disease Management Health Outcomes, 11*(8), 489-498.

Albanese, C. V. (2003). Clinical applications of body composition measurements using DXA. *Journal of Clinical Densitometry, 6*(2), 75-85.

Aldoori, W. H., Giovannucci, E. L., Rockett, H. R., Sampson, L., Rimm, E. B., & Willett, W. C. (1998). A prospective study of dietary fiber types and symptomatic diverticular disease in men. *Journal of Nutrition, 128,* 714-719.

Aldoori, W. H., & Rahman, S. H. (1998). Smoking and stroke: A causative role. *British Medical Journal, 317,* 962-963.

Alén, M., Reinilä, M., & Vihko, R. (1985). Response of serum hormones to androgen administration in power athletes. *Medicine & Science in Sports & Exercise, 17*(3), 354-359.

Alfieri, M. A., Pomerleau, J., Grace, D. M., & Anderson, L. (1995). Fiber intake of normal weight, moderately obese and severely obese subjects. *Obesity Research, 3*(6), 541-547.

Alonso, J., Buron, A., Bruffaerts, R., He, Y., Posada-Villa, J., Lepine, J. P., et al. [The World Mental Health Consortium]. (2008, August). Association of Perceived Stigma and Mood and Anxiety Disorders: Results from the World Mental Health Surveys. *Acta Psychiatrica Scandinavica, 118*(4), 305-314.

Alternative. (2008). In *Dictionary.com unabridged (v. 1.1)*. Retrieved October 19, 2008, from Dictionary.com Web site: http://dictionary.reference.com/search?q=alternative

Altmaier, E. M., Lehmann, T. R., Russell, D. W., Weinstein, J. N., & Kao, C. F. (1991). The effectiveness of psychological interventions for the rehabilitation of low back pain: A randomized controlled trial evaluation. *Pain, 49*, 329-335.

Alu, D. (2006). Taking a holistic approach to treatment. *News-Line: For Physical Therapists and Physical Therapy Assistants, 11*, 4-5.

American Academy of Pediatrics. (2008). *Teen Q&A: Steroids.* Retrieved May 30, 2009, from http://www.aap.org/publiced/BR_Teen_Steroids.htm

American College of Sports Medicine. (2000). *ACSM's guidelines for exercise testing and prescription* (6th ed.). Philadelphia: Lippincott Williams & Wilkins.

American College of Sports Medicine. (2001). *ACSM health/fitness instructor.* Retrieved May 6, 2004, from http://www.lww.com/acsmcrc/hfinstr.html

American College of Sports Medicine. (2004). *ACSM certification and registry programs.* Retrieved May 6, 2004, from http://www.acsm.org/certification/getcertified.htm

American College of Sports Medicine. (2006). *ACSM's guidelines for exercise testing and prescription* (7th ed.). Philadelphia: Lippincott Williams & Wilkins.

American College of Sports Medicine. (2007). *ACSM's health-related physical fitness assessment manual.* Philadelphia: Lippincott Williams & Wilkins.

American Council on Exercise. (2006). *Abdominal curl.* Retrieved July 10, 2006, from http://www.acefitness.org/getfit/exercise_display.aspx?pageID=434

American Diabetes Association. (n.d.). *Total prevalence of diabetes & pre-diabetes.* Retrieved August 30, 2009, from http://www.diabetes.org/diabetes-statistics/prevalence.jsp

American Dietetic Association. (2003, June). Vegetarian diets. *Journal of the American Dietetic Association, 103*(6), 748-765.

American Heart Association. (2008a). *African Americans and cardiovascular diseases: Statistics.* Retrieved May 30, 2009, from http://www.americanheart.org/downloadable/heart/1197933296813FS01AF08.pdf

American Heart Association. (2008b). *Whites and cardiovascular diseases: Statistics.* Retrieved May 30, 2009, from http://www.americanheart.org/downloadable/heart/1199827443697FS09WHT08.DOC

American Heart Association. (2009a). *Cigarette smoking statistics.* Retrieved May 30, 2009, from http://www.americanheart.org/presenter.jhtml?identifier=4559

American Heart Association. (2009b). *Know your fats.* Retrieved May 30, 2009, from http://www.americanheart.org/presenter.jhtml?identifier=532

American Heart Association. (2009c). *Fat.* Retrieved July 30, 2009, from http://www.americanheart.org/presenter.jhtml?identifier=4582

American Journal of Health Promotion. (n.d.). *Definition of health promotion.* Retrieved May 30, 2009, from http://www.healthpromotionjournal.com/

American Lung Association. (2009). *Smoking and women fact sheet.* Retrieved May 30, 2009, from http://www.lungusa.org/site/c.dvLUK9O0E/b.33572/

American Medical Association. (2008). *AMA: Helping doctors help patients.* Retrieved June 30, 2008, from http://www.ama-assn.org/ama/pub/category/1810.html

American Occupational Therapy Association. (2000). Occupational therapy in the promotion of health and the prevention of disease and disability statement. *American Journal of Occupational Therapy, 55*(6), 656-660.

American Occupational Therapy Association. (2002). *Occupational therapy practice framework domain and process.* Bethesda, MD: Author.

American Physical Therapy Association. (1993). *Health promotion and wellness by physical therapists and physical therapist assistants*: *HOD 06-93-25-50.* Retrieved August 6, 2004, from http://www.apta.org/governance/HOD/policies/HoDPolicies/Section_I/HEALTH,-_SOCIAL,_AND,_ENVI/HOD_06932550

American Physical Therapy Association. (1996). Evaluative criteria for accreditation of education programs for the preparation of physical therapists. *Accreditation Handbook: PT criteria.* Retrieved September 1, 2004, from http://www.apta.org/pdfs/-accreditation/AppendixB-PT-Criteria.pdf

American Physical Therapy Association. (1997). *Guide to physical therapist practice.* Alexandria, VA: Author.

American Physical Therapy Association. (2001a). *Fitness and wellness consultation course.* Retrieved August 8, 2004, from http://www.apta.org/PT_Practice/prevention_wellness/fit_and_well/fitwell_outline

American Physical Therapy Association. (2001b). *Guide to physical therapist practice* (2nd ed.). *Journal of the American Physical Therapy Association, 81*(1), 1-768.

American Physical Therapy Association. (2003a). *Goals that represent the 2003 priorities of the American Physical Therapy Association.* Retrieved July 10, 2009, from http://www.apta.org/AM/Template.cfm?Section=Home&CONTENTID=43122&TEMPLATE=/CM/ContentDisplay.cfm

American Physical Therapy Association. (2003b). Wellness programs serve the "whole" patient with chronic pain, presenter says. *PT 2003 news and highlights.* Retrieved June 30, 2003, from http://www.apta.org/Meetings/past_events/pt2003/news_pt2003/june19

American Physical Therapy Association. (2004a). *APTA mission statement.* Retrieved August 14, 2004, from http://www.apta.org/About/aptamissiongoals/aptamissionstatement

American Physical Therapy Association. (2004b). *A historical perspective.* Retrieved August 8, 2004, from http://www.apta.org/About/apta_history/history

American Physical Therapy Association. (2004d). *Policies.* Retrieved August 18, 2004, from http://www.apta.org/governance/HOD/policies/HoDPolicies/hodExplanation

American Physical Therapy Association. (2004e). *Search.* Retrieved August 31, 2004, from http://www.apta.org/membership/Members_Directory

American Physical Therapy Association. (2006a). *2006–2020 education strategic plan.* Alexandria, VA: Author.

American Physical Therapy Association. (2006b). *Goals that represent the priorities of the American Physical Therapy Association.* Retrieved May 30, 2009, from http://www.apta.org/AM/Template.cfm?Section=Policies_and_Bylaws&TEMPLATE=/CM/ContentDisplay.cfm&CONTENTID=25270

American Physical Therapy Association. (2007a). *Vision 2020.* Retrieved May 30, 2009, from http://www.apta.org/AM/Template.cfm?Section=Vision_20201&Template=/TaggedPage/TaggedPageDisplay.cfm&TPLID=285&ContentID=32061

American Physical Therapy Association. (2007b). *Working operational definitions of elements of Vision 2020 from the Task Force on Strategic Plan to achieve Vision 2020.* Retrieved May 30, 2009, from http://www.apta.org/AM/Template.cfm?Section=Vision_20201&CONTENTID=39951&TEMPLATE=/CM/ContentDisplay.cfm

American Physical Therapy Association. (2008a). *ABPTS online directory of certified clinical specialists in physical therapy.* Retrieved May 30, 2008, from http://www.apta.org/AM/Template.cfm?Section=ABPTS1&TEMPLATE=/CM/ContentDisplay.cfm&CONTENTID=38100

American Physical Therapy Association. (2008b). *APTA sections.* Retrieved May 30, 2008, from http://www.apta.org/AM/Template.cfm?Section=Chapters&Template=/CM/ContentDisplay.cfm&CONTENTID=36890

American Physical Therapy Association. (2008c). *Directory of state practice acts.* Retrieved December 15, 2008, from http://www.apta.org/AM/Template.cfm?Section=Home&Template=/TaggedPage/TaggedPageDisplay.cfm&TPLID=163&ContentID=24096

American Physical Therapy Association. (2008d). *Professionalism in physical therapy: Core Values BOD P05-04-02-03.* Retrieved June 30, 2008, from http://www.apta.org/AM/Template.cfm?Section=Logout&CONTENTID=36073&TEMPLATE=/CM/ContentDisplay.cfm

American Psychiatric Association. (2004). *Diagnostic and statistical manual of mental disorders* (4th ed.). Washington, DC: Author.

American Psychological Association. (2005). *New definition: Hypnosis.* Retrieved May 30, 2009, from http://www.apa.org/divisions/div30/define_hypnosis.html

Anderson, A. S., & Caswell, S. (2008). Obesity and cancer risk: A weighty problem for the 21st century. *Biologist, 55*(2), 100-104.

Anderson, D., Brink, S., & Courtney, T. D. (1995). The health risk on medical costs. *Medical Interface, 8*(12), 121-122.

Anderson, G. (n.d.). *Quotationsbook.* Retrieved July 10, 2009, from http://quotationsbook.com/quote/18678/

Andrews, F. M. (1984). Construct validity and error components of survey measures: A structural modeling approach. *Public Opinion Quarterly, 48*, 409-442.

Andrews, G., & Hunt, C. (1998). Treatments that work in anxiety disorders. *Medical Journal of Australia, 168*(12), 628-634.

Anspaugh, D., & Ezell, G. (2007). *Teaching today's health* (8th ed.). San Francisco: Benjamin Cummings.

Antonovsky, A. (1987). *Unraveling the mystery of health.* San Francisco: Jossey-Bass.

Apps, J. W. (1991). *Mastering the teaching of adults.* Malabar, FL: Krieger.

Aquinas, T. (n.d.). *On the principles of nature* (Gyula Klima, Trans.). Retrieved May 30, 2009, from http://www.fordham.edu/gsas/phil/klima/principles.htm

Ardell, D. B. (1977). *High level wellness.* Berkeley, CA: Ten Speed Press.

Ardell, D. B. (1982). *14 days to high level wellness.* Novato, CA: New World Library.

Ardell, D. B. (1985). Definition of wellness. *Ardell Wellness Report, 37,* 1-5.

Ardell, D. B. (1986a). Definition of wellness. *Ardell Wellness Report, 18,* 1-5.

Ardell, D. B. (1986b). *High level wellness.* Berkeley, CA: Ten Speed Press.

Ardell, D. B. (1990). *Ardell Wellness Report, 23,* 8.

Ardell, D. B. (1999). Definition of wellness. *Ardell Wellness Report, 18,* 1: 1-5.

Ardell, D. B. (2001). *Wellness models.* Retrieved May 30, 2009, from http://www.seekwellness.com/wellness/daily_reports/show_report.htm?reportdate=2001-05-10

Ardell, D. B. (2009a). *The nature of DBRU equivalents.* Retrieved May 30, 2009, from http://www.seekwellness.com/wellness/articles/DRBUs.htm

Ardell, D. B. (2009b). *Wellness models.* Retrieved May 30, 2009, from http://www.seekwellness.com/wellness/articles/wellness_models.htm

Arnett, P. A., Barwick, F. H., Beeney, J. E. (2008). Depression in multiple sclerosis: Review and theoretical proposal. *Journal of the International Neuropsychological Society, 14*(5), 691-724.

Asimov, I. (1982). *Asimov's biographical encyclopedia of science and technology* (2nd ed.). Garden City, NY: Doubleday.

Atkins "nightmare" diet. (2004). Retrieved May 30, 2009, from http://www.atkinsexposed.org/

Awakenings. (n.d.). *Burnout inventory.* Retrieved August 18, 2006, from http://www.lessons4living.com/burnout_inventory2.htm

Axler, C. T., & McGill, S. M. (1997). Low back loads over a variety of abdominal exercising: Searching for the safest abdominal exercise. *Medicine & Science in Sports & Exercise, 29*(6), 804-811.

Ayse, S., Fusan, A., Ozgen, M., Topuz, O., & Semez, Y. (2006). The effects of aerobics and resistance exercise in obese women. *Clinical Rehabilitation, 20*, 773-784.

Bachko, K. (2007). Eater's digest. *Dance Spirit, 11*(4), 34-37.

Bacurau, R. F., Monteiro, G. A., Ugrinowitsch, C., Tricoli, V., Cabral, L. F., & Aoki, M. S. (2009). Acute effect of a ballistic and a static stretching exercise bout on flexibility and maximal strength. *Journal of Strength and Conditioning Research, 23*(1), 304-308.

Baechle, T. R., & Earle, R. W. (Eds.). (2000). *Essentials of strength and conditioning* (2nd ed.). Champaign, IL: Human Kinetics.

Baecke, J. A., Burema, J., & Frijters, J. E. (1982). A short questionnaire for the measurement of habitual physical activity in epidemiological studies. *American Journal of Clinical Nutrition, 36*, 936-942.

Bagatell, C., Knopp, R., Vale, W., Rivier, J., & Bremner, W. (1992). Physiologic testosterone levels in normal men suppress high-density lipoprotein cholesterol levels. *Annals of Internal Medicine, 116*, 967-973.

Bailey, K. G., & Nava, G. (1989). Psychological kinship, love, and liking: Preliminary validity data. *Journal of Clinical Psychology, 45*(4), 587-594.

Bailey, L. T., & Lehigh, U. (1998). The wellness, positive psychological attitudes, and perceived faculty support of counseling psychology doctoral students. *Dissertation Abstracts International, 58*(11-b), 5883.

Ball, S. D. (2005). Interdevice variability in percent fat estimates using the BOD POD. *European Journal of Clinical Nutrition, 59*(9), 996-1001.

Bandura, A. (2004). Health promotion by social cognitive means. *Health Education Behavior, 31*(2), 143-164.

Bandura, A., Adams, N. E., & Beyer, J. (1977). Cognitive processes mediating behavioral change. *Journal of Personality and Social Psychology, 35*(3), 125-139.

Bandura, A., Barbaranelli, C., Caprara, G. V., & Pastorelli, C. (1996). Multifaceted impact of self-efficacy beliefs on academic functioning. *Child Development, 67*(3), 1206-1222.

Bandura, A., Caprara, G. V., Barbaranelli, C., Pastorelli, C., & Regalia, C. (2001). Sociocognitive self-regulatory mechanisms governing transgressive behavior. *Journal of Personality and Social Psychology, 80*(1), 125-135.

Bandura, A., & Locke, E. A. (2003). Negative self-efficacy and goal effects revisited. *Journal of Applied Psychology, 88*(1), 87-89.

Barack Obama's Inaugural Address [Transcript]. (2009, January 20). *New York Times.* Retrieved May 30, 2009, from http://www.nytimes.com/2009/01/20/us/politics/20text-obama.html?pagewanted=2&sq=obama%20inaugural%20address&st=cse&scp=1

Barber, B. (2000, April). Niche practices in geriatrics. *Magazine of Physical Therapy.* Retrieved June 30, 2003, from http://www.apta.org /pt_magazine/April00/geriatrics.html

Barnard, R. J., Grimditch, G. K., & Wilmore, J. H. (1979). Physiological characteristics of sprint and endurance masters runners. *Medicine & Science in Sports & Exercise, 11*(2), 167-171.

Barnes, P. (2007). *Physical activity among adults: United States, 2000 and 2005.* Retrieved May 30, 2009, from National Center for Health Statistics Web site: http://www.cdc.gov/nchs/products/pubs/pubd/hestats/physicalactivity/physicalactivity.htm

Barnett, L. D., & MacDonald, R. H. (1976). A study of the membership of the National Organization for Non-Parents. *Social Biology, 23*(4), 297-310.

Barrett-Connor, E. (1995). Testosterone and risk factors for cardiovascular disease in men. *Diabetes and Metabolism, 21*(3), 156-161.

Barriball, K. L., & While, A. E. (1999). Non-response in survey research: A methodological discussion and development of an explanatory model. *Journal of Advanced Nursing, 30*(3), 677-687.

Bas, M., & Donmez, S. (2009). Self-efficacy and restrained eating in relation to weight loss among overweight men and women in Turkey. *Appetite, 52*(1), 209-216.

Bass, C. (2007). Conversion syndrome. *Oxford Medical School Gazette, 57*(1). Retrieved May 30, 2009, from http://www.medsci.ox.ac.uk/gazette/previousissues/55vol2/Part6

Bassett, J. (2000, June 26). *Handling inappropriate patient behavior.* Retrieved May 30, 2009, from Advance for Physical Therapists & PT Assistants Web site: http://physical-therapy.advanceweb.com/Editorial/Content/Editorial.aspx?CC=9708

Bassett, J. (2001). Wellness and everyday practice. *Advance for Physical Therapists & PT Assistants, 12*(5), 6-7, 36.

Baume, P., O'Malley, E., & Bauman, A. (1995). Professed religious affiliation and the practice of euthanasia. *Journal of Medical Ethics, 21*(1), 49-54.

Baxter, J. D., & Rosseau, G. G. (1979). Glucocorticoid hormone action. *Endocrinology, 12*, 1-26.

BBC News. (1999). *Health: Steroid aid for kidney disease and HIV.* Retrieved March 20, 2009, from http://news.bbc.co.uk/1/hi/health/319016.stm

BBC News. (2004a). *UK among most secular nations.* Retrieved May 30, 2009, from http://news.bbc.co.uk/1/hi/programmes/wtwtgod/3518375.stm

BBC News. (2004b). What the world thinks of God. Retrieved May 30, 2009, from http://news.bbc.co.uk/1/shared/spl/hi/programmes/wtwtgod/pdf/wtwtogod.pdf

Bean, S. W., Bezner, J. R., & Otterback, H. H. (1998, May). PL-RR-190-SA: The relationship between perceived wellness, perceived physical function and traditional medical outcomes in physical therapy [Abstract]. *Physical Therapy, 78*(5), S64.

Beauregard, M., Courtemanche, J., Paquette, V., & St. Pierre, E. L. (2009). The neural basis of unconditional love. *Psychiatry Research, 172*(2), 93-98.

Becker, M. H. (n.d.). The health belief model and personal health behavior. *Health Education Monographs, 2*(4).

Becker, M. H., Radius, S. M., & Rosenstock, I. M. (1978). Compliance with a medical regimen for asthma: A test of the health belief model. *Public Health Reports, 93*, 268-277.

Beedle, B. B., Leydig, S. N., & Carnucci, J. M. (2007). No difference in pre- and postexercise stretching on flexibility. *Journal of Strength Conditioning and Research, 21*(3), 780-783.

Begley, C. M. (1996). Triangulation of communication skills in qualitative research instruments. *Journal of Advanced Nursing, 24*(4), 688-694.

Bellis, M. (2008). *Anton Van Leeuwenhoek.* Retrieved May 30, 2009, from http://inventors.about.com/library/inventors/blleeuwenhoek.htm

Bennet, W., & Gurin, J. (1982). *The dieter's dilemma: Eating less and weighing more.* New York: Basic Books.

Bennett, N., Greco, D. D., Peterson, M. E., Kirk, C., Mathes, M., & Fettman, M. J. (2006). Comparison of a low carbohydrate–low fiber diet and a moderate carbohydrate–high fiber diet in the management of feline mellitus. *Journal of Feline Medical Surgery, 8*(2), 73-84.

Bente, R. D., Hiza, H., & Fungwe, T. (2008). *Dietary fiber in the U.S. food supply.* Retrieved July 30, 2009, from http://www.cnpp.usda.gov/Publications/FoodSupply/DietaryFiberPPT1-23-08.ppt

Bentzur, K. M., Kravitz, L., & Lockner, D. W. (2008). Evaluation of the BOD POD for estimating percent body fat in collegiate track and field athletes: A comparison of four methods. *Journal of Strength and Conditioning Research, 22*(6), 1985-1991.

Berardi, J. M., Price, T. B., Noreen, E. E., & Lemon, P. W. (2006). Postexercise muscle glycogen recovery enhanced with a carbohydrate–protein supplement. *Medicine & Science in Sports & Exercise, 38*(6), 1106-1113.

Berg, C. (1952). Amended definition of anxiety. *British Journal of Medical Psychology, 12*(2-3), 158.

Bernacki, E. J., & Baun, W. B. (1984). The relationship of job performance to exercise adherence in a corporate fitness program. *Journal of Occupational Medicine, 26*(7), 529-531.

Best, J. W., & Kahn, V. (1989). *Research in education* (6th ed.). New York: Prentice-Hall.

Bingham, S. A., Everhart, J. E., Newman, A. B., Tylavsky, F. A. (2004). Water turnover in 458 American adults 40-79 yr of age. *American Journal of Renal Physiology, 286*, F394-F401.

Biomedical model. (n.d.). In *Wikipedia.org.* (2005). Retrieved May 30, 2008, from http://encyclopedia.thefreedictionary.com/biomedical+model

Biopsychosocial model. (n.d.). In *Wikipedia.org.* (2005). Retrieved May 30, 2008, from http://encyclopedia.thefreedictionary.com/biopsychosocial+model

Blair, S. N., & Nichaman, M. Z. (2002). The public health problem of increasing prevalence rates of obesity and what should be done about it. *Mayo Clinical Proceedings, 77*(2), 109-113.

Blatny, M., & Adam, Z. (2008). Type C personality (cancer personality): Current view and implications for future research. *Vnitrni Lekarstvi, 54*(6), 638-645.

Bloom, B. S. (1956). *Taxonomy of educational objectives, handbook I: The cognitive domain.* New York: David McKay.

Bloom, B. S. (1984). *Taxonomy of educational objectives.* Boston: Allyn and Bacon Pearson Education.

Blumenthal, J. A., Williams, R. B., Kong, R., Schanberg, S. M., & Thompson, L. W. (1978). Type A behavior pattern and coronary atherosclerosis. *Circulation, 58*(4), 634-639.

Bly, J. L., Jones, R. C., & Richardson, J. E. (1986). Impact of worksite promotion on health care costs and utilization: Evaluation of Johnson & Johnson's Live for Life program. *JAMA, 256*(23), 3235-3240.

Body Building Pro. (n.d.). *Body type information.* Retrieved May 30, 2009, from http://bodybuilding pro.com/bodytypeinformation.html

Bond, M. (1988a). Assertiveness training. Number 1. Understanding assertiveness. *Nursing Times, 84*(9), 61-64.

Bond, M. (1988b). Assertiveness training. Number 2. When and why non-assertive? *Nursing Times, 84*(11), 67-70.

Bond, M. (1988c). Assertiveness training. Number 3. Assertiveness rights and body language. *Nursing Times, 84*(10), 69-72.

Bond, M. (1988d). Assertiveness training. Number 5. Making requests assertively. *Nursing Times, 84*(13), 77-80.

Bond, M. (1988e). Assertiveness training. Number 8. Responding to feedback. *Nursing Times, 84*(16), 75-78.

Bonnar, B. P., Deivert, R. G., & Gould, T. E. (2004). The relationship between isometric contraction durations during hold-relax stretching and improvement of hamstring flexibility. *Journal of Sports Medicine and Physical Fitness, 44*(3), 258-261.

Borstatd, J. D., & Ludewig, P. M. (2006). Comparison of three stretches for the pectoralis muscle. *Journal Shoulder and Elbow Surgery, 15*(3), 324-330.

Boulier, A., Fricker, J., Thomasset, A., & Apfelbaum, M. (1990). Fat-free mass estimation by the two-electrode impedance method. *American Journal of Clinical Nutrition, 52,* 581-585.

Braun-Lewensohn, O., Celestin-Westreich, S., Celestin, L. P., Verleye, G., Verté, D., & Ponjaert-Kristoffersen, I. (2008). Coping styles as moderating the relationships between terrorist attacks and well-being outcomes. *Journal of Adolescence, 32*(3), 585-599.

Brearley, M. B., & Zhou, S. (2001). Mitochondrial DNA and maximum oxygen consumption. *Sportscience, 5*(2). Retrieved May 30, 2009, from http://sportsci.org/jour/0102/mbb.htm

Brehm, B. J., Seeley, R. J., Daniels, S. R., & D'Alessio, D. (1993). A randomized trial comparing a very low carbohydrate diet and a calorie-restricted low fat diet on body weight and cardio-vascular risk factors in healthy women. *Journal of Clinical Endocrinology and Metabolism, 88*(4), 1617-1623.

Brenner, B. M., Meter, T. W., & Hosteler, D. (1982). Protein intake and the progressive nature of kidney disease. *New England Journal of Medicine, 307,* 652-657.

Breuleux, C., Heck, S. K., Hollenback, J., & Kinzer, S. (1993). Preliminary comparison of medical care costs between fitness center members and nonmembers. *American Journal of Health Promotion, 7*(6), 405-407.

Briefel, R. R., & Johnson, C. L. (2004). Secular trends in dietary intake in the United States. *Annual Review of Nutrition, 24,* 401-431.

Broeder, C. E., Burrhus, K. A., Svanevik, L. S., Volpe, J., & Wilmore, J. H. (1997). Assessing body composition before and after resistance or endurance training. *Medicine & Science in Sports & Exercise, 29,* 705.

Brown, L., Rosner, B., Willett, W. W., & Sacks, F. M. (1999). Cholesterol-lowering effects of dietary fiber: A meta-analysis. *American Journal of Clinical Nutrition, 69,* 30-42.

Brown, M. A., Goldstein-Shirley, J., Robinson, J., & Casey, S. (2001). The effects of a multi-modal intervention trial of light, exercise, and vitamins on women's mood. *Women's Health, 34*(3), 93-112.

Brozek, J., Grande, F., & Anderson, J. T. (1963). Densitometric analysis of body composition: Revision of some quantitative assumptions. *Annals of the New York Academy of Sciences, 110,* 113-140.

Bruce, J., & Chambers, W. A. (2002). Questionnaire surveys. *Anaesthesia, 57,* 1050-1051.

Bruce, R. A. (1971). Exercise testing of patients with coronary artery disease. *Annuals of Clinical Research, 3,* 323-330.

Bruce, R. A., Blackmon, J. R., Jones, J. W., & Strait, G. (1963). Exercising testing in adult normal subjects and cardiac patients. *Pediatrics, 32,* S742-S756.

Bruce, T. A., & McKane, S. U. (Eds.). (2000). *Community-based public health: A partnership model.* Washington, DC: American Public Health Association.

Bucci, L. (1995). *Nutrition applied to injury prevention and sports medicine.* Boca Raton, FL: CRC.

Buchner, D., & Miles, R. (2002). Seeking a contemporary understanding of factors that influence physical activity. *American Journal of Preventative Medicine, 23*(2S), 3-4.

Bulik, C. M., Slof-Op't Landt, S., van Furth, E. F., & Sullivan, P. F. (2007). The genetics of anorexia nervosa. *Annual Review of Nutrition, 27,* 263-275.

Bull, F. C., Armstrong, T., Dixon, T., Ham, S., Neiman, A. B., & Pratt, M. (2002). Physical inactivity. In M. Ezzati, A. Lopez, A. Rodgers, & C. Murray (Eds.). *Comparative quantification of health risks: Global and regional burden of disease due to selected major risk factors.* Geneva: World Health Organization.

Bull, F. C., Armstrong, T., Dixon, T., Ham, S., Neiman, A. B., & Pratt, M. (2003). Commentary: Defining physical inactivity. *Lancet, 361,* 258-259.

Burns, K. J., Camaione, D. N., & Chatteron, C. T. (2000). Prescription of physical activity by adult nurse practitioners: A national survey. *Nursing Outlook, 48*(1), 28-33.

Butler, P. E. (1976). Techniques of assertive training in groups. *International Journal of Group Psychotherapy, 26*(3), 361-371.

Byrne, D. G., & Rosenman, R. H. (1986). The Type A behavior pattern as a precursor to stressful life-events: A confluence of coronary risks. *British Journal of Medical Psychology, 59,* 75-82.

Cade, B., & O'Hanlon, W. H. (1993). *A brief guide to brief therapy.* New York: W. W. Norton.

Cahill, H. (2005). *Case 3: Greek medicine from Galen to Aetius.* Retrieved May 30, 2009, from Kings College London Web site: http://www.kcl.ac.uk/depsta/iss/library/speccoll/exhibitions/gsci/med2.html

Campbell, B., Rohle, D., Taylor, L., Thomas, A., Vacanti, A., Wilborn C. et al. (2005). Effects of the Curves(r) fitness & weight loss program III: Training adaptations. *Journal of the Federation of American Societies for Experimental Biology.* LBA, 55.

Campbell, M. K., McLerran, D., Turner-McGrievey, G., Feng, Z., Havas, S., Sorensen, G., et al. (2008). Mediation of adult fruit and vegetable consumption in the National 5 A Day for Better Health community studies. *Annals of Behavioral Medicine, 35*(1), 49-60.

Canadian Society for Exercise Physiology. (2002). *Par-Q and you.* Retrieved May 30, 2009, from University of Waterloo Web site: http://uwfitness.uwaterloo.ca/PDF/par-q.pdf

Canadian Society for Exercise Physiology. (2007). *Par-Q and you.* Retrieved May 30, 2009, from http://www.lcsd.gov.hk/en/forms/parq.pdf

Canetti, L., Berry, E. M., & Elizur Y. (2009). Psychosocial predictors of weight loss and psychological adjustment following bariatric surgery and a weight-loss program: The mediating role of emotional eating. *International Journal of Obesity, 42*(2), 109-117.

Carels, R. A., Young, K. M., Coit, C., Clayton, A. M., Spencer, A., & Wagner, M. (2008). Skipping meals and alcohol consumption: The regulation of energy intake and expenditure among weight loss participants. *Appetite, 51*(3), 538-545.

Carels, R. A., Young, K. M., Coit, C., Clayton, A. M., Spencer, A., Wagner, M., et al. (2005). Short-term effect of eggs on satiety in overweight and obese subjects. *Journal of the American College of Nutrition, 24*(6), 510-515.

Carlson, L. E., & Bultz, B. D. (2008, August). Mind-body interventions in oncology. *Current Treatment Options in Oncology, 9*(2-3), 127-134.

Carpenter, P. J., & Coleman, R. (1998). A longitudinal study of elite youth cricketers' commitment. *International Journal of Sport Psychology, 29,* 195-210.

Carter-Su, C., & Okamoto, K. (1987). Effect of insulin and glucocorticoids on glucose transporters in rat adipocytes. *American Journal of Physiology, 252,* E441-E453.

Carver, J., & Tamlyn, D. (1985). Sources of stress in third year baccalaureate nursing students. *Nursing Papers, 17*(3), 7-15.

Centers for Disease Control and Prevention. (1999). *Physical activity and health: A report of the Surgeon General.* Retrieved May 30, 2009, from http://www.cdc.gov/nccdphp/sgr/sgr.htm

Centers for Disease Control and Prevention. (2003). Prevalence of physical activity including lifestyle activities among adults: United States, 2000–2001. *Morbidity and Mortality Weekly Reports (MMWR), 52,* 764-769.

Centers for Disease Control and Prevention. (2006a). *Prevalence of overweight and obesity among adults: Unites States, 2003–2004.* Retrieved July 30, 2009, from http://www.cdc.gov/nchs/products/pubs/pubd/hestats/overweight/overwght_adult_03.htm

Centers for Disease Control and Prevention. (2006b). Tobacco using among adults, 2005. *Morbidity and Mortality Weekly Report, 55,* 1145-1148.

Centers for Disease Control and Prevention. (2007a). *Health promotion.* Retrieved March 5, 2007, from http://www.cdc.gov/healthpromotion/

Centers for Disease Control and Prevention. (2007b). *Health United States 2007.* Retrieved May 30, 2009, from http://www.cdc.gov/nchs/data/hus/hus07.pdf#066

Centers for Disease Control and Prevention. (2008). *Alcohol: Frequently asked questions.* Retrieved May 30, 2009, from http://www.cdc.gov/alcohol/faqs.htm

Centers for Disease Control and Prevention. (2009a). *Health related behaviors.* Retrieved June 30, 2009, from http://www.cdc.gov/Aging/info.htm

Centers for Disease Control and Prevention. (2009b). *Overweight and obesity: Frequently asked questions (FAQs).* Retrieved May 20, 2009, from http://www.cdc.gov/nccdphp/dnpa/obesity/faq.htm

Centers for Disease Control and Prevention. (2009c). *Perceived exertion (Borg rating of perceived exertion scale).* Retrieved July 30, 2009, from http://www.cdc.gov/physicalactivity/everyone/measuring/exertion.html

Centers for Disease Control and Prevention finds that Americans are not very active. (2003). *Journal of Physical Education, Recreation, and Dance.* Retrieved May 30, 2009, from http://www.highbeam.com/doc/1G1-108550003.html

Champion, V. L. (1984). Instrument development for health belief model constructs. *Advances in Nursing Science, 6,* 73-85.

Chang, M. W., Brown, R. L., Baumann, L. J., & Nitzke, S. A. (2008). Self-efficacy and dietary fat reduction behaviors in obese African-American and white mothers. *Obesity, 16*(5), 992-1001.

Chapter three: Interventions provided by physical therapists. (1995, August). *Physical Therapy, 75*(8), 739-749.

Cheema, B., Abas, H., Smith, B., O'Sullivan, A., Chan, M., Patwardhan, A., et al. (2007). Progressive exercise for anabolism in kidney disease (PEAK): A randomized controlled trial of resistance training during hemodialysis. *Journal of the American Society of Nephrology, 18,* 1594-1601.

Chen, K. M., Lin, J. N., Lin, H. S., Wu, H. C., Chen, WT, Li, C.H., et al. (2008). The effects of a Simplified Tai-Chi Exercise Program (STEP) on the physical health of older adults living in long-term care facilities: A single group design with multiple time points. *International Journal of Nursing Studies, 45*(4), 501-507.

Chen, Y., Dales, R., Tang, M., & Krewski, D. (2002). Obesity may increase the incidence of asthma in women but not in men: Longitudinal observations from the Canadian National Population Health Services. *American Journal of Epidemiology, 155*(3), 191-197.

Cheuvront, S. N. (2000, April). The Zone diet and athletic performance. *Sports Medicine, 27*(4), 289-294.

Chumlea, W. C., Guo, S., Baumgartner, R. N., & Siervogel, R. M. (1993). Determination of body fluid compartments with multiple frequency bioelectrical impedance. In K. J. Ellis & J. D. Eastman (Eds.), *Human body composition* (pp. 23-26). New York: Plenum.

Cigolini, M., & Smith, U. (1979). Human adipose tissue in culture, VIII: Studies on the insulin-antagonistic effect of glucocorticoids. *Metabolism, 28,* 502-510.

Cink, R. E., & Thomas, T. R. (1981). Validity of the Astrand-Ryhming nomogram for predicting maximal oxygen intake. *British Journal of Sports Medicine, 15*(3), 182-185. Retrieved May 30, 2009, from http://bjsm.bmjjournals.com/cgi/content/abstract/15/3/182

Claire, C. (2005). Addressing spirituality issues in patient interventions. *Magazine of Physical Therapy* [Online], *13*(7), 1. Retrieved March 5, 2007, from http://www.apta.org/AM/Template.cfm?Section=Archives3&TEMPLATE=/CM/HTMLDisplay.cfm&CONTENTID=23188

Clark, C. C. (1996). *Wellness practitioner concepts, research, and strategies.* New York: Springer.

Clark, R. R., et al. (1993). A comparison of methods to predict minimal weight in high school wrestlers. *Medicine & Science in Sports & Exercise, 25,* 1541.

Clarkson, H. M., & Gilewich, G. B. (1999). Musculoskeletal assessment: Joint range of motion and manual muscle test and muscles. Baltimore: Lippincott Williams & Wilkins.

Clarkson University students offer wellness program to musician and dance majors. (2004, March). *Magazine of Physical Therapy, 12*(3), 12.

Cobb, S. (1976). Presidential address—1976. Social support as a moderator of life stress. *Psychosomatic Medicine, 38*(5), 300-314.

Cochran, W. J., Fiorotto, M. L., Sheng, H. P., & Klish, W. J. (1989). Reliability of fat-free mass estimates derived from total body electrical conductivity measurements as influenced by changes in extracellular fluid volume. *American Journal of Clinical Nutrition, 49,* 29-32.

Cochrane, G. (2008). Role for a sense of self-worth in weight-loss treatments: Helping patients develop self-efficacy. *Canadian Family Physician, 54*(4), 543-547.

Colby, K. M. (1951). On the disagreement between Freud and Adler. *American Imago, 8*(3), 229-238.

Colles, S. L., Dixon, J. B., & O'Brien, P. E. (2007). Night eating syndrome and nocturnal snacking: Association with obesity, binge eating and psychological distress. *International Journal of Obesity, 31*(11), 1722-1730.

Collier, P. F. (n.d.). *Oath and law of Hippocrates (1910)*. Harvard Classics, 38. Retrieved November 30, 2007, from gopher.//ftp.std.com//00/obi/book/Hippocrates/Hippocratic.Oath

Collins, A. L., & McCarthy, H. D. (2003). Evaluation of factors determining the precision of body composition measurements by air displacement plethysmography. *European Journal of Clinical Nutrition, 57,* 770-776.

Collins, M. A., Millard-Stafford, M. L., Evans, E. M., Snow, T. K., Cureton, K. J., & Rossopf, L. B. (2004). Effect of race and musculoskeletal development on the accuracy of air plethysmography. *Medicine & Science in Sports & Exercise, 36*(6), 1070-1077.

Commission on Accreditation of Physical Therapist Education (CAPTE). (2000a). *Normative model of physical therapist education*. Alexandria, VA: Author.

Commission on Accreditation of Physical Therapist Education (CAPTE). (2000b). *Normative model of physical therapist education: Supplement to the 2000 version*. Alexandria, VA: Author.

Commission on Accreditation of Physical Therapist Education (CAPTE). (2004). *Normative model of physical therapist education*. Alexandria, VA: Author.

Complement. (n.d.). In *Dictionary.com unabridged (v. 1.1)*. Retrieved October 19, 2008, from Dictionary.com Web site: http://dictionary.reference.com/browse/complement

Conner, M., & Norman, P. (1996). *Predicting health behaviour: Research practice with social cognition models*. Buckingham: Open University Press.

Conover, W. J. (1999). *Practical nonparametric statistics* (3rd ed.). New York: John Wiley & Sons.

Conrad, A., Isaac, L., & Roth, W. T. (2008). The psychophysiology of generalized anxiety disorder: 2. Effects of applied relaxation. *Psychophysiology, 45*(3), 377-388.

Converse, J. M. (1984). Strong arguments and weak evidence: The open/closed questioning controversy of the 1940s. *Public Opinion Quarterly, 48,* 267-282.

Cooper, K. H. (1968). A means of assessing maximal oxygen intake. *JAMA, 203,* 201-204.

Cooper, K. H. (1982). *The aerobics way*. New York: Bantam Books.

Cooper, K. H. (2008). *Dr. Kenneth H. Cooper: The father of aerobics*. Retrieved June 30, 2008, from http://www.cooperaerobics.com/corporate/BioKenCooper.aspx

Copeland, J., Peters, R., & Dillon, P. (1998). A study of 100 anabolic-androgenic steroid users. *Medical Journal of Australia, 168*(6), 311-312.

Cornish, B. H., Thomas, B. J., & Ward, L. C. (1993). Improved prediction of extracellular and total body water using impedance loci generated by multiple frequency bioelectrical impedance analysis. *Physics in Medicine and Biology, 38,* 337-346.

Corrado, C., & Loperfido, N. (2004). The relationship of the Six-Minute Walk Test to maximal oxygen consumption under the assumption of skew-normality. *Quaderni DSEMS, 18.* Retrieved May 30, 2009, from http://ideas.repec.org/p/ufg/qdsems/18-2004.html#abstract

Correa, M., Conde, J., & Santini, N. (1989). A physical fitness program for health professionals and students. *Boletin de la Asociacion Medica de Puerto Rico, 81*(12), 471-474.

Corry, J. M. (1990). MetLife's experience with fitness and wellness programming. *Statistical Bulletin: Metropolitan Life Insurance Company, 71*(4), 19-20.

Corsini, R. J., & Wedding, D. (Eds.). (2007). *Current Psychotherapies* (8th ed.). Illinois: F. E. Peacock.

Corti, M. C., & Rigon, C. (2003). Epidemiology of osteoarthritis: Prevalence, risk factors and functional impact. *Aging Clinical and Experimental Research, 15*(5), 359-363.

CPT-Plus! (2009). A comprehensive guide to current procedural terminology. Los Angeles: PMIC.

Craig, C. L., Marshall, A. L., Sjostrom, M., Bauman, A. E., Booth, M. L., Ainsworth, B. E., et al. (2003). International physical activity questionnaire: 12-country reliability and validity. *Medicine & Science in Sports & Exercise, 35*(8), 1381-1395.

Crespi, I. (1996). Ethical considerations when establishing survey standards. *International Journal of Public Opinion Research, 10*(1), 75-82.

Croft, J. B., Strogatz, D. S., & Keenan, N. L. (1993). The independent effects of obesity and body fat distribution on blood pressure in black adults: The Pitt County Study. *International Journal of Obesity, 17*, 391-397.

Cromie, W. J. (1999). An egg a day is OK, nutritionists say. *Harvard University Gazette.* Retrieved May 30, 2009, from http://www.hno.harvard.edu/gazette/1999/04.22/eggs.html

Cullum, I. D., Ell, P. J., & Ryder, J. R. (1989). X-ray dual photon absorptiometry: A new method for the measurement of bone density. *British Journal of Radiology, 62*, 587-592.

Culver, L. (2007). Physical fitness for special populations. *Magazine of Physical Therapy, 14*(10). Retrieved March 5, 2007, from http://www.apta.org/AM/Template.cfm?Section=Archives3&CONTENTID=34954&TEMPLATE=/CM/HTMLDisplay.cfm

Daley, A. J., Copeland, R. J., Wright, N. P., Roalfe, A., & Wales, J. K. (2006). Exercise therapy as a treatment for psychopathologic conditions in obese and morbidly obese adolescents: A randomized, controlled trial. *Pediatrics, 118*(5), 2126-2134.

Dallard, I., Cathebras, P., Sauron, C., & Massoubre, C. (2001). Is cocoa a psychotropic drug? Psychopathologic study of population of subjects self-identified as chocolate addicts [French]. *Encephale, 27*(2), 181-186.

Dallman, M. F., Pecoraro, N. C., & la Fleur, S. E. (2005). Chronic stress and comfort foods: Self-medication and abdominal obesity. *Brain, Behaviors and Immunity, 19*(4), 275-280.

D'Anci, K. E., Watts, K. L., Kanarek, R. B., & Taylor, H. A. (2009). Low-carbohydrate weight-loss diets: Effects on cognition and mood. *Appetite, 52*(1), 96-103.

Daughton, C. G. (2007). Pharmaceuticals in the environment: Sources and their management. In D. Barcelo (Series Ed.) & M. Petrovic and D. Barcelo (Vol. Eds.), *Wilson & Wilson's comprehensive analytical chemistry: Vol. 50. Analysis, fate and removal of pharmaceuticals in the water cycle* (pp. 1-58). New York: Elsevier Science.

Davies, P. S. W., Preece, M. A., & Hicks, C. J. (1988). The prediction of total body water using bioelectrical impedance in children and adolescents. *Annals of Human Biology, 15*, 237-240.

Davis, C., & Saltos, E. (2002). *Dietary recommendations and how they have changed over time.* U.S. Department of Agriculture, Publication AIB-70 (pp. 33-50). Retrieved May 30, 2009, from http://www.ers.usda.gov/publications/aib750/aib750b.pdf

Davis, C. M. (Ed.). (1997). *Complementary therapies in rehabilitation.* Thorofare, NJ: Slack.

Davis, M., Eshelman, E. R., & McKay, M. (2008). *The relaxation and stress reduction workbook* (6th ed.). Oakland, CA: New Harbinger. Retrieved May 30, 2009, from http://books.google.com/books?hl=en&lr=&id=ruFxYAgSUjQC&oi=fnd&pg=PP12&dq=stress+reduction+exercises&ots=w9OYbGTsiu&sig=2uI5uhGRkqUN7ieY2ZeHYU0A2BE#PPP1,M1

Davis, M. P., Dreicer, R., Walsh, D., Lagman, R., & LeGrand, S. B. (2004). Appetite and cancer-associated anorexia: A review. *Journal of Clinical Oncology, 22*(8), 1510-1517.

Davolt, S., & Woods, E. N. (1998, December). Profiles in wellness. *Magazine of Physical Therapy, 6*(12).

Dawkins, R. (2007). *The God delusion.* New York: Houghton Mifflin.

DeBate, R. D., Topping, M. S., & Sargent, R. G. (2001). Racial and gender differences in weight status and dietary practices among college students. *Adolescence, 36*, 819-834.

Debus, A. G. (1968). *World who's who in science: A biographical dictionary of notable scientists from antiquity to the present.* Chicago: Marquis.

DeCesaris, R., Ranieri, G., Filitti, V., Bonfantino, M. V., & Andriani, A. (1981). Cardiovascular effects of cigarette smoking. *Cardiology, 81,* 233-237.

Dehart, M. M. (1999). *Relationship between the Talk Test and ventilatory threshold.* Unpublished master's thesis, University of Wisconsin–La Crosse.

De Matos, M. G., Calmeiro, L., & Da Fonseca, D. (2009). Effect of physical activity on anxiety and depression [French]. *Presse Medicale, 38*(5), 734-739.

den Besten, C., Vansant, G., Weststrate, J. A., & Deurenberg, P. (1988). Resting metabolic rate and diet-induced thermogenesis in abdominal and gluteal-femoral obese women before and after weight reduction. *American Journal of Clinical Nutrition, 47*(5), 840-847.

Denollet, J. (2005). DS14: Standard assessment of negative affectivity, social inhibition, and type D personality. *Psychosomatic Medicine, 67,* 89-97.

De Piccoli, B., Giada, F., Benettin, A., Sartori, F., & Piccolo, E. (1991). Anabolic steroid use in body builders: An echocardiographic study of left ventricle morphology and function. *International Journal of Sports Medicine, 12*(4), 408-412.

Derogatis, L. R., Lipman, R. S., Rickels, K., Uhlenhuth, E. H., & Covi, L. (1974). Hopkins Symptom Checklist (HSCL): A self-report symptom inventory. *Behavioral Science, 19*(1): 1-15. Abstract published January 3, 2007, and retrieved November 28, 2008, from http://www3.interscience.wiley.com/journal/114034742/abstract?CRETRY=1&SRETRY=0

Deurenberg, P., & Schouten, F. J. M. (1992). Loss of total body water and extracellular water assessed by multifrequency impedance. *European Journal of Clinical Nutrition, 46,* 247-255.

Deurenberg, P., van der Kooy, K., & Leenen, R. (1991). Sex and age specific prediction formulas for estimating body composition from bioelectrical impedance: A cross-validation study. *International Journal of Obesity, 15,* 17-25.

Devereux, J. M., Hastings, R. P., Noone, S. J., Firth, A., & Totsika, V. (2009). Social support and coping as mediators or moderators of the impact of work stressors on burnout in intellectual disability support staff. *Research in Developmental Disabilities, 30*(2), 367-377.

DeVito, J. A. (1998). *Human communication: The basic course* (8th ed.). New York: HarperCollins.

de Vreede, P. L., van Meeteren, N. L., Samson, M. M., Wittink, H. M., Duursma, S. A., Verhaar, H. J. (2007). The effect of functional tasks and exercise and resistance exercise on health-related quality of life and physical activity. *International Journal of Experimental, Clinical, Behavioral, Regenerative and Technological Gerontology, 53*(1): 12-20.

Dicker, D., Belnic, Y., Goldsmith, R., & Kaluski, D. N. (2008). Relationship between dietary calcium intake, body mass index, and waist circumference in MABAT—the Israeli National Health and Nutrition Study. *Israel Medical Association Journal, 10*(7), 512-515.

Diener, E. (1984). Subjective well-being. *Psychological Bulletin, 95,* 542-575.

Diener, E., Lucas, R. E., & Schimmack, U. (2008). *National accounts of well-being.* Oxford: Oxford University Press.

Dietary reference intakes. (2001). Retrieved May 30, 2009, from the Institute of Medicine of the National Academies Web site: http://www.iom.edu/Object.File/Master/7/296/0.pdf

DiGiacomo, M. (2005). PREVIEW 2020: What you need today to prepare for your future. *Magazine of Physical Therapy, 13*(5). Retrieved November 30, 2008, from http://www.apta.org/AM/Template.cfm?Section=Archives3&CONTENTID=24878&TEMPLATE=/CM/HTMLDisplay.cfm

Dimitroulis, G. (1998). Temporomandibular disorders: A clinical update. *British Medical Journal, 317*(7152), 190-194.

Dinger, M. K. (1999). Physical activity and dietary intake among college students. *American Journal of Health Studies, 15*(3), 139-145.

Dinger, M. K., Massie, J., & Ransdell, L. (2000). Physical activity among certified health education specialists. *Journal of Health Education, 31*(2), 98-104.

Dioum, A., Gartner, A., Maire, B., Delpeuch, F., & Wade, S. (2005). Body composition predicted from skinfolds in African women: A cross-validation study using air-displacement plethysmography and a black-specific equation. *British Journal of Nutrition, 93*(6), 973-979.

Divertie, G., Jensen, M., & Miles, J. (1991). Stimulation of lipolysis in humans by physiological hypercortisolemia. *Diabetes, 40,* 1228-1232.

Dolgener, F. A., Hensey, L. D., Marsh, J. J., & Fjelstul, J. K. (1994). Validation of the Rockport Fitness Walking Test in college males and females. *Research Quarterly for Exercise and Sport, 65*(2), 152-158.

Donnelly, G. F. (2009). Depression, alcohol abuse, and healthy living strategies. *Holistic Nursing Practices, 23*(1), 1.

Dootson, S. (1995, July). An in-depth study of triangulation. *Journal of Advanced Nursing, 22*(1), 183-188.

Dorant, E., van den Brandt, P. A., & Goldbohm, R. A. (1996). Consumption of onions and a reduced risk of stomach carcinoma. *Gastroenterology, 110*(1), 12-20.

Doucet, E., St-Pierre, S., Alméras, N., & Tremblay, A, (2003). Relation between appetite ratings before and after a standard meal and estimates of daily energy intake in obese and reduced obese individuals. *Appetite, 40*(2), 137-143.

Dozza, M., Chiari, L., Chan, B., Rocchi, L., Horak, F. B., & Cappello, A. (2005). Influence of a portable audio-biofeedback device on structural properties of postural sway. *Journal of Neuro-engineering Rehabilitation, 2,* 13.

Drysdale, C. L., Earl, J. E., & Hertel, J. (2004). Surface electromyographic activity of the abdominal muscles during pelvic-tilt and abdominal-hollowing exercises. *Journal of Athletic Training. 39*(1), 32-36.

Dunn, H. L. (1961). *High level wellness.* Washington, DC: Mt. Vernon.

Dunn, H. L. (1973). *High level wellness.* Washington, DC: Mt. Vernon.

Dunnagan, T. (2003). Gender differences in selected dietary intakes and eating behaviors in rural communities in Wyoming, Montana, and Idaho. *Nutrition Research, 23*(8), 991-1002.

Dworkin, B., Miller, N. E., Dworkin, S., Birbaumer, N., Brines, M. L., Jonas, S., et al. (1985). Behavioral method for the treatment of idiopathic scoliosis. *Proceedings of the National Academies Science USA, 82*(8), 2493-2497.

Dylan, B. (1991). The times they are a changing. Retrieved May 30, 2009, from http://www.bobdylan.com/songs/times.html

Edgill, P. (2006). Atheists identified as America's most distrusted minority, according to new U of M study. *University of Minnesota News.* Retrieved December 18, 2007, from http://www.ur.umn.edu/FMPro?-db=releases&-lay=web&-format=umnnewsreleases/releasesdetail.html&ID=2816&-Find

Edland, L. M., MacDougall, J. D., Tarnopolsky, M. A., Elorriaga, A., & Borgmann, A. (1997). Effected of oral creatine supplementation on muscle [PCr] and short-term maximum power output. *Medicine & Science in Sports & Exercise, 29*(2), 216-219.

EEG biofeedback frequently asked questions. (1996). Retrieved November 15, 2005, from http://users.aol.com/eegspectrm/articles/faq.htm

Effect of dietary protein intake on kidney function in women with normal or mildly abnormal kidneys [Summaries for Patients]. (2003). *Annals of Internal Medicine, 183*(6), 51.

Eisen, M., Zellman, G. L., & McAlister, A. L. (1992). A health belief model—Social learning theory approach to adolescents' fertility control: Findings from a controlled field trial. *Health Education Quarterly, 19*(2), 249-262.

Elfhag, K., & Rössner, S. (2005). Who succeeds in maintaining weight loss? A conceptual review of factors associated with weight loss maintenance and weight regain. *Obesity Review, 6*(1), 67-85.

Eliakim, A., Ish-Shalom, S., Giladi, A., Falk, B., & Constantini, N. (2000). Assessment of body composition in ballet dancers: Correlation among anthropometric measurements, bio-electrical impedance analysis, and dual-energy X-ray absorpitometry. *International Journal of Sports Medicine, 21,* 598-601.

Ellis, A. (1993). Reflections on rational–emotive therapy. *Journal of Consulting and Clinical Psychology, 61*(2), 199-201.

Ellis, J. B., & Smith, P. C. (1991). Spiritual well-being, social desirability and reasons for living: Is there a connection? *International Journal of Social Psychiatry, 37*(1), 57-63.

Engel, G. L. (1977). The need for a new medical model. *Science, 196*, 129-136.

Engel, P. A. (2001). George L. Engel, MD, 1913–1999: Remembering his life and work: Rediscovering his soul. *Psychosomatics, 42*, 94-99. Retrieved May 30, 2009, from http://psy.psychiatryonline.org/cgi/content/full/42/2/94

Enzi, G., Gasparo, M., & Biondetti, P. R. (1986). Subcutaneous and visceral fat distribution according to sex, age, and overweight, evaluated by computed tomography. *American Journal of Clinical Nutrition, 44*, 739-746.

Erzberger, C., & Prein, G. (1997, May). Triangulation: Validity and empirically-based hypothesis construction. *Quality & Quantity, 31*(2), 141-155.

Esch, T., & Stefano, G. B. (2005). The neurobiology of love. *Neuro Endocrinology Letters, 26*(3), 175-192.

Exercise and reduce heart disease risk. (2008). *Ethnicity & Disease, 18*(4), 519.

Expert Panel on the Identification, Evaluation, and Treatment of Overweight in Adults. (1998). Clinical guidelines on the identification, evaluation, and treatment of overweight and obesity in adults: Executive summary. *American Journal of Clinical Nutrition, 68*, 899-917.

Fain, J. N., Kovacev, V. P., & Scow, R. O. (1965). Effect of growth hormone and dexamethasone on lipolysis and metabolism in isolated fat cells of the rat. *Journal of Biological Chemistry, 240*, 3522-3529.

Fair, S. E. (1987). *The effects of moderate versus a modest exercise regimen on the quality of weight loss of obese women on a very low calorie diet.* Paper for the Maryland Metabolic Institute, Baltimore, MD.

Fair, S. E. (2002a). *The efficacy of the 420 calorie Optifast diet in one hospital-based clinic.* Paper for the Southern California University for Professional Studies, Palo Alto, CA.

Fair, S. E. (2002b). *The humanistic model of wellness.* Paper for the Southern California University for Professional Studies, Palo Alto, CA.

Fair, S. E. (2003). A comparison of the perception of self-wellness of graduate and PT students [Abstract]. The Florida Physical Therapy Association, Orlando, FL.

Fair, S. E. (2004a). A comparison of the perception of self-wellness of female and male physical therapy students [Abstract]. The Florida Physical Therapy Association, Orlando, FL.

Fair, S. E. (2004b). A comparison of the self-wellness of female and male students in one entry-level physical therapy program. *American Physical Therapy Association: Journal of the Section on Women's Health, 28*(3), 15-21.

Fair, S. E. (2004c). Health promotion and physical therapy: The fitness and nutritional dimensions of wellness [Abstract]. APTA Preview 2020, Las Vegas, NV.

Fair, S. E. (2004d). Health promotion and physical therapy: The psychological dimension of wellness and literature relating to PT and wellness [Abstract]. APTA Preview 2020, Las Vegas, NV.

Fair, S. E. (2004e). An online seminar in wellness for physical therapists. In Program and abstracts of the XIV International Conference on College Teaching and Learning, March 29–April 2, 2004, Jacksonville, FL.

Fair, S. E. (2005). The fitness self-wellness of physical therapists. ProQuest Information and Learning (formerly UMI) No. 3162726. *Dissertation Abstracts International, 66*(1), 236.

Fair, S. E. (2007). A comparison of the aerobic capacity wellness of female and male physical therapy members of the American Physical Therapy Association. *American Physical Therapy Association: Journal of the Section on Women's Health, 31*(1), 6-10.

Fair, S. E. (2007b). *Wellness and Physical Therapy.* St. Augustine, FL: Embury.

Falvo, M. J., Hoffman, J. R., Ratamess, N. A., Kang, J., Wendell, M., Faigenbaum, A., et al. (2005). Effect of protein supplementation on strength, power and body composition changes in experienced resistance trained men. *Medicine & Science in Sports & Exercise, 37*(5), S45.

Fasen, J. M., O'Connor, A. M., Schwartz, S. L., Watson, J. O., Plastaras, C. T., Garvan, C. W., et al. (2009). A randomized controlled trial of hamstring stretching: Comparison of four techniques. *Journal of Strength and Conditioning Research, 23*(2), 660-667.

Fehring, R. J., Brennan, P. F., & Keller, M. L. (1987). Psychological and spiritual well-being in college students. *Research in Nursing and Health, 19*(6), 391-398.

Feland, J. B. (2001). The effect of duration of stretching of the hamstring muscle group for increasing ROM in people aged 65 yrs or older. *Journal of the American Physical Therapy Association, 81*(5), 1110-1117.

Feldman, D., & Loose, G. (1977). Glucocorticoid receptors in adipose tissue. *Endocrinology, 100,* 389-405.

Fenstermaker, K. L., Plowman, S. A., & Looney, M. A. (1992). Validation of the Rockport Fitness Walking Test in females 65 years and older. *Research Quarterly for Exercise and Sport, 63*(3), 322-327.

Fenton, K. (2004, May). [Editorial.] *Nursing Management–United Kingdom, 11*(2), 3.

Fergusson, D. M., Bodden, J. M., & Horwood, L. G. (2009). Tests of causal links between alcohol abuse or dependence and major depression. *Archives of General Psychiatry, 66*(3), 260-236.

Fern, P. A. (2008). Hypnosis to alleviate perioperative anxiety and stress: A journey to challenge ideas. *Journal of Perioperative Practice, 18*(1), 14-16.

Fielding, J. E., Husten, C. G., & Eriksen, M. P. (1998). Tobacco: Health effects and control. In: Maxcy, K. F., Rosenau, M. J., Last, J. M., Wallace, R. B., Doebbling, B. N. (eds.). *Public Health and Preventive Medicine.* New York: McGraw-Hill; pp. 817-845.

Fielding, R. A., & Parkington, J. (2002). What are the dietary protein requirements of physically active individuals? *Nutrition in Clinical Care, 5*(4), 191-196.

Fields, D. A., Higgins, P. B., & Radley, D. (2005). Air-displacement plethysmography: Here to stay. *Current Opinion in Clinical Nutrition and Metabolic Care, 8*(6), 624-629.

52 proven stress reducers. (1997). Retrieved November 30, 2008, from Texas Women's University Web site: http://www.twu.edu/o-sl/counseling/SelfHelp001.html

Findlay, I. N., Taylor, R. S., Dargie, H. J., Grant, S., Pettigrew, A. R., Wilson, J. T., et al. (1987, August). Cardiovascular effects of training for a marathon run in unfit middle aged men. *British Medical Journal (Clinical Research Education), 295*(6597), 521-524.

Flegal, K. M., Carroll, M. D., Ogden, C. L., & Johnson, C. L. (2002). Prevalence and trends in obesity among U.S. adults, 1999–2000. *JAMA, 288*(14), 1195-1200.

Fogelholm, M. (2003). Dairy products, meat and sport performance. *Sports Medicine, 333*(8), 615-631.

Folkins, C. H. (1976). Effects of physical training on mood. *Journal of Clinical Psychology, 32*(2), 385-388.

Food and Nutrition Board, Institute of Medicine. (1997). *Dietary reference intakes for calcium, phosphorus, magnesium, vitamin D, and fluoride.* Retrieved May 30, 2009, from the National Academies Press Web site: http://www.nap.edu/books/0309063507/html/index.html

Food and Nutrition Board, Institute of Medicine. (1998). *Dietary reference intakes for thiamin, riboflavin, niacin, vitamin B6, folate, vitamin B12, pantothenic acid, biotin, and choline.* Retrieved May 30, 2009, from the National Academies Press Web site: http://www.nap.edu/books/0309065542/html/index.html

Food and Nutrition Board, Institute of Medicine. (2000a). *Dietary reference intakes for vitamin A, vitamin K, arsenic, boron, chromium, copper, iodine, iron, manganese, molybdenum, nickel, silicon, vanadium, and zinc.* Retrieved May 30, 2009, from the National Academies Press Web site: http://www.nap.edu/books/0309072794/html/

Food and Nutrition Board, Institute of Medicine. (2000b). *Dietary reference intakes for vitamin C, vitamin E, selenium, and carotenoids.* Retrieved May 30, 2009, from the National Academies Press Web site: http://www.nap.edu/books/0309069351/html/

Food and Nutrition Board, Institute of Medicine. (2004). *Dietary reference intakes for water, potassium, sodium, chloride, and sulfate.* Retrieved May 30, 2009, from the National Academies Press Web site: http://www.nap.edu/books/0309091691/html/

Food and Nutrition Board, Institute of Medicine. (2005). *Dietary reference intakes for energy, carbohydrate, fiber, fat, fatty acids, cholesterol, protein, and amino acids (macronutrients).* Retrieved May 30, 2009, from the National Academies Web site: http://www.nap.edu/openbook. php?isbn=0309085373

Ford, H. T., Pucket, J. R., Blessing, D. L., & Tucker, L. A. (1989). Effects of selected physical activities on health-related fitness and psychological well-being. *Psychological Report, 64*(1), 203-208.

Foster, G. D., Phelan, S., Wadden, T. A., Gill, D., Ermold, J., & Didie, E. (2004). Promoting more modest weight losses: A pilot study. *Obesity Research. 12*(8), 1271-1277.

Fox, K. R. (1999). The influence of physical activity on mental well-being. *Public Health Nutrition, 2*(3A), 411-418.

Frank, E., Dell, M. L., & Chopp, R. (1999). Religious characteristics of U.S. women physicians. *Social Science Medicine, 49*(12), 1717-1722.

Franken, P. A. & Page, D. G. (1972). Noise in the environment. *Environmental Science & Technology, 6*(2), 124-129.

Frankenfield, D. C., Muth, E. R., & Rowe, W. A. (1998). The Harris-Benedict studies of human basal metabolism: History and limitations. *Journal of the American Dietetic Association, 98*(9), 970-971.

Frankle, R. T., & Yang, M. (Eds.). (1988). *Obesity and weight control: The health professionals guide to understanding and treatment.* Rockville, MD: Aspen.

Freedberg, E. J., & Johnston, W. E. (1979). Behavioral change in a short-term, intensive multimodal alcoholism treatment program. *Psychological Reports, 44,* 791-797.

Freeman, A., Mahoney, M. J., Devito, P., & Martin, D. (Eds.). (2004). *Cognition and Psychotherapy* (2nd ed.). New York: Springer.

Freeman, L. W., & Lawlis, G. F. (2001). *Complementary and alternative medicine: A research-based approach.* Philadelphia: Mosby.

Frident, J., & Lieber, R. L. (1992). Structural and mechanical basis of exercise-induced muscle injury. *Medicine Science Sports Exercise, 24*(5), 521-530.

Friedman, K. E., Reichmann, S. K., Costanzo, P. R., & Musante, G. J. (2002). Body image partially mediates the relationship the relationship between obesity and psychological distress. *Obesity Research, 10*(1), 33-41.

Friedman, M. (1996). *Type A behavior: Its diagnosis and treatment.* New York: Springer.

Frisard, M. I., Greenway, F. L., & Delany, J. P. (2005). Comparison of methods to assess body composition changes during a period of weight loss. *Obesity Research, 13*(5), 845-854.

Froelicher, V. F., Thompson, A. J., Davis, G., Stewart, A. J., & Triebwasser, J. H. (1975). Prediction of maximal oxygen consumption: Comparison of the Bruce and Balke protocols. *Chest, 68,* 331-336. Retrieved May 30, 2009, from http://www.chestjournal.org/cgi/reprint/68/3/331.pdf

Fuchs, C. S., Giovannucci, E. L., & Colditz, G. A. (1999). Dietary fiber and the risk of colorectal cancer and adenoma in women. *New England Journal of Medicine, 340,* 169-176.

Fuimano, J. (2004, May). Add coaching to your leadership repertoire. *Nursing Management, 35*(1):16-17.

Fung, T. T., Hu, F. B., & Pereira, M. A. (2002). Whole-grain intake and the risk of type 2 diabetes: A prospective study in men. *American Journal of Clinical Nutrition, 76,* 535-540.

Gale Group. (2001). Locus of control. In *Encyclopedia of Psychology* (2nd ed.) [Online]. Retrieved May 30, 2009, from www.findarticles.com/cf_dls/g2699/0005/2699000535/p1/article.jhtml

Gall, M. D., Gall, J. P., & Borg, W. R. (2003). *Educational research: An introduction* (7th ed.). New York: Pearson Education.

Gamboa, J. M., & White, N. T. (2008). *Cash practice: Strategies for integrating rehabilitation, health promotion, and fitness.* Presented at the APTA Annual Conference, San Antonio, TX.

Gebhardt, S. E., & Thomas, R. G. (2002). *Nutritive value of foods.* Beltsville, MD: U.S. Department of Agriculture. Retrieved May 30, 2009, from the U.S. Department of Agriculture Web site: http://www.nal.usda.gov/fnic/foodcomp/Data/HG72/hg72_2002.pdf

George, J. D., Fellington, G. W., & Fisher, A. G. (1998). A modified version of the Rockport Fitness Walking Test for college men and women. *Research Quarterly for Exercise and Sport, 69*(2), 205-209.

Gersh, M., & Echternach, J. (1996, December). Management of individual with pain: Parts 1 and 2. *Magazine of Physical Therapy.* Retrieved June 30, 2003, from http://www.apta.org-/Education/Continuing_ Education/onLine_ceu_List/electro_text_intro/electro_pain_exc

Gettman, L. R., Pollock, M. L., Durstine, J. L., Ward, A., Ayres, J., & Linnerud, A. C. (1976). Physiological responses to men of 1, 3, and 5 day per week training programs. *Research Quarterly for Exercise and Sport, 47,* 638-646.

Gibson, E. L. (2006). Emotional influences on food choice: Sensory, physiological and psychological pathways. *Physiology and Behavior, 89*(1), 53-61.

Gillett, P. A. (1988). Self-reported factors influencing exercise adherence in overweight women. *Nursing Research, 37*(1), 25-29.

Gillman, M. W., Cupples, L. A., & Gagnon, D. (1995). Protective effect of fruits and vegetables on development of stroke in men. *JAMA, 273*(14), 1113-1117.

Ginde, S. R., Geliebter, A., Rubiano, F., Silva, A. M., Wang, J., Heshka, S., et al. (2005). Air displacement plethysmography: Validation in overweight and obese subjects. *Obesity Research, 13*(7), 1232-1237.

Giovannucci, E., Ascherio, A., & Rimm, E. B. (1995). Intake of carotenoids and retinol in relation to risk of prostate cancer. *Journal of the National Cancer Institute, 87*(23), 1767-1776.

Girdin, D. A., Everly, G. S., & Dusek, D. E. (1996). *Controlling stress and tension.* Needham Heights, MA: Allyn & Bacon.

Gisolfi, C. V. (1983). Temperature regulation during exercise: Directions—1983. *Medicine & Science in Sports & Exercise, 15*(1), 15-20.

Glanz, K., Lewis, F. M., & Rimer, B. K. (1997). *Theory at a glance: A guide for health promotion practice.* Washington, DC: National Institutes of Health.

Glanz, K., & Rimer, B. K. (2005). *Theory at a glance: A guide for health promotion practice* (2nd ed.). NIH Publication No. 05-3896. Bethesda, MD: National Institutes of Health. Retrieved May 30, 2009, from http://www.cancer.gov/PDF/481f5d53-63df-41bc-bfaf-5aa48ee1da4d/TAAG3.pdf

Glanz, K., Rimer, B. K., & Lewis, F. M. (2002). *Health behavior and health education. Theory, research and practice.* San Francisco: Wiley & Sons.

Glass, D. C. (1977). Stress, behavior patterns and coronary disease. *American Scientist, 65*(2), 177-187.

Glasser, W., & Zunin, L. M. (1972). Reality therapy. *Current Psychiatric Therapies, 12,* 58-61.

Glick, I. D., & Horsfall, J. L. (2005). Diagnosis and psychiatric treatment of athletes. *Clinical Sports Medicine, 24*(4), 771-781, vii.

Gluck, M. E., Geliebter, A., & Satov, T. (2001). Night eating syndrome is associated with depression, low self-esteem, reduced daytime hunger, and less weight loss in obese outpatients. *Obesity Research, 9*(4), 264-267.

Gluconeogenesis. (n.d.). *Interactive Concepts in Biochemistry.* Retrieved May 30, 2009, from Wiley & Sons Web site: http://www.wiley.com/legacy/college/boyer/0470003790/animations/gluconeogenesis/gluconeogenesis.htm

Godfrey, R. J., Ingham, S. A., Pedlar, C. R., & Whyte, G. P. (2005). The detraining and retraining of an elite rower: A case study. *Journal of Science and Medicine in Sport, 8*(3), 314-320.

Going, S. B., Massett, M. P., & Hall, M. C. (1993). Detection of small changes in body composition by dual-energy x-ray absorptiometry. *American Journal of Clinical Nutrition, 57,* 845-850.

Golbasi, Z., Kelleci, M., & Dogan, S. (2008, August 12). Relationships between coping strategies, individual characteristics and job satisfaction in a sample of hospital nurses: Cross-sectional questionnaire survey. *International Journal of Nursing Studies, 45*(12), 1800-1806. Retrieved May 30, 2009, from http://www.ncbi.nlm.nih.gov/sites/entrez

Goldberg, L., Elliot, D. L., & Kuehl, K. S. (1988). Assessment of exercise intensity formulas by use of ventilatory threshold. *Chest, 94*(1), 95-98.

Goodhand, J., & Rampton, D. (2008). Psychological stress and coping in IBD. *Gut, 57*(10), 1345-1347.

Goodman, E., Hinden, B. R., & Khandelwal, S. (2000). Accuracy of teen and parental reports of obesity and body mass index. *Pediatrics, 106*(1), 52-59.

Goodstein, L. (2009, April 26). More atheists shout it from the rooftops. *New York Times.* Retrieved May 30, 2009, from http://www.nytimes.com/2009/04/27/us/27atheist.html?_r=2

Gore, A. (2006). *An inconvenient truth: A planetary emergence of global warming and what we can do.* New York: Rodale.

Grace, F., Sculthorpe, N., Baker, J., & Davies, B. (2003). Blood pressure and rate pressure product response in males using high-dose anabolic-androgenic steroids (AAS). *Journal of Sports and Science in Medicine, 6*(3), 307-312.

Greenhaus, A. (1997). A catch 22 situation [Letter to the Editor]. *Magazine of Physical Therapy.* Retrieved September 30, 2003, from http://www.apta.org/pt_magazine/Sept97/letters.htm

Greenwood, M., Kreider, R., Rasmussen, C., Kerksick, C., Magrans, T., Marcello, B., et al. (2004). Effects of the Curves(r) fitness program on muscular strength, muscular endurance, and maximal aerobic capacity [Abstract]. *Medicine & Science in Sport & Exercise, 36*(5), S80.

Gremmen, T., Van den Boom, F. M., & Witlox, R. (1992). Self-help groups for PWA's show positive results. *International Conference on AIDS, 24*(8):B224. Retrieved May 30, 2009, from http://gateway.nlm.nih.gov/MeetingAbstracts/ma?f=102199245.html

Grepmair, L., Mitterlehner, F., Loew, T., Bachler, E., Rother, W., & Nickel, M. (2007). Promoting mindfulness in psychotherapists in training influences the treatment results of their patients: A randomized, double-blind, controlled study. *Psychotherapy and Psychosomatics, 76*(6), 332-338.

Grieger, J. A., Nowson, C. A., & Ackland, L. M. (2009). Nutritional and functional status indicators in residents of a long-term care facility. *Journal of Nutrition for the Elderly, 28*(1), 47-60.

Grodjinovsky, A., & Magel, J. R. (1970). Effect of warm-up on running performance. *Research Quarterly, 41*(1), 116-119.

Groesz, L. M., Levine, M. P., & Murnen, S. K. (2002). The effect of experimental presentation of thin media images on body satisfaction: A meta-analytic review. *International Journal of Eating Disorders, 31*, 1-16.

Guccione, A. (1999). What is a physical therapist? *Magazine of Physical Therapy.* Retrieved August 8, 2004, from http://www.apta.org/pt_magazine/oct99/closer.html

Guillaume-Gentil, C., Assimacopoulos-Jeannet, F., & Jeanrenaud, B. (1993). Involvement of non-esterified fatty acid oxidation in glucocorticoid-induced peripheral insulin resistance in vivo in rats. *Diabetologia, 36*, 899-906.

Gutek, B. A. (1978). On the accuracy of retrospective attitudinal data. *Public Opinion Quarterly*, 390-401.

Guyton, A. C., & Hall, J. E. (2005). *Textbook of Medical Physiology* (11th ed.). Philadelphia: Elsevier Saunders.

Haarbo, J., Marskew, U., Gottfredsen, A., & Christiansen, C. (1991). Postmenopausal hormone replacement therapy prevents central distribution of body fat after menopause. *Metabolism, 40*, 323-326.

Hall, J. F. (1979). Book review. *Quality and Quantity, 13*, 183-184.

Hans, T. (2000). A meta-analysis of the effects of adventure programming on locus of control. *Journal of Contemporary Psychotherapy, 30*(1), 33-60. Retrieved May 30, 2009, from http://www.wilderdom.com/pdf/Hans2000AdventureTherapyLOCMetaanalysis.pdf

Hansen, N. J., Lohman, T. G., & Going, S. B. (1993). Prediction of body composition in premenopausal females from dual-energy x-ray absorptiometry. *Journal of Applied Physiology, 75*, 1637-1641.

Hanson, A. E. (n.d.). Hippocrates: The "Greek Miracle" in medicine. In *Medicina Antiqua.* Retrieved May 30, 2009, from http://www.medicinaantiqua.org.uk/sa_hippint.html

Hanson, P. (1984). *Clinical exercise training.* In R. Strauss (Ed.), *Sport medicine* (pp. 13-40). Philadelphia: W. B. Saunders.

Harari, M. J., Waehler, C. A., & Rogers, J. R. (2005). An empirical investigation of a theoretically based measure of perceived wellness. *Journal of Counseling Psychology, 52*(1), 93-103. Retrieved May 30, 2009, from http://www.eric.ed.gov/ERICWebPortal/custom/portlets/recordDetails/detailmini.jsp?_nfpb=true&_&ERICExtSearch_SearchValue_0=EJ684905&ERICExtSearch_SearchType_0=no&accno=EJ684905

Hardinge, M. G., & Shroyck, H. (1991). *Family medical guide to health and fitness, Vol. 1: Lifestyle.* Indianapolis: Pacific Press.

Harris, R., & Veinot, T. (2004). The Empowerment Model and using e-health to distribute information. Retrieved May 30, 2009, from Action for Health Web site: http://www.sfu.ca/act4hlth/pub/working/Empowerment.pdf

Harrison, M. H., Bruce, D. L., Brown, G. A., & Cochrane, L. A. (1980). A comparison of some indirect methods for predicting maximal oxygen uptake. *Aviation Space Environmental Medicine, 51*(10), 1128-1133.

Hart, J. (1998, August 15). The perils of polling and how to avoid them. *Editor & Publisher, 131*(33), 5-7.

Hartz, A. J., Fischer, M. E., Bril, G., Kelber, S., Rupley, D., Oken, B., et al. (1986). The association of obesity with joint pain and osteoarthritis. *Journal of Chronic Diseases, 39*(4), 311-319.

Harvard College. (2007). *The early history of Harvard University.* Retrieved May 30, 2009, from the Harvard Guide Web site: http://www.hno.harvard.edu/guide/intro/index.html

Harvard Health Publications. (2009). *Water, sodium & potassium: Guidelines to water, sodium & potassium intake.* Retrieved August 30, 2009, from https://www.health.harvard.edu/press_releases/water_sodium_potassium_intake

Harvard Medical School history. (2002). Retrieved May 30, 2009, from http://www.hms.harvard.edu/about/history.html

Harvard School of Public Health. (2008). *The nutrition source: Daily fiber requirements.* Retrieved May 30, 2009, from http://www.hsph.harvard.edu/nutritionsource/what-should-you-eat/fiber-table/index.html

Harvard School of Public Health. (2009a). *The nutrition source: Fats and cholesterol: Out with the bad and in with the good.* Retrieved May 30, 2009, from http://www.hsph.harvard.edu/nutritionsource/what-should-you-eat/fats-full-story/index.html

Harvard School of Public Health. (2009b). *The nutrition source: Fiber: Start roughing it!* Retrieved May 30, 2009, from http://www.hsph.harvard.edu/nutritionsource/what-should-you-eat/fiber-full-story/index.html

Harvard School of Public Health. (2009c). *The nutrition source: Food pyramids: What should you really eat?* Retrieved May 30, 2009, from http://www.hsph.harvard.edu/nutritionsource/what-should-you-eat/pyramid-full-story/index.html

Harvard School of Public Health. (2009d). *The nutrition source: Healthy eating pyramid.* Retrieved May 30, 2009, from http://www.hsph.harvard.edu/nutritionsource/what-should-you-eat/pyramid/

Harvard School of Public Health. (2009e). *The nutrition source: The bottom line.* Retrieved May 30, 2009, from http://www.hsph.harvard.edu/nutritionsource/what-should-you-eat/alcohol/

Harvard School of Public Health, Department of Nutrition. (n.d.) *The nutrition source.* Retrieved August 10, 2009, from http://www.thenutritionsource.org.

Harvard University. (2008). *The healthy eating food pyramid.* Retrieved July 30, 2009, from http://www.hsph.harvard.edu/nutritionsource/what-should-you-eat/pyramid/

Harvey, T., Beckham, H., Campbell, B., Galbreath, M., Kerksick, C., LaBounty, P., et al. (2005). Effects of the Curves(r) fitness & weight loss program I: Body composition [Abstract]. *Journal of the American Societies for Experimental Biology,* LBA:54.

Hash, R. (2002, February). Practicing what we preach: Are we role models? *Journal of Family Practice, 51*(2), 185.

Hattie, J. A., Marsh, H. W., Neill, J. T. & Richards, G. E. (1997). Adventure Education and Outward Bound: Out-of-class experiences that have a lasting effect. *Review of Educational Research, 67,* 43-87. Retrieved March 30, 2009, from http://www.wilderdom.com/pdf/HattieAdvEdMA1997.pdf

Hauge, A. (2000). Thomas H. Huxley: The naval doctor who became Darwin's bulldog [Norwegian]. *Tidsskr Nor Laegeforen, 120*(30), 3708-3713.

Hawk, C. (2001). Toward a wellness model for chiropractic: The role of prevention and health promotion. *Topics in Clinical Chiropractic, 8*(4), 1-7.

Hawley, J. A., Myburgh, K. H., & Noakes, T. D. (1999). Maximal oxygen consumption: A contemporary perspective. In *Encyclopedia of Sports Medicine and Science* [Online]. Retrieved May 20, 2009, from http://www.sportsci.org/encyc/drafts/VO2max.doc

Health Care Communication Group. (2001). *Writing, speaking, and communication skills for health professionals.* New Haven, CT: Yale University Press.

Health Goods. (2007). *Omron HBF 400 Body Fat & Weight Scale.* Retrieved May 30, 2009, from http://www.healthgoods.com/Shopping/Health_and_Fitness_Products/Omron_Body_Fat_Weight_Scale_HBF_400.asp

Heath, G. W. (2003). Behavioral approaches to physical activity promotion. In J. K. Ehrman, P. M. Gordon, P. S. Visich, & S. J. Keteyian (Eds.). *Clinical exercise physiology* (pp. 11-25). Champaign, IL: Human Kinetics.

Heitmann, B. L. (1991). Body fat distribution in the adult Danish population aged 35-65 years: An epidemiological study. *International Journal of Obesity, 15*, 535-545.

Herman, C. J., Alen, P., Hunt, W. C., & Brady, T. J. (2004). Use of complementary therapies among primary care clinic patients with arthritis. *Preventing Chronic Disease, 1*(4). Retrieved June 26, 2006, from http://www.pubmedcentral.nih.gov/articlerender

Hettler, W. (1979). *Six dimensional model of wellness.* Retrieved May 30, 2009, from National Wellness Institute Web site: http://www.nationalwellness.org/index.php?id_tier=2&id_c=25

Hettler, W. (1980). Wellness promotion on a university campus. *Family and Community Health, 3,* 77-95.

Hettler, W. (1984). Wellness: Encouraging a lifetime pursuit of excellence. *Health Values, 8*(4), 13-17.

Hicks, V. L., et al. (2000). Validation of near-infrared interactance and skinfold methods for estimating body composition of American Indian women. *Medicine & Science in Sports & Exercise, 32,* 531.

Hickson, R., Czerwinski, S., Falduto, M., & Young, A. (1990). Glucocorticoid antagonism by exercise and androgenic–anabolic steroids. *Medicine & Science in Sports & Exercise, 22*(3), 331-340.

Hickson, R. C., Kanakis, C., Davis, J. R., Moore, A. M., & Rich, S. (1982). Reduced training duration effects on aerobic power, endurance and cardiac growth. *Journal of Applied Physiology, 53*(1), 225-229.

Hickson, R. C., & Rosenkoetter, M. A. (1981). Reduced training frequencies and maintenance of increased aerobic power. *Medicine & Science in Sports & Exercise, 13*(1), 13-16.

Higdon, J. V., & Frei, B. (2006). Coffee and health: A review of recent human research. *Critical Reviews in Food and Science Nutrition, 46,* 101-123.

Hippocrates. (1997). Asclepeion Hospital—Athens. Retrieved July 15, 2007, from http://www.forthnet.gr.asclepeion/hippo/htm

Hippocrates. (n.d.). In *Encyclopedia Britannica* [Online]. Retrieved May 30, 2009, from http://www.eb.com/Hippocrates

Hippocrates: The "Greek Miracle" in medicine. (1997). In *Ancient Medicine.* Retrieved July 15, 2007, from http://web1.ea.pvt.K12.pa.us/medant/hippint.htm#history

Hirsh, J. (1987, February). *The set point theory.* Symposium at the City University of New York Queens College, Flushing, NY.

Hoffman, E. J., & Mathew, S. J. (2008). Anxiety disorders: A comprehensive review of pharmacotherapies. *Mount Sinai Journal of Medicine, 75*(3), 248-262.

Hoffman, J. R., & Ratamess, N. A. (2006, June 1). Medical issues associated with anabolic steroid use: Are they exaggerated? *Journal of Sports Science and Medicine, 5,* 182-193.

Holahan, C. J., & Moos, R. H. (1985). Life stress and health: Personality, coping, and family support in stress resistance. *Journal of Personality and Social Psychology, 49*(3), 739-747.

Holahan, C. J., & Moos, R. H. (1986). Personality, coping, and family resources in stress resistance: A longitudinal analysis. *Journal of Personality and Social Psychology, 51*(2), 389-395.

Holahan, C. J., & Moos, R. H. (1987). Risk, resistance, and psychological distress: A longitudinal analysis with adults and children. *Journal of Abnormal Psychology, 96*(1), 3-13.

Horgan, C., Skwara, K. C., & Strickler, G. (2001, February). *Substance abuse: The nation's number one health problem, 2001.* Princeton, NJ: Robert Wood Johnson Foundation.

Howard, G. E., Blyth, C. S., & Thornton, W. E. (1966). Effects of warm-up on the heart rate during exercise. *Research Quarterly for Exercise and Sport, 37*(3), 360-367.

Hu, F. B., Manson, J. E., Stampfer, M. J., Colditz, G., & Liu, S. (2001). Diet, lifestyle and the risk of type 2 diabetes mellitus in women. *New England Journal of Medicine, 345*(11), 790-797.

Hubert, H. B., Feinleib, M., McNamara, P. M., & Castelli, W. P. (1983). Obesity as an independent risk factor for cardiovascular disease: A 26-year follow-up of the participants in the Framingham Heart Study. *Circulation, 67*(5), 968-977.

Huberty, J. L., Ransdell, L. B., Sidman, C., Flohr, J. A., Shultz, B., Grosshans, O., et al. (2008). Explaining long-term exercise adherence in women who complete a structured exercise program. *Research Quarterly for Exercise and Sport, 79*(3), 374-84.

Huffman, Carl. (2008, Winter). Alcmaeon. In E. N. Zalta (Ed.), *The Stanford Encyclopedia of Philosophy.* Retrieved May 30, 2009, from http://plato.stanford.edu/entries/alcmaeon/

Hunsaker, P. L., Alessandra, T., Alessandra, A. J. (1986). *The art of managing people.* New York: Simon and Schuster.

International Food Information Council (IFIC). (2007). *Fact sheet: Caffeine and health.* Retrieved May 30, 2009, from http://www.ific.org/publications/factsheets/upload/Caffeine-and-Health-formatted.pdf

International Olympic Committee. (2008). Retrieved May 30, 2009, from http://www.olympic.org/uk/index_uk.asp

Irving, L., Wall, M., Neumark-Sztainer, D., & Story, M. (2002). Steroid use among adolescents: Findings from Project EAT. *Journal of Adolescent Health, 30*(4), 243-252.

Iso-Ahola, S. (1989). Motivation for leisure. In E. L. Jackson & T. L. Burton (Eds.), *Understanding leisure and recreation: Mapping the past, charting the future* (pp. 247-279). State College, PA: Venture.

Iso-Ahola, S. (1999). Motivational foundations of leisure. In E. L. Jackson & T. L. Burton (Eds.), *Leisure studies: Prospects for the twenty-first century* (pp. 35-51). State College, PA: Venture.

Iwasaki, Y., & Mannell, R. (1999). Situational and personality influences on intrinsically motivated leisure behavior: Interaction effects and cognitive processes. *Leisure Sciences, 21,* 287-306.

Jackson, A. S., & Pollock, M. L. (1978). Generalized equations for predicting body density of men. *British Journal of Nutrition, 40,* 497-504.

Jackson, A. S., Pollock, M. L., & Ward, A. (1980). Generalized equations for predicting body density of women. *Medicine & Science in Sports & Exercise, 12,* 175-182. Retrieved May 30, 2009, from http://www.exrx.net/Calculators/BodyComp.html

Jackson, Y., Dietz, W. H., Sanders, C., Kolbe, L. J., Whyte, J. J., Wechsler, H., et al. (2002). Summary of the 2000 Surgeon General's listening session: Toward a national action plan on overweight and obesity. *Obesity Research, 10,* 1299-1305.

Jacobs, P. (1979). Analyzing environmental health hazards. *Environmental Science & Technology, 13*(5), 526-529.

Jacobson, E. (1938). Yoga: A scientific evaluation. *Psychological Bulletin, 35*(1), 46-50.

Jayne, D. (1925). *Medical almanac and guide to health.* New York: Dr. D. Jayne & Son.

Jenab, M., & Thompson, L. U. (1998). The influence of phytic acid in wheat bran on early biomarkers of colon carcinogenesis. *Carcinogenesis, 19*(6), 1087-1092.

Jewell, D. V. (2006). The role of fitness in physical therapy patient management: Applications across the continuum of care. *Cardiopulmonary Physical Therapy Journal, 17*(2), 47-62.

Johnson, C. K. (2007, July 3). Study: Over 30 pct report alcohol abuse. Retrieved May 30, 2009, from http://www.bookrags.com/news/study-over-30-pct-report-alcohol-moc/

Johnson, P. B., Glassman, M. (1998). The relationship between ethnicity, gender, and alcohol consumption. *Addiction, 93*(4), 583-589.

Jonas, S. (2000). *Talking about health and wellness with your patients.* New York: Springer.

Jones, D., Tanegawa, T., Weiss, S. M. (2003). Stress management and workplace disability in the US, Europe, and Japan: A review. *Journal of Occupational Health, 45,* 1-7.

Jones, F., Harris, P., Waller, H., & Coggins, A. (2005). Adherence to an exercise prescription scheme: The role of expectations, self-efficacy, stage of change and psychological well-being. *British Journal of Health Psychology, 3,* 359-378.

Jones, J. P., & Frazier, S. E. (1994). Assessment of self-esteem and wellness in health promotion professionals. *Psychological Reports, 75,* 833-834.

Joshipura, K. J., Hung, H. C., Li, T. Y., Hu, F. B., Rimm, E. B., Stampfer, M. J., et al. (2008). Intakes of fruits, vegetables and carbohydrates and the risk of CVD. *Public Health Nutrition, 12*(1), 115-121.

Juchmès-Férir, A. M., Juchmès, J., Frankignoul, M., Cession-Fossion, A., Volon, G., & Bottin, R. (1971). Comparison of physiological responses to moderate muscular exercise in normal subjects in relation to the degree of anxiety [French]. *Pathologic Biologie, 19*(5), 697-703.

Juhn, M. (2003). Popular sports supplements and ergogenic aids. *Sports Medicine, 23*(12), 921-940.

Kanayama, G., Barry, S., Hudson, J. I., & Pope, H. G. (2006). Body image and attitudes toward male roles in anabolic–androgenic steroid users. *American Journal of Psychiatry, 163*(4), 697-703.

Kant, A. (2000). Consumption of energy-dense, nutrient-poor foods by adult Americans: Nutritional and health implications. The third National Health and Nutrition Examination Survey, 1988-1994. *American Journal of Clinical Nutrition, 72,* 929-936.

Kanter, J. W., Rusch, L. C., & Brondino, M. J. (2008). Depression self-stigma: A new measure and preliminary findings. *Journal of Nervous and Mental Disorders, 196*(9), 663-670. Retrieved May 30, 2009, from http://www.ncbi.nlm.nih.gov/pubmed/18791427?ordinalpos=3&itool=EntrezSystem2.PEntrez.Pubmed.Pubmed_ResultsPanel.Pubmed_DefaultReportPanel.Pubmed_RVDocSum

Karpov, V. (2002, June). Religiosity and tolerance in the United States and Poland. *Journal for the Scientific Study of Religion, 41*(2), 267-288 .

Karvonen, J., & Vuorimaa, T. (1988). Heart rate and exercise intensity during sports activities. Practical application. *Sports Medicine, 5*(5), 303-311.

Karvonen, M. J., Kentala, E., & Mustala, O. (1957). The effects of training on heart rate: A longitudinal study. *Annales Medicinae Experimentalis et Biologiae Fenniae, 35*(3), 307-315.

Kawano, Y., Ishizaki, S., Sasamoto, S., Katoh, Y., & Kobayashi, S. (2002). Effect of meals with milk on body iron stores and improvement of dietary habit during weight loss in female rhythmic gymnasts [Japanese]. *Journal of Nutrition Science and Vitaminology* [Tokyo], *48*(5), 395-400.

Kaye, S. A., Folsom, A. R., & Jacobs, D. R. (1993). Psychosocial correlates of body fat distribution in black and white young adults. *International Journal of Obesity, 17,* 271-277.

Keefe, F. J., Block, A. R., Williams, R. B., & Surwit, R. S. (1981). Behavioral treatment of chronic low back pain: Clinical outcome and individual differences in pain relief. *Pain, 11,* 221-231.

Keesey, R. E. (1986). A set-point theory of obesity. In K. D. Brownell & J. P. Foreyt (Eds.), *Handbook of Eating Disorders* (pp. 63-87). New York: Basic Books.

Keim, N. L., Canty, D. J., Barbieri, T. F., & Wu, M. M. (1996). Effect of exercise and dietary restraint on energy intake of reduced-obese women. *Appetite, 26*(1), 55-70.

Kelley, K., Clark, B., Brown, V., & Sitzia, J. (2003). Good practice in the conduct and reporting of survey research. *Journal for Quality in Health Care, 15*(30), 261-266.

Kelly, D. F. (2004). *Contemporary Catholic health ethics.* Washington, DC: Georgetown University Press.

Kendall, F., McCreary, E., & Provance, P. (2005). *Muscle testing and function with posture and pain* (5th ed.). Baltimore: Lippincott Williams & Wilkins.

Kilkus, S. P. (1993). Assertiveness among professional nurses. *Journal of Advanced Nursing, 18*(8), 1324-1330.

Kline, G. M., Porcari, J. P., Hintermeister, R., Freedson, P. S., Ward, A., McCarron, R. F., et al. (1987). Estimation of VO$_2$max from a one-mile track walk, gender, age, and body weight. *Medicine Science in Sport & Exercise, 19*(3), 253-259.

Ko, J. Y., Brown, D. R., Galuska, D. A., Zhang, J., Blanck, H. M., Ainsworth, B. E. (2008). Weight loss advice U.S. obese adults receive from health care professionals. *Preventative Medicine, 47*(6), 587-592.

Kobasa, S. C. (1979). Personality and resistance to illness. *American Journal of Community Psychology, 7*(4), 413-423.

Kobasa, S. C., Maddi, S. R., & Puccetti, M. C. (1982). Personality and exercise as buffers in the stress-illness relationship. *Journal of Behavioral Medicine, 5*(4), 391-404.

Kobasa, S. C., Maddi, S. R., Puccetti, M. C., & Zola, M. A. (1985). Effectiveness of hardiness, exercise and social support as resources against illness. *Journal of Psychosomatic Research, 29*(5), 525-528.

Kobasa, S. C., Maddi, S. R., & Zola, M. A. (1983). Type A and hardiness. *Journal of Behavioral Medicine, 6*(1), 41-51.

Kobasa, S. C., & Puccetti, M. C. (1983). Personality and social resources in stress resistance. *Journal of Personality and Social Psychology, 45*(4), 839-850.

Kohrt, W. M. (1995). Body composition by DXA: Tried and true? *Medicine & Science in Sports & Exercise, 27*(10), 1349-1353.

Kopinak, J. K. (1999, May). The use of triangulation in a study of refugee well-being. *Quality & Quantity, 33*(2), 169-184.

Korzenik, J. R. (2006). Case closed? Diverticulitis: Epidemiology and fiber. *Journal of Clinical Gastroenterology, 40*(Suppl 3), S112-S116.

Kosmin, B. A., & Keysar, A. (2008). *American Religious Identification Survey (ARIS 2008) Summary Report.* Retrieved May 30, 2009, from http://livinginliminality.files.wordpress.com/2009/03/aris_report_2008.pdf

Kosmin, B. A., & Keysar, A. (2009). *American religious identification survey (ARIS 2008).* Retrieved May 30, 2009, from http://livinginliminality.files.wordpress.com/2009/03/aris_report_2008.pdf

Krasnopolsky-Levine, E., & Olender-Russo, L. (1992). Nutrition in health and wellness: Planning and services. In J. Rothman & R. E. Levine (Eds.), *Prevention practice: Strategies for physical therapy and occupational therapy.* Philadelphia: Saunders.

Krathwohl, D. R., Bloom, B. S., & Bertram, B. M. (1973). *Taxonomy of educational objectives, the classification of educational goals. Handbook II: Affective domain.* New York: McKay.

Krefutler, P. A. (1980). *Nutrition in perspective.* Englewood Cliffs, NJ: Prentice-Hall.

Kreider, R. B. (1999). Dietary supplements and the promotion of growth with resistance exercise. *Sports Medicine, 27*(2), 97-111.

Kreider, R. B. (2005). Effects of the Curves(r) fitness & weight loss program I: Body composition [Abstract]. *Journal of the American Societies for Experimental Biology,* LBA:54.

Kreider, R. B., Rasmussen, C., Kerksick, C., Magrans, T., Marcello, B., Taylor, L., et al. (2004). Effects of the Curves(r) fitness program on weight loss and resting energy expenditure [Abstract]. *Medicine & Science in Sport & Exercise, 36*(5), S81.

Kriska, A. M., & Caspersen, C. J. (Eds.). (1997). A collection of physical activity questionnaires for health-related research. *Medicine & Science in Sports & Exercise, 29,* S1-S205.

Krista, L. (2004). New insights into protein intake and progression of renal disease. *Current Opinion in Nephrology & Hypertension, 13*(3), 333-337.

Krotkiewski, M., Blohme, B., Lindholm, N., & Björntorp, P. (1976). The effects of adrenal corticosteroids on regional adipocyte size in man. *Journal of Clinical Endocrinology & Metabolism, 42,* 91-97.

Kruger, J. (2007, November 23). Prevalence of regular physical activity among adults—United States, 2001 and 2005. *MMWR Weekly, 56*(46), 1209-1212. Retrieved October 30, 2008, from http://www.cdc.gov/mmwr/preview/mmwrhtml/mm5646a1.htm

Kurata, S., Nawata, K., Nawata, S., Hongo, H., Suto, R., Nagashima, H., et al. (1998). Surgery for abdominal aortic aneurysms associate with malignancy. *Surgery Today, 28,* 895-899.

Kurup, R. K., & Kurup, P. A. (2001). Hypothalamic digoxin, hemispheric dominance and the acquired immunodeficiency syndrome. *NeuroImmunoModulation, 9*(5), 286-294. Retrieved May 30, 2009, from http://content.karger.com/ProdukteDB/produkte.asp?Aktion=ShowPDF&ProduktNr=224176&Ausgabe=228055&ArtikelNr=54291

Kushner, R. F. (1992). Bioelectric impedance analysis: A review of principles and applications. *Journal of the American College of Nutrition, 11,* 199-209.

Kushner, R. F. (1993). Body weight and mortality. *Nutrition Review, 51,* 1-10.

Kushner, R. F., & Schoeller, D. A. (1986). Estimation of total body water by bioelectrical impedance analysis. *American Journal of Clinical Nutrition, 44,* 417-424.

Kushner, R. F., Schoeller, D. A., Fjeld, C. R., & Danford, L. (1992). Is the impedance index (ht2/R) significant in predicting total body water? *American Journal of Clinical Nutrition, 56,* 835-839.

Landers, D. M. (n.d.). *The influence of exercise on mental health.* Retrieved May 30, 2009, from http://www.fitness.gov/mentalhealth.htm

Landry, J. (2004, May). Reflections on responsibility. *Magazine of Physical Therapy, 12*(1), 9.

Lanza, E. (1987). Dietary fiber intake in the U.S. population. *American Journal of Clinical Nutrition, 46,* 490.

Large, E. (2005, December). Incorporating yoga therapy into rehabilitation for chronic low back pain. *Annals of Internal Medicine.*

Largest atheist/agnostic populations. (1999). Retrieved May 30, 2009, from http://www.adherents.com/largecom/com_atheist.html

Larsen, J. (2008). *Caffeine, coffee, tea, cola & energy drinks.* Retrieved May 30, 2009, from http://www.dietitian.com/caffeine.html

Larson, E. J., & Witham, L. (1998). Leading scientists still reject God. *Nature, 394*(6691), 313. Retrieved May 30, 2009, from http://www.stephenjaygould.org/ctrl/news/file002.html

Lasater, J. (1997). Untying the knot: Yoga as physical therapy. In C. M. Davis (Ed.), *Complementary therapies in rehabilitation* (pp. 125-131). Thorofare, NJ: Slack.

Laughlin, J. (2000, May). AWAA offers water system basics. *Waterworld, 16*(5). Retrieved May 30, 2009, from http://ww.pennnet.com/articles/print_toc.cfm?p=41&v=16&i=5

Lawrence, R. C., Helmick, C. G., Arnett, F. C., Deyo, R. A., Felson, D. T., Giannini, E. H., et al. (1998). Estimates of the prevalence of arthritis and selected musculoskeletal disorders in the United States. *Arthritis Rheumatology, 43,* 778-799.

Layman, D. K. (2004). Protein quantity and quality at levels above the RDA improves adult weight loss. *Journal of the American College of Nutrition, 23*(Suppl 6), 631S-636S.

Lazarus, A. A. (1973), Multimodal behavior therapy: Treating the BASIC ID. *Journal of Nervous and Mental Disease, 156,* 404-411.

Lazarus, A. A. (1976). *Multimodal behavior therapy.* New York: Springer.

Lazarus, A. A., & Rachman, S. S. (1957). The use of systematic desensitization in psychotherapy. *South African Medical Journal, 31*(37), 934-937.

Lazarus, R. S., & Launier, R. (1978). Stress-related transactions between person and environment. In L. A. Pervin & M. Lewis (Eds.). *Perspectives in interactional psychology* (pp. 287-327). New York: Plenum.

Lee, C. (2004). *Yoga teacher and studio owner Cyndi Lee answers your frequently asked questions.* Retrieved May 30, 2009, from http://www.yogajournal.com/newtoyoga/820.cfm

Léger, L. A., & Lambert, J. (1982). A maximal multistage 20-m shuttle run test to predict VO2 max. *European Journal of Applied Physiology and Occupational Physiology, 49*(1), 1-12.

Legge, B. J., & Banister, E. W. (1986). The Astrand-ryhming nomogram revisited. *Journal of Applied Physiology, 61*(3), 1203-1209.

Lejeune, M. P., Kovacs, E. M., & Westerterp-Plantenga, M. S. (2005). Additional protein intake limits weight regain after weight loss in humans. *British Journal of Nutrition, 93*(2), 281-289.

Lemon, P. W. (1998). Effects of exercise on dietary protein requirements. *International Journal of Sport Nutrition, 8,* 426-447.

Lemon, P. W., Tarnopolsky, M. A., MacDougall, J. D., & Atkinson, S. A. (1992). Protein requirements and muscle mass/strength changes during intensive training in novice bodybuilders. *Journal of Applied Physiology, 73*, 767-775.

Leshner, A. I. (2000, March). Addressing the medical consequences of drug abuse. *NIDA Notes, 15*(1). Retrieved May 30, 2008, from the National Institute on Drug Abuse Web site: http://www.drugabuse.gov/NIDA_Notes/NNVol15N1/DirRepVol15N1.html

Leskowitz, E. (2003). *Complementary and alternative medicine in rehabilitation.* New York: Churchill Livingstone.

Leuba, J. H. (1916). *The belief in God and immorality: A psychological, anthropological and statistical study.* Boston: Sherman, French, & Co.

Leuba, J. H. (1921). *The belief in God and immorality: A psychological, anthropological and statistical study* (2nd ed.) [PDF format]. Boston: Sherman, French, & Co. Retrieved May 30, 2009, from http://www.archive.org/details/beliefingodimmor00leubuoft

Leuba, J. H. (1934, August). Religious beliefs of American scientists. *Harper's Magazine,* 291-300. Retrieved May 30, 2009, from http://www.harpers.org/archive/1934/08/0018789

Ley, C. J., Lees, B., & Stevenson, J. C. (1992). Sex- and menopause-associated changes in body fat distribution. *American Journal of Clinical Nutrition, 55,* 950-954.

Li, F., Harmer, P., & Fisher, J. (2005). Tai chi and fall reductions in older adults: A randomized controlled trial. *Journal of Gerontology, 60A,* 187-194.

Li, J., Kaneko, T., Oin, L. Q., Wang, J., Wang, Y., & Sato, A. (2003). Long-term effects of high dietary fiber intake on glucose tolerance and lipid metabolism in GK rats: Comparison among barley, rice, and cornstarch. *Metabolism, 52*(9), 1206-1210.

Lieberman, A., Bruning, N. (1990). *The real vitamin and mineral book.* New York: Avery Group.

Lightman, B. (2002). Huxley and scientific agnosticism: The strange history of a failed rhetorical strategy. *British Journal of Historical Science, 35*(126), 271-289.

Liu, S., Willett, W. C., & Stampfer, M. J. (2000). A prospective study of dietary glycemic load, carbohydrate intake, and risk of coronary heart disease in U.S. women. *American Journal of Clinical Nutrition, 71,* 1455-1461.

Long, L., Lanning, B., Bowden, R., Nassar, E., Zimmerman, A., Campbell, B., et al. (2005). Effects of the Curves(r) fitness & weight loss program VI: Body image. *Journal of the American Societies for Experimental Biology, LBA,* 58.

Low, M. R., & Kral, T. V. (2006). Stress-induced eating in restrained eaters may not be caused by stress or restraint. *Appetite, 46*(1), 16-21.

Lowry, R., Wechsler, H., Galuska, D. A., Fulton, J. E., & Kann, L. (2002). Television viewing and its association with overweight, sedentary lifestyle, and insufficient consumption of fruits and vegetables among U.S. high-school students: Differences by race, ethnicity, and gender. *Journal of School Health, 72,* 413-421.

Lukaski, H. C., & Bolonchuk, W. W. (1988). Estimation of body fluid volumes using tetrapolar bioelectrical impedance measurements. *Aviation Space & Environmental Medicine, 59,* 1163-1169.

Lukaski, H. C., & Bolonchuk, W. W. (1989). Maintenance of aerobic capacity and body composition of volunteers residing on a metabolic research unit. *Journal of Sports Medicine of Physical Fitness, 29*(3), 273-278.

Lukaski, H. C., Bolonchuk, W. W., Hall, C. B., & Siders, W. A. (1986). Validation of tetrapolar bioelectrical impedance method to assess human body composition. *Journal of Applied Physiology, 60,* 1327-1332.

Mac, B. (2006). *Multi-stage fitness test.* Retrieved May 30, 2009, from http://www.brianmac.demon.co.uk/beep.htm

MacArthur, J. D., & MacArthur, C. T. (1997). *Body composition.* Retrieved December 18, 2007, from http://www.macses.ucsf.edu/Research/Allostatic/notebook/body.html

Macková, E., Macková, E., Melichna, J., Havlíčková, L., Placheta, Z., Blahová, D., et al. (1986). Skeletal muscle characteristics of sprint cyclists and nonathletes. *International Journal of Sports Medicine, 7*(5), 295-297.

Maddalozzo, G. F., Cardinal, B. J., & Snow, C. M. (2002). Concurrent validity of the BOD POD and dual energy x-ray absorptiometry techniques for assessing body composition in young women. *Journal of the American Dietetic Association, 102*, 1677-1679.

Malina, R. M., & Stern, M. P. (1992). [The San Antonio Heart Study]. Unpublished raw data.

Manjarrez, C., & Birrer, R. (1983). Nutrition and athletic performance. *American Family Physician, 28*(5), 105-115.

Manson, J. E., Willett, W. C., & Stampfer, M. J. (1994). Vegetable and fruit consumption and incidence of stroke in women [Abstract]. *Circulation, 89*(2), 932.

Manzari, S., Ruddy, T., Woycik, T., & Pfalzer, L. (2001). The optimal length of time (1, 2, 20, and 50 minutes) to stretch the hamstring muscle group in a seated position using a discomfort scale in individuals 50–54 years of age. In J. M. Rothstein (Ed.)., PT 2001: The annual conference and exposition of the APTA abstracts of papers accepted for presentation. *Physical Therapy, 81*(5).

Manzoni, G. M., Pagnini, F., Castelnuovo, G., & Molinari, E. (2008). Relaxation training for anxiety: a ten-years systematic review with meta-analysis. *BMC Psychiatry, 2*(8), 41.

Marin, P., Darin, N., & Amemiya, T. (1992). Cortisol secretion in relation to body fat distribution in obese premenopausal women. *Metabolism, 41*, 882-886.

Marlett, J. A., McBurney, M. I., Slavin, J. L., & American Dietetic Association. (2002). Position of the American Dietetic Association: Health implications of dietary fiber. *Journal of the American Dietetic Association, 102*(7), 993-1000.

Marsh, H. W., & Richards, G. E. (1986). The Rotter Locus of Control Scale: The comparison of alternative response formats and implications for reliability, validity and dimensionality. *Journal of Research in Personality, 20*, 509-558.

Marston, A. R., & Criss, J. (1984). Maintenance of successful weight loss: Incidence and prediction. *International Journal of Obesity, 8*(5), 435-439.

Martin, C. K., Church, T. S., Thompson, A.M., Earnest, C. P., & Blair, S. N. (2009). Exercise dose and quality of life: A randomized controlled trial. *Archives of Internal Medicine, 169*(3), 269-278.

Martinsen, E. W. (2008). Physical activity in the prevention and treatment of anxiety and depression. *Nordic Journal of Psychiatry, 62*(Suppl 47), 25-29.

Masheb, R. M., & Grilo, C. M. (2006). Eating patterns and breakfast consumption in obese patients with binge eating disorder. *Behavior Research Therapy, 44*(11), 1545-1553.

Masse, L. C., Heech, K. C., Fulton, J. E., & Watson, K. B. (2002). Raters objectivity in using the compendium of physical activities to code physical activity diaries. *Measurement Physical Education Exercise Science, 6*, 207-224.

Massey, F. P. (2002, December 5). APTA's letter to the editor of *The Washington Post* regarding "who trained the trainer?" *Physical Therapy* [Online]. Retrieved September 1, 2003, from http://www.apta.org/news/letters/trainer

Matsumoto, A. (1990). Effects of chronic testosterone administration in normal men: Safety and efficacy of high dosage testosterone and parallel dose-dependent suppression of luteinizing hormone, follicle-stimulating hormone, and sperm production. *Journal of Clinical Endocrinology and Metabolism, 70*(1), 282-287.

Mattes, R. D. (2002). Ready-to-eat cereal used as a meal replacement promotes weight loss in humans. *Journal of American College of Nutrition, 21*(6), 570-577.

Matthews, K. A., & Krantz, D. S. (1976). Resemblances of twins and their parents in pattern A behavior. *Psychosomatic Medicine, 38*, 140-144.

Maximal oxygen consumption. (n.d.). Retrieved May 30, 2009, from San Diego State University Web site: http://www-rohan.sdsu.edu/course/ens304/public_html/section1/maxoxygen consumption.htm

May, W. W., Morgan, B. J., Lemke, J. C., Karsi, G. M., & Stone, H. L. (1993). Model for ability-based assessment in physical therapy education. *Journal of Physical Therapy Education, 9*, 3-6.

Mayo Clinic. (2008a). *Dehydration.* Retrieved May 30, 2009, from http://www.mayoclinic.com/health/dehydration/DS00561/DSECTION=2

Mayo Clinic. (2008b). *Exercise: Rev up your routine to reduce stress.* Retrieved May 30, 2009, from http://www.mayoclinic.com/health/exercise-and-stress/SR00036

Mayo Clinic. (2009a). *Dietary fats: Know which types to choose.* Retrieved May 30, 2009, from http://www.mayoclinic.com/health/fat/NU00262

Mayo Clinic. (2009b). *Self-esteem: Boost your self-image with these 5 steps.* Retrieved May 30, 2009, from http://www.mayoclinic.com/health/self-esteem/MH00129

Mazess, R. B., Peppler, W. W., & Chestnut, C. H., III. (1981). Total body bone mineral and lean body mass by dual-photon absorptiometry, II: Comparison with total body calcium by neutron activisceral adipose tissue ion analysis. *Calcified Tissue International, 33,* 361-363.

Mazess, R. B., Peppler, W. W., & Gibbons, M. (1984). Total body composition by dual-photon (153Gd) absorptiometry. *American Journal of Clinical Journal, 40,* 834-839.

Mazess, R. B., Trempe, J. A., Bisek, J. P., Hanson, J. A., & Hans, D. (1991). Calibration of dual-energy x-ray absorptiometry for bone density. *Journal of Bone and Mineral Research, 6,* 799-806.

McAllister, M. (2008). Looking below the surface: developing critical literacy skills to reduce the stigma of mental disorders. *Journal of Nursing Education, 47*(9), 426-430.

McArdle, W. D., Katch, F. I., & Katch, V. L. (2006). *Exercise physiology: Energy, nutrition, and human performance* (7th ed.). Philadelphia: Lippincott Williams & Wilkins.

McCabe, S. E., Brower, K. J., West, B. T., Nelson, T. F., & Wechsler, H. (2007). Trends in non-medical use of anabolic steroids by U.S. college students: Results from four national surveys. *Drug and Alcohol Dependence, 90*(2-3), 243-251.

McDaniel, A., & Hammond, M. (1997a). *Alexandrian medicine.* Retrieved May 30, 2009, from Claude Moore Health Sciences Library, University of Virginia Health System Web site: http://www.hsl.virginia.edu/historical/artifacts/antiqua/alexandrian.cfm

McDaniel, A., & Hammond, M. (1997b). *Byzantine.* Retrieved May 30, 2009, from Claude Moore Health Sciences Library, University of Virginia Health System Web site: http://www.hsl.virginia.edu/historical/artifacts/antiqua/byzantine.cfm

McDaniel, A., & Hammond, M. (1997c). *From Homer to Hippocrates.* Retrieved May 30, 2009, from Claude Moore Health Sciences Library, University of Virginia Health System Web site: http://www.hsl.virginia.edu/historical/artifacts/antiqua/homer.cfm

McDaniel, A., & Hammond, M. (1997d). *Hippocrates.* Retrieved May 30, 2009, from Claude Moore Health Sciences Library, University of Virginia Health System Web site: http://www.hsl.virginia.edu/historical/artifacts/antiqua/hippocrates.cfm

McDowell, I., & Newell, C. (1987). *Measuring health: A guide to rating scales and questionnaires.* New York: Oxford University Press.

McGlynn, F. D. (1971). Individual versus standardized hierarchies in the systematic desensitization of snake-avoidance. *Behavior Research Therapy, 9*(1), 1-5.

McGlynn, F. D., & Walls, R. (1976). Credibility ratings for desensitization and pseudotherapy among moderately and mildly snake-avoidant college students. *Journal of Clinical Psychology, 32*(1), 140-145.

McKeown, N. M., Meigs, J. B., Liu, S., Saltzman, E., Wilson, P. W., & Jacques, P. F. (2004). Carbohydrate nutrition, insulin resistance, and the prevalence of the metabolic syndrome in the Framingham Offspring Cohort. *Diabetes Care, 27,* 538-546.

McKeown, N. M., Meigs, J. B., Liu, S., Wilson, P. W., & Jacques, P. F. (2002). Whole-grain intake is favorably associated with metabolic risk factors for type 2 diabetes and cardiovascular disease in the Framingham Offspring Study. *American Journal of Clinical Nutrition, 76,* 390-398.

Mclean, W. (1992). Validity of Futrex-5000 for body composition. *Medicine & Exercise in Sports & Exercise, 2*(2), 253-257.

McLoughlin, C. S., & Kubick, R. J. (2004). Wellness promotion as a life-long endeavor: Promoting and developing life competencies from childhood. *Psychology in the Schools, 41*(1), 131-142.

McMahon, M., Gerich, J., & Rizza, J. (1988). Effects of glucocorticoids on carbohydrate metabolism. *Diabetes & Metabolic Reviews, 4,* 17-30.

McManus, C. (2003, June 19). Wellness programs serve the "whole" patient with chronic pain. *PT 2003 News and Highlights.* Retrieved June 30, 2003, from http://www.apta.org-/Meetings/past_ events/pt2003/news_pt2003/june19

McNaughton, S. A., Dunstan, D. W., Ball, K., Shaw, J., & Crawford, D. (2009, February 11). Dietary quality is associated with diabetes and cardio-metabolic risk factors. *Journal of Nutrition, 139*(4), 734-742.

Megnien, J. L., & Simon, A. (2008). Exercise tolerance test for predicting coronary heart disease in asymptomatic individuals: A review [e-pub ahead of print]. *Atherosclerosis.*

Meijer, P. C., Verloop, N., & Beijaard, D. (2002, May). Multi-method triangulation in a qualitative study on teachers' practical knowledge: An attempt to increase internal validity. *Quality & Quantity, 36*(2), 145-168.

Members on the move. (2002, May). *Magazine of Physical Therapy, 10*(5), 12.

Meredith, C. N., Zackin, M. J., Frontera, W. R., & Evans, W. J. (1989). Dietary protein requirements and body protein metabolism in endurance-trained men. *Journal of Applied Physiology, 66*(6), 2850-2856.

Meriggiola, M., Costantino, A., Bremner, W., & Morselli-Labate, A. (2002). Higher testosterone dose impairs sperm suppression induced by a combined androgen-progestin regimen. *Journal of Andrology, 23*(5), 684-690.

Mewis, C., Spyridopoulos, I., Kühlkamp, V., & Seipel, L. (1996). Manifestation of severe coronary heart disease after anabolic drug abuse. *Clinical Cardiology, 19*(2), 153-155.

Middaugh, S. J. (1978). EMG feedback as a muscle reeducation technique: A controlled study. *Physical Therapy, 58*(1), 15-21.

Miller, M. C. (2005). Questions and answers: What is Type D personality? *Harvard Health Letter, 22*(5), 8.

Miller, K. D. (1991). Body-image therapy. *Nursing Clinics of North America, 26*(3), 727-736.

Miller, N. W. (2002). *What is medical necessity?* Retrieved May 30, 2009, from Physician's News Digest Web site: http://www.physiciansnews.com/law/802.miller.html

Mills, D. W. (2002). *Applying what we know student learning styles.* Retrieved March 30, 2009, from http://www.csrnet.org/csrnet/articles/student-learning-styles.html

Minami, J., Toshihiko, I., & Matsuoka, H. (1999). Effects of smoking cession on blood pressure and heart rate variability in habitual smokers. *Hypertension, 33*(5), 586-590.

Miovic, M. (2004). An introduction to spiritual psychology: Overview of the literature, east and west. *Harvard Review of Psychiatry, 12*(2), 105-115.

Mirabella, J. (2003a). *How not to write a survey.* Unpublished manuscript, Capella University, Minneapolis, Minnesota.

Mirabella, J. (2003b). *Sampling scenarios for survey success.* Unpublished manuscript, Capella University, Minneapolis, Minnesota.

Misquita, N. A., Davis, D. C., Dobrovolny, C. L., Ryan, A. S., Dennis, K. E., & Bicklas, B. J. (2001). Applicability of maximal oxygen consumption criteria in obese, menopausal women. *Journal of Women's Health & Gender-Based Medicine, 10*(9), 879-885. Retrieved May 30, 2009, from http://www.liebertonline.com/doi/abs/10.1089/152460901753285787

Miyatkake, N., Takename, E., Kawasaki, Y., & Fujii, M. (2005). Comparison of air displacement plethysmograph and bioelectrical impedance for assessing body composition changes during weight loss in Japanese women. *Diabetes, Obesity, and Metabolism, 7*(3), 268-272.

Moffat, M. (1996). The 1996 APTA presidential address: Three quarters of a century of healing generations. *Physical Therapy, 76,* 1242-1252.

Montgomery, A. C., & Crittenden, K. S. (1977). Improving coding reliability for open-ended questions. *Public Opinion Quarterly, 41*(2), 235-243.

Montoye, H. M., Kemper, H. C. J., Saris, W. H. N., & Washburn, R. A. (1996). *Measuring physical activity and energy expenditure.* Champaign, IL: Human Kinetics.

Moos, R. H., & Holahan, C. J. (2003). Dispositional and contextual perspectives on coping: Toward an integrative framework. *Journal of Clinical Psychology, 59*(12), 1387-1403.

Morrow, J. R., Jackson, A. W., Bazzarre, T. L., Milne, D., & Blair, S. N. (1999). A one-year follow-up to physical activity and health: A report of the Surgeon General. *American Journal of Preventative Medicine, 17*(1), 24-30.

Morton, A. R., & Holmick, E. V. (1985). The effects of cigarette smoking on maximal oxygen consumption and selected physiological responses of elite team sportsmen. *European Journal of Applied Physiology, 53*(4), 348-352. Retrieved May 30, 2009, from http://www.springerlink.com/content/v6p9415643j5q43n/

Mukamal, K. J., Hallqvist, J., Hammar, N., Ljung, R., Gemes, K., Ahlbom, A., et al. (2009). Coffee consumption and mortality after acute myocardial infarction: The Stockholm Heart Epidemiology Program. *American Heart Journal, 157*(3), 495-501.

Murphy, W. (1995). *Healing the generations: A history of physical therapy and the American Physical Therapy Association.* Alexandria, VA: American Physical Therapy Association.

Myers, J. E., Mobley, A. K., & Booth, C. S. (2003). Wellness of counseling students: Practicing what we preach. *Counselor Education & Supervision, 42,* 264-274.

Myers, J. E., Sweeney, T. J., & Witmer, J. M. (2000). The wheel of wellness counseling for wellness: A holistic model for treatment planning. *Journal of Counseling & Development, 78*(3), 251-266.

Myers, J. E., Sweeney, T. J., & Witmer, J. M. (2005). *Wellness evaluation lifestyle.* Mento Park, CA: Mindset. Retrieved February 15, 2008, from http://www.mindgarden.com/products/wells.htm#workbook

National Cancer Institute. (2004). *Cigarette smoking and cancer: Questions and answers.* Retrieved May 30, 2009, from http://www.cancer.gov/cancertopics/factsheet/tobacco/cancer

National Center for Chronic Disease Prevention and Health Promotion. (1999). *Physical activity and health: A report of the Surgeon General.* Retrieved May 30, 2009, from http://www.cdc.gov/nccdphp/sgr/ataglan.htm

National Center for Health Statistics. (2008). *Prevalence of overweight and obesity among adults: United States, 2003–2004.* Retrieved February 20, 2009, from http://www.cdc.gov/nchs/products/pubs/pubd/hestats/overweight/overwght_adult_03.htm

National Institute of Alcohol Abuse and Alcoholism. (2004). NIAAA council approves definition of binge drinking (PDF–1.6Mb). *NIAAA Newsletter, 3,* 3.

National Institute on Drug Abuse. (2008a). *Marijuana.* Retrieved February 20, 2009, from http://www.nida.nih.gov/DrugPages/Marijuana.html

National Institute on Drug Abuse. (2008b). *Prescription drug abuse.* Retrieved February 20, 2009, from http://www.drugabuse.gov/pdf/tib/prescription.pdf

National Institute of Mental Health. (2000). *Depression.* Retrieved August 1, 2008, from http://www.nimh.nih.gov/healthinformation/depressionmenu.cfm

National Institute of Sports Medicine and Athletic Trauma. (2008). *NISMAT exercise physiology corner: Maximum oxygen consumption primer.* Retrieved May 30, 2009, from http://www.nismat.org/physcor/max_o2.html

National Institute on Alcohol Abuse and Alcoholism. (2004, June 10). *Alcohol abuse increases, dependence declines across decade: Young minorities emerge as high-risk subgroups.* Retrieved May 30, 2009, from http://www.niaaa.nih.gov/NewsEvents/NewsReleases/NESARCNews.htm

National Institutes of Health. (2001). *Gastric surgery for severe obesity.* Retrieved May 30, 2009, from the National Institute of Diabetes and Digestive and Kidney Diseases Web site:http://www.niddk.nih.gov/health/nutrit/pubs/gastric/gastricsurgery.htm

National Institutes of Health. (2003). *Very low calorie diets.* Retrieved May 30, 2009, from the National Institute of Diabetes and Digestive and Kidney Diseases Web site: http://www.niddk.nih.gov/health/nutrit/pubs/vlcd.htm

National Institutes of Health. (2009). *Greek medicine.* Retrieved May 30, 2009, from http://www.nlm.nih.gov/hmd/greek/greek_galen.html

National Mental Health Information Center. (n.d.). *Building self-esteem: A self-help guide.* Retrieved April 30, 2009, from http://mentalhealth.samhsa.gov/publications/allpubs/sma-3715/activities.asp

National Strength and Conditioning Association (NSCA). (2009). *Position statement: Plyometric exercises.* Retrieved March 20, 2009, from http://www.nsca.com/Publications/PLYOforWeb.pdf

National Wellness Institute. (n.d.). *Defining wellness.* Retrieved May 30, 2009, from http://www.nationalwellness.org/index.php?id_tier=2&id_c=26

National Wellness Institute. (n.d.). *National Wellness Institute 6 Dimensional Wellness Model.* Retrieved March 6, 2007, from http://www.nationalwellness.org/index.php?id=390&id_tier=81

National Wellness Institute. (1999). The testwell wellness inventory. Retrieved July 30, 2009, from http://www.testwell.org/pdf/QSetSA100Sample.pdf

National Wellness Institute. (2004). *National Wellness Institute history.* Retrieved May 6, 2004, from http://www.nationalwellness.org/index2.php

National Wellness Institute. (2006). *Wellness dimensions.* Retrieved May 30, 2009, from http://www.friendly-ware.com/wellness/WellnessDimensions.html

Naughton, J. (1978). The National Exercise and Heart Disease Project: The pre-randomization exercise program. Report number 2. *Cardiology, 63*(6), 352-367.

Neil, J. (2006). *What is locus of control?* Retrieved March 30, 2009, from http://wilderdom.com/psychology/loc/LocusOfControlWhatIs.html

Neilson, E. A. (1988). Health Values: Achieving high level wellness—Origin, philosophy, purpose. *Health Values, 12*(3), 3-5.

Nemours Foundation. (2007, August). *What's an osteopath?* Retrieved May 30, 2009, from the Kids Health Web site: http://kidshealth.org/parent/system/doctor/osteopath.html

Nespor, K. (2000). *Yoga and health. A course for Swedish yoga teachers.* Retrieved June 26, 2006, from http:/www.mujweb.cz/veda/Nespor

Newell-Morris, L., Moceri, V., & Fujimoto, W, (2005). Gynoid and android fat patterning in Japanese-American men: Body build and glucose metabolism. *American Journal of Human Biology, 1*(1), 73-86.

Nieman, D. C., Trone, G. A., & Austin, M. D. (2003). A new handheld device for measuring resting metabolic rate and oxygen consumption. *Journal of the American Dietetic Association, 103*(5), 588-593.

Noelle-Neumann, E. (1996). Quality criteria in survey research. *International Journal of Public Opinion Research, 9*(1), 29-32.

Norris, S. L., Zhang, X., Avenell, A., Gregg, E., Bowman, B., Schmid, C. H., et al. (2005). Long-term effectiveness of weight-loss interventions in adults with pre-diabetes: A review. *American Journal of Preventative Medicine, 28*(1), 126-139.

Nouwen, A., & Solinger, J. W. (1979). The effectiveness of EMG biofeedback training in low back pain. *Biofeedback and Self-Regulation, 4*(2), 103-111.

Ntoumanis, N., Edmunds, J., & Duda, J. L. (2009). Understanding the coping process from a self-determination theory perspective. *British Journal of Health Psychology, 14*(Pt. 2), 249-260.

Nunes, D. F., Rodriguez, A. L., da Silva Hoffmann, F., Luz, C., Braga Filho, A. P., Muller, M. C., et al. (2007). Relaxation and guided imagery program in patients with breast cancer undergoing radiotherapy is not associated with neuroimmunomodulatory effects. *Journal of Psychosomatic Research, 63*(6), 647-655.

Nunnally, J. (1978). *Psychometric theory.* New York: McGraw-Hill.

Nutrition and exercise: What your body needs. (1993, May). *University of California at Berkeley Wellness Letter, 9*(8), 4-6.

Nutrition infocenter. (2007). *What is U.S. daily allowances?* Retrieved May 30, 2009, from http://1stholistic.com/Nutrition/hol_nutrition-RDA.htm

O'Connell, K. A., & Skevington, S. M. (2005). The relevance of spirituality, religion and personal beliefs to health-related quality of life: Themes from focus groups in Britain. *British Journal of Health Psychology, 10*(Pt. 3), 379-398.

O'Connor, R. M., Farrow, S., & Colder, C. R. (2001). Clarifying the anxiety sensitivity and alcohol use relation: Considering alcohol expectancies as moderators. *Journal of the Studies of Alcohol and Drugs, 69*(5), 765-772.

O'Dea, J. A., & Abraham, S. (2001). Knowledge, beliefs, attitudes, and behaviors related to weight control, eating disorders, and body image in Australian trainee home economics and physical education teachers. *Journal of Nutrition Education, 33*(6), 332-340.

O'Donnell, M. P. (1986). Definition of health promotion. *American Journal of Health Promotion, 5*(101), 1.

O'Donovan, G., Owen, A., Bird, S., Kearney, E., Nevill, M., Jones, D., et al. (2005). Changes in cardiorespiratory fitness and coronary heart disease risk factors following 24 wk of moderate- or high-intensity exercise of equal energy cost. *Journal of Applied Physiology, 98*, 1619-1625. Retrieved June 3, 2008, from http://jap.physiology.org/cgi/content/full/98/5/1619

Office of Naval Research. (n.d.). *Science & technology focus.* Retrieved March 30, 2009, from http://www.onr.navy.mil/focus/blowballast/sub/work2.htm

Ogden, C. L., Carroll, M. D., Curtin, L. R., McDowell, M. A., Tabak, C. J., & Flegal, K. M. (2006). Prevalence of overweight and obesity in the United States, 1999–2004. *JAMA, 295*, 1549-1555.

Ogden, C. L., Carroll, M. D., McDowell, M. A., & Flegal, K. M. (2007). *Obesity among adults in the United States—No change since 2003–2004.* NCHS data brief no 1. Hyattsville, MD: National Center for Health Statistics.

Ogden, J. (2007). *Health psychology* (3rd ed.). Buckingham, United Kingdom: Open University Press.

Oldridge, N. B., & Stoedefalke, K. G. (1984). Compliance and motivation in cardiac exercise programs. *Clinical Sports Medicine, 3*(2), 443-454.

Oliveira, P. V., Baptista, L., Moreira, F., Vieira, P., & Landna, A. H. (2005). Correlation among muscle mass, strength, and cross-sectional muscle area according to carbohydrate and protein supplementation. *Medicine & Science in Sports & Exercise, 37*(5), S38.

Olsen, D., & Ferin, M. (1987). Corticotropin-releasing hormone inhibits gonadotropin secretion in ovariectomized Rhesus monkey. *Journal of Clinical Endocrinology and Metabolism, 65*, 262-267.

Ost, L. G. (1978). Fading vs systematic desensitization in the treatment of snake and spider phobia. *Behavioral Research and Therapy, 16*(6), 379-389.

Ottosson, M., Lönnroth, P., Björntorp, P., & Edén, S. (1995). Effects of cortisol and growth hormone on lipolysis in human adipose tissue. *Journal of Clinical Endocrinology and Metabolism, 85*(2), 799-803. Retrieved May 30, 2009, from http://jcem.endojournals.org/cgi/reprint/85/2/799.pdf

Ottoson, A. (2005). *Sjukgymnasten-Vart Tog Han Vågen?* Doctoral dissertation. Göteborg, Sweden: Historiska Institutionen, Göteborgs Universitet.

Ourania, M., Yvoni, H., Christos, K., & Ionannis, T. (2003). Effects of a physical activity program: The study of selected physical abilities among elderly women. *Journal of Gernotological Nursing, 29*(7), 50-55.

Overholser, W. (1951). The meaning of Freud for our time. *International Record of Medicine and General Practice Clinics, 164*(5), 249-257.

Paeratakul, S., York-Crowe, E. E., Williamson, D. A., Ryan, D. H., & Bray, G. A. (2002). Americans on diet: Results from the 1994–1996 continuing survey of food intakes by individuals. *Journal of the American Dietetic Association, 102*(9),1247-1251.

Paffenbarger, R. S., Wing, A. L., & Hyde, R. T. (1978). Physical activity as an index of heart attack risk in college alumni. *American Journal of Epidemiology, 108*, 161-175.

Pafnote, M., Vaida, I., & Luchian, O. (1979). Physical fitness in different groups of industrial workers. *Physiologie, 16*(2), 129-131.

Parkinson, A., & Evans, N. A. (2006). Anabolic–androgenic steroids: A survey of 500 users. *Medicine & Science in Sports & Exercise, 38*(4), 644-651.

Parra-Blanco, A. (2006). Colonic diverticular disease: Pathophysiology and clinical picture. *Digestion, 73*(1), S47-S57.

Pascal, G. R. (1949). The effect of relaxation upon recall. *American Journal of Psychology, 62*(1), 32-47.

Pate, R. R., Pratt, M., Blair, S. N., Haskell, W. L., Macera, C. A., Bouchard, C., et al. (1995). Physical activity and public health: A recommendation from the Centers for Disease Control and Prevention and the American College of Sports Medicine. *JAMA. 273*(5), 402-407. Retrieved February 20, 2009, from http://jama.ama-assn.org/cgi/content/abstract/273/5/402

Pearcy, L. T. (n.d.). Dreams in ancient medicine. In *Medicina Antiqua*. Retrieved May 30, 2009, from the Wellcome Trust Centre for the History of Medicine at UCL Web site: http://www.ucl.ac.uk/~ucgajpd/medicina%20antiqua/sa_dreams.html

Pearcy, L. T. (n.d.). Galen: A biographical sketch. In *Medicina Antiqua*. Retrieved May 30, 2009, from the Wellcome Trust Centre for the History of Medicine at UCL Web site: http://www.ucl.ac.uk/~ucgajpd/medicina%20antiqua/bio_gal.html

Penland, J. G. (2005). *Dietary reference intakes (DRIs)—New dietary guidelines really are new!* Retrieved May 30, 2009, from the U.S. Department of Agriculture, Agricultural Research Service Web site: http://www.ars.usda.gov/News/docs.htm?docid=10870

Pereira, M. A., O'Reilly, E., & Augustsson, K., et al. (2004). Dietary fiber and risk of coronary heart disease: A pooled analysis of cohort studies. *Archives of Internal Medicine, 164*, 370-376.

Perryman, B. E. (1980). Developing an employee cardiovascular fitness program. *Physiotherapy Canada, 32*(3), 157-159.

Phillips, S. M., Tarnopolsky, M. A., Tipton, K. D., Yarasheski, K. E., Hambraeus, L., & Campbell, W. W. (1999). Protein metabolism and requirements in exercising humans: Recent advances. *Medicine & Science in Sports & Exercise, 31*(5), S235.

The physical fitness specialist certification manual. (1997). Dallas, TX: The Cooper Institute for Aerobics Research.

Physiology and psychology. (1998). Retrieved May 30, 2009, from the Montana State University Web site: http://btc.montana.edu/olympics/physiology/pb02.html

Pierson, C. A. (2000, August). Expanding the nurse practitioner horizons. *Journal of American Academy of Nursing Practice, 12*, 302.

Pippenger, W. S., & Scalzitti, D. A. (2004). What are the effects, if any, of lower-extremity strength training on gait in children with cerebral palsy? *Physical Therapy, 84*(9), 849-858.

Pizer, A. (2006). *Your guide to yoga.* Retrieved July 10, 2006, from www.yoga.about.com

Plautz, P. (1997). *Wellness works.* Santa Fe, NM: Words With Wings.

Pollock, M. L., Bohannon, R. L., Cooper, K. H., Ayres, J. J., Ward, A., White, S. R., et al. (1976). A comparative analysis of four protocols for maximal treadmill stress testing. *American Heart Journal, 92*(1), 39-46.

Pollock, M. L., Schmidt, D. H., Jackson, A. S. (1980). Measurement of cardio-respiratory fitness and body composition in the clinical setting. *Comprehensive Therapy, 6*(9), 12-27.

Pope, H. G., Kanayama, G., Ionescu-Pioggia, M., & Hudson, J. I. (2004). Anabolic steroid users' attitudes towards physicians. *Addiction, 99*(9), 1189-1194.

Popescu, E., Badica, C., & Trigano, P. (2007). *Rules for learner modeling and adaptation provisioning in an education hypermedia system.* International Symposium on Symbolic and Numeric Algorithms for Scientific Computing, Syna, SC.

Porter, R. (1994). *The biographical dictionary of scientists* (2nd ed.). New York: Oxford University Press.

Powers, E. A., Morrow, P., Goudy, W. J., & Keith, P. M. (1977). Serial order preference in survey research. *Public Opinion Quarterly, 41*(1), 80-85.

Prentice, W. E. (2006). Impaired mobility: Restoring range of motion and improving flexibility. In M. J. Voight, B. J. Hoogenboom, & W. E. Prentice (Eds.), *Musculoskeletal interventions: Techniques for therapeutic exercise* (pp. 165-180). New York: McGraw-Hill Professional.

Presser, S. (1984). Is accuracy on factual survey items item-specific or respondent-specific? *Public Opinion Quarterly, 48*, 344-355.

Pressman, A. H., & Buff, S. (1997). *The Complete Idiot's Guide to Vitamins and Minerals.* New York: Alpha Books.

Pronk, N. P. (2004). Active physically fit employees have better work performance. *Journal of Occupational & Environmental Medicine (ACOEM).* Retrieved April 14, 2004, from http://www.acoem.org/news/news/default.asp?NEWS_ID=212

Purtilo, R. (1999). *Ethical dimensions in the health professions* (3rd ed.). Philadelphia: W. B. Saunders.

Pyle, R. L. (1979a). Corporate fitness programs: How do they shape up? *Personnel, 56*(1), 58-67.

Pyle, R. L. (1979b). Fitness development programs: Strengthening the corporate body. *Manage World, 8*(7), 8-11.

Quintana, J. M., Arsotegui, I., Escobar, A., Azkarate, J., Goenaga, J. I., & Lafuente, I. (2008). Prevalence of knee and hip osteoarthritis and the appropriateness of joint replacement in an older population. *Archives of Internal Medicine, 168*(14), 1576-1584.

Quotes: Fat, obesity. (n.d.). Retrieved May 30, 2009, from http://www.wordinfo.info/words/index/info/view_unit/2999

Raben, A., Jensen, N. D., Marckmann, P., Sandstrom, B., & Astrup, A. (1995). Spontaneous weight loss during 11 weeks' ad libitum intake of a low fat/high fiber diet in young, normal weight subjects. *International Journal of Obesity Related Medical Disorders 19*(12), 916-923.

Racette, S. B., Deusinger, S. S., & Deusinger, R. H. (2003). Obesity: Overview of prevalence, etiology, and treatment. *Physical Therapy, 83*(3), 276-285.

Ratzlaff, C. R., Gillies, J. H., & Koehoorn, M. W. (2007). Work-related repetitive strain injury and leisure-time physical activity. *Arthritis Care & Research*. Retrieved May 30, 2009, from http://www3.interscience.wiley.com/cgi-bin/abstract/114204212/ABSTRACT

Ray, J. J., & Bozek, R. (1980). Dissecting the A–B personality type. *The British Journal of Medical Psychology, 53*(2), 181-186.

Raymond, C. (1991, November 20). Debate on survey research continues as center marks 50th anniversary. *The Chronicle of Higher Education, 38*(13), A12.

Rea, B. L., Marshak, H. H., Neish, C., & Davis, N. (2004). The role of health promotion in physical therapy in California, New York, and Tennessee. *Physical Therapy, 84*(6), 510-515. Retrieved May 30, 2009, from http://www.ptjournal.org/cgi/content/full/84/6/510?maxtoshow=&HITS=10&hits=10&RESULTFORMAT=&author1=Rea&andorexactfulltext=and&searchid=1&FIRSTINDEX=0&sortspec=relevance&resourcetype=HWCIT

Rebuffé-Scrive, M., Brönnegard, M., & Nilsson, A. (1990). Steroid hormone receptors in human adipose tissues. *Journal of Clinical Endocrinology and Metabolism, 71,* 1215-1219.

Rebuffé-Scrive, M., Eldh, J., Hafström, L. O., & Björntorp, P. (1986). Metabolism of mammary, abdominal and femoral adipocytes in women before and after menopause. *Metabolism, 35,* 792-797.

Rebuffé-Scrive, M., Enk, L., & Crona, N. (1985). Fat cell metabolism in different regions in women: Effect of menstrual cycle, pregnancy, and lactation. *Journal of Clinical Investigation, 75,* 1973-1976.

Rebuffé-Scrive, M., Krotkiewski, M., Elfverson, J., & Björntorp, P. (1988). Muscle and adipose tissue morphology and metabolism in Cushing's syndrome. *Journal of Clinical Endocrinology and Metabolism, 67,* 1122-1128.

Rebuffé-Scrive, M., Lundholm, K., & Björntorp, P. (1985). Glucocorticoid hormone binding to human adipose tissue. *European Journal of Clinical Investigation, 15,* 267-272.

Reel, J. J., Greenleaf, C., Baker, W. K., Aragon, S., Bishop, D., Cachaper, C., et al. (2007). Relations of body concerns and exercise behavior: A meta-analysis. *Psychological Reports, 101*(3), 927-942.

Rejeski, W. J., Thompson, A., Brubaker, P. H., & Miller, H. S. (1992). Acute exercise: Buffering psychosocial stress responses in women. *Health Psychology, 11,* 355-362.

Relaxing. (2008). In *Merriam-Webster Online*. Retrieved October 30, 2008, from http://www.merriam-webster.com/dictionary/relaxing

Resnick, B., Magaziner, J., Orwig, D., & Zimmerman, S. (2002). Evaluating the components of the exercise plus program: Rationale, theory, and implementation. *Health Education Research, 17*(5), 648-658.

Retief, F. P., & Cilliers, L. (n.d.). Poisons, poisoning, and poisoners in Ancient Rome. In *Medicina Antiqua*. Retrieved May 30, 2009, from the Wellcome Trust Centre for the History of Medicine at UCL Web site: http://www.ucl.ac.uk/~ucgajpd/medicina%20antiqua/sa_poisons.html

Revel Sports.com. (2007). *VO2 max calculator.* Retrieved May 30, 2009, from http://revelsports. com/Articles/VO2_Max.htm

Ribisl, P. M., Lang, W., Jaramillo, S. A., Jakicic, J. M., Stewart, K. J., Bahnson, J., et al. (2007). Exercise capacity and cardiovascular/metabolic characteristics of overweight and obese individuals with type 2 diabetes. *Diabetes Care, 30*(10), 2679-2684.

Richards, D. K. (1968). A two-factor theory of the warm-up effect in jumping performance. *Research Quarterly, 39*(3), 668-673.

Richardson, J. K. (1999, October). President's perspective: Thought's from APTA's president: Health, balance, and the future. *Magazine of Physical Therapy.* Retrieved June 30, 2003, from http://www.apta.org/pt_magazine/oct99/president.html

Ries, E. (2003, September). In sickness and in wellness. *Magazine of Physical Therapy, 11*(9), 44-50.

Ries, E. (2006). Improving women's health across the lifespan. *Magazine of Physical Therapy* [Online], *14*(6), 1. Retrieved May 30, 2009, from http://www.apta.org/AM/Template.cfm? Section=Archives3&TEMPLATE=/CM/HTMLDisplay.cfm&CONTENTID=33350

Rimm, E. B., Ascherio, A., Giovannucci, E., Spiegelman, D., Stampfer, M. J., & Willett, W. C. (1996). Vegetable, fruit, and cereal fiber intake and risk of coronary heart disease among men. *JAMA, 275,* 447-451.

Rimmer, J. H. (1999, May). Health promotion for people with disabilities: The emerging paradigm shift from disability prevention to prevention of secondary conditions. *Physical Therapy, 79*(5), 495-502. Retrieved June 30, 2003, from http://www.ptjournal.org/pt_journal/-PTJournal/ May1999/May99/v79n5p495.cfm

Roach, J. B., Yadrick, M. K., Johnson, J. T., Boudreaux, L. J., Forsythe, W. A., III, & Billon, W. (2003). Using self-efficacy to predict weight loss among young adults. *Journal of the American Dietetic Association, 103*(10), 1357-1359.

Roberts, R. E., Kaplan, G. A., Shema, S. J., & Strawbridge, W. F. (2000). Are the obese at greater risk for depression? *American Journal of Epidemiology, 152*(2), 163-170.

Roberts, S. (2004). Self-experimentation as a source of new ideas: Ten examples about sleep, mood, health, and weight. *Behavioral Brain Science, 27*(2), 227-262.

Rodrigues, S. C., Dutra de Oliverira, J. E., de Souza, R. A., & Silva, H. C. (2005). Effect of a rice bran fiber diet on serum glucose levels of diabetic patients in Brazil. *Archives of Latino American Nutrition, 55*(1), 23-27.

Roebuck, C. (1998). *Effective communication: The essential guide to thinking and working smarter.* New York: Amacon.

Role models for mental health. (2004, May 28). *Nursing Standard, 18*(20), 4.

Rosenstock, I. (1974). Historical origins of the health belief model. *Health Education Monographs, 2,* 4.

Rosenstock, I. M., Strecher, V. J., & Becker, M. H. (1988). Social learning theory and the Health Belief Model. *Health Education Quarterly, 15*(2), 175-183.

Rothacker, D. Q., & Watemberg, S. (2004). Short-term hunger intensity changes following ingestion of a meal replacement bar for weight control. *International Journal of Food Science Nutrition, 55*(3), 223-226.

Rothman, J., & Levine, R. (1992). *Prevention practice: Strategies for physical therapy and occupational therapy.* Philadelphia: W. B. Saunders.

Rotter, J. B. (1982). *The development and applications of social learning theory.* New York: Praeger.

Runck, B. (n.d.) *What is biofeedback?* DHHS Pub. No. (ADM) 83-1273. Retrieved May 30, 2009, from http://www.psychotherapy.com/bio.html

Rungreangkulkij, S., & Wongtakee, W. (2008). The psychological impact of Buddhist counseling for patients suffering from symptoms of anxiety. *Archives of Psychiatric Nursing, 22*(3), 127-134.

Russell, P. J. (1972). Transcendental meditation. *Lancet, 1*(7760), 1125.

Sallis, J. F., & Saelens, B. E. (2000). Assessment of physical activity by self-report: Status, limitations, and future directions. *Research Quarterly for Exercise and Sport, 71*(2), 1-14.

Salzman, A. P. (2001a). Removing professional stereotypes, part II: Understanding the clinical exercise physiologist. *Advance for Physical Therapists & PT Assistants.* Retrieved February 5, 2001, from http://www.advanceforpt.com/PTfeature4.html

Salzman, A. P. (2001b). Removing professional stereotypes, part IV: Understanding the massage professional. *Advance for Physical Therapists & PT Assistants.* Retrieved February 5, 2001, from http://www.advanceforpt.com/PTfeature4.html

Salzman, A. P. (2001c). Removing professional stereotypes, part V: Understanding the occupational therapist. *Advance for Physical Therapists & PT Assistants.* Retrieved February 5, 2001, from http://www.advanceforpt.com/PTfeature4.html

Samaha, A. A., Nasser-Eddine, W., Shatila, E., Haddad, J. J., Wazne, J., & Eid, A. H. (2008). Multi-organ damage induced by anabolic steroid supplements: A case report and literature review. *Journal of Medical Case Reports, 2,* 340.

Sarafino, E. P. (2002). *Health psychology biopsychosocial interactions* (4th ed.). New York: John Wiley & Sons.

Sarafino, E. P. (2008). *Health psychology biopsychosocial interaction* (6th ed.). New York: John Wiley & Sons.

Sawka, M. N., Francesconi, R. P., Pimental, N. A., & Pandolf, K. B. (1984). Hydration and vascular fluid shifts during exercise in the heat. *Journal of Applied Physiology, 56*(1), 91-96.

Schlienger, J. L., & Pradiqnac, A. (2009). Nutrition approaches to prevent chronic disease. *La Revue du Praticien, 59*(1), 61-65.

Schlundt, D. G., Hill, J. O., Sbrocco, T., Pope-Cordle, J., & Sharp, T. (1992). The role of breakfast in the treatment of obesity: A randomized clinical trial. *American Journal of Clinical Nutrition, 55*(3), 645-651.

Schmied, L. A., & Lawler, K. A. (1986). Hardiness, type A behavior, and the stress-illness relation in working women. *Journal of Personality and Social Psychology, 51*(6), 1218-1223.

Schmitz, F., & Folsch, U. R. (2000). High fiber diet or not, that is the question here—Comments on prevention of colorectal carcinoma by dietary fiber. *American Journal of Gastroenterology, 38*(1), 137-139.

Schnirring, L. (2004). The South Beach Diet. *Physician and Sports Medicine, 32*(1), 9-10.

Schuckit, M. A. (2009). Alcohol-use disorders. *Lancet, 373*(9662), 492-501.

Schulze, M. B., Liu, S., Rimm, E. B., Manson, J. E., Willett, W. C., & Hu, F. B. (2004). Glycemic index, glycemic load, and dietary fiber intake and incidence of type 2 diabetes in younger and middle-aged women. *American Journal of Clinical Nutrition, 80,* 348-356.

Schwetschenau, H. M., O'Brien, W. H., Cunningham, C. J., & Jex, S. M. (2008). Barriers to physical activity in an on-site corporate fitness center. *Journal of Occupational Health Psychology, 13*(4), 371-380.

Seiler, S. (2005). *Maximal oxygen consumption: The VO$_2$ max.* Retrieved March 20, 2009, from http://home.hia.no/~stephens/vo2max.htm

Seiler, S. (2006). *Principles of training: Revisited.* Retrieved March 20, 2009, from http://home.hia.no/~stephens/traprin.htm

Serfass, R. C., & Gerberich, S. G. (1984). Exercise for optimal health: Strategies and motivational considerations. *Preventative Medicine, 13*(1), 79-99.

Shaikh, A. R., Yaroch, A. L., Nebeling, L., Yeh, M. C., & Resnicow, K. (2008). Psychosocial predictors of fruit and vegetable consumption in adults a review of the literature. *American Journal of Preventative Medicine, 34*(6), 535-543.

Shapiro, C. M. (1997, May). PL-SI-252-S: Vibro-tactile stimulation: The use of drums and percussion instruments in rehabilitation and wellness [Abstract]. *Physical Therapy, 77*(5), S81.

Shearer, J. (2007). *Coffee & caffeine: Considerations in health, exercise & performance* [PowerPoint format]. Paper presented at the Canadian Society for Exercise Physiology 2007 Annual Meeting. Retrieved June 10, 2009, from http://coffeescience.org/csep

Shepard, R. J. (1992). A critical analysis of work-site fitness programs and their postulated economic benefits. *Medicine & Science in Sports & Exercise, 24*(3), 354-370.

Shephard, R. J. (1984). Tests of maximum oxygen intake: A critical review. *Sports Medicine, 1*(2), 99-124.

Sheridan, C. L., & Radmacher, S. A. (1991). Health psychology: Challenging the biomedical model. San Francisco: John Wiley & Sons.

Sherman, K. J., Cherkin, D. C., Erro, J., Miglioretti, D. L., & Deyo, R. A. (2005). Comparing yoga, exercise, and self-care book for chronic low back pain: A randomized, controlled trial. *Annals of Internal Medicine, 143,* 849-856.

Shih, F. J. (1998, September). Triangulation in nursing research: Issues of conceptual clarity and purpose. *Journal of Advanced Nursing, 28*(3), 631-642.

Shvartz, E., & Reibold, R. C. (1990). Aerobic fitness norms for males and females aged 6-75: A review. *Aviation, Space and Environmental Medicine. 61,* 3-11.

Simoneau, J. A., & Bouchard, C. (1989). Human variation in skeletal muscle fiber-type proportion and enzyme activities. *American Journal of Physiology, 257*(4), E567-E572.

Simopoulos, A. P., & Van Itallie, T. B. (1984). Body weight, health and longevity. *Annuals of Internal Medicine, 100*(2), 285-295.

Simpson, E. J. (1972). *The classification of educational objectives in the psychomotor domain.* Washington, DC: Gryphon House.

Singh, A. S., Chin, A., Paw, M. J., Bosscher, R. J., & van Mechelen, W. (2006). Cross-sectional relationship between physical fitness components and functional performance in older persons living in long-term care facilities. *BMC Geriatrics, 7*(6), 4.

Sinokki, M., Hinkka, K., Ahola, K., Koskinen, S., Kivimäki, M., Honkonen, T., et al. (2009). The association of social support at work and in private life with mental health and antidepressant use: The Health 2000 Study. *Journal of Affective Disorders, 115*(1-2), 36-45.

Siri, W. E. (1956). The gross composition of the body. In C. A. Tobias & J. H. Lawrence (Eds.), *Advances in biological and medical physics, vol. 4* (pp. 239-280). New York: Academic Press.

Siri, W. E. (1961). Body composition from fluid spaces and density: Analysis of methods. In J. Brozek & A. Henschel (Eds.), *Techniques for measuring body composition* (pp. 223-224). Washington, DC: National Academy of Sciences, National Research Council.

Sitzman, K. (2006). Eating breakfast helps sustain weight loss. *American Association of Occupational Health Nurses Journal, 54*(3), 136.

Sjögren, J., Weck, M., Nilsson, A., Ottosson, M., & Björntorp, P. (1994). Glucocorticoid binding to rat adipocytes. *Biochimical Biophysical Acta, 1224,* 17-21.

Sjöqvist, F., Garle, M., & Rane, A. (2008). Use of doping agents, particularly anabolic steroids, in sports and society. *Lancet, 31*(371), 1872-1882.

Slater, J. (1990). Effecting personal effectiveness: Assertiveness training for nurses. *Journal of Advanced Nursing, 15*(3), 337-356.

Slattery, M. L., McDonald, A., & Bild, D. E. (1992). Associations of body fat and its distribution with dietary intake, physical activity, alcohol, and smoking in blacks and whites. *American Journal of Clinical Nutrition, 55,* 943-949.

Smart, M., Smith, M., Hearn, E., Brown, A., Dodge, B., & Jackson, T. J. (2006). Occupational Wellness. Unpublished manuscript as presented during a Wellness and Prevention course at the University of St. Augustine for Health Sciences, St. Augustine, Florida.

Smith, L. C. (2000, December). Risk management: The hot topics. *Magazine of Physical Therapy, 8*(12), 26-34.

Smith, M. A., Garbharran, H., Edwards, M. J., & O'Hara-Murdock, P. (2004, May). Health promotion and disease prevention through sanitation education in South African Zulu and Xhosa women. *Journal of Transcultural Nursing, 15*(1), 62-69.

Socas, L., Zumbado, M., Pérez-Luzardo, O., Ramos, A., Perez, C., Hernandez, J. R., et al. (2005). Hepatocellular adenomas associated with anabolic androgenic steroid abuse in bodybuilders: A report of two cases and a review of the literature. *British Journal of Sports Medicine, 39*(5), e27.

Somerset-Butler, R. (2004, April 21). Romini Somerset-Butler learns how to be a role model for patients. *Nursing Standard, 18*(32), 25.

Sonnenschein, E. G., Kim, M. Y., Pasternack, B. S., & Toniolo, P. G. (1993). Sources of variability in waist and hip measurements in middle-aged women. *American Journal of Epidemiology, 138,* 301-309.

Sophia, E. D., Tavares, H., & Zilberman, M. L. (2007). Pathological love: Is it a new psychiatric disorder [Portuguese]? *Revista Brasileira de Psiquitria, 29*(1), 55-62.

Sorenson, G., Jacobs, D. R., Pirie, P., Folsom, A., Luepker, R., & Gillum, R. (1987). Relationships among type A behavior, employment experiences, and gender: The Minnesota Heart Survey. *Journal of Behavioral Medicine, 10,* 323-336.

The South Beach Diet can also help you achieve your weight goal. (2005). Retrieved June 23, 2006, from the Heart Health Online Web site: http://www.heart-health-diets-and-exercises.com/South_Beach_diet.html?OVRAW=south%20beach%20diet&OVKEY=south%20beach%20diet&OVMTC=standard

The South Beach Diet Online. (2006). *About the diet.* Retrieved May 30, 2009, from http://www.southbeachdiet.com/public/about-the-south-beach-diet/about-the-south-beach-diet.asp?GID=201

Sowan, N. A., Moffatt, S. G., & Canales, M. K. (2004) Creating a mentoring partnership model: A university-department of health experience. *Family Community Health, 27*(4), 326-337.

Sparling, P. B., Millard-Stafford, M., & Snow, T. K. (1997). Development of a cadence curl-up test for college students. *Research Quarterly for Exercise and Sport.* Retrieved November 30, 2008, from http://findarticles.com/p/articles/mi_hb3397/is_n4_v68/ai_n28697442/pg_1?tag=artBody;col1

Special Olympics Nevada (SONV). (2004). *Principles of training.* Retrieved June 16, 2006, from: http://72.14.209.104/search?q=cache:l257k6NwQ1QJ:www.sonv.org/intro/pdfs/training_principles.pdf+Principles%2Bof%2BTraining&hl=en&gl=u&ct=clnk&cd=12

Speer, K. P. (Ed.). (2005). *Injury prevention and rehabilitation for active older adults.* Champaign, IL: Human Kinetics.

Spiga, R. (1986). Social interaction and cardiovascular response of boys exhibiting the coronary-prone behavior patterns. *Journal of Pediatric Psychology, 11,* 59-69.

Spotlight on wellness and fitness. (2000, September). *Magazine of Physical Therapy, 8*(9), 112-116.

Start, K. B. (1963). Relation of warm-up to spontaneous muscle injury. *New York State Journal of Medicine, 15*(63), 3530-3532.

Start, K. B., & Hines, J. (1963). The effect of warm-up on the incidence of muscle injury during activities involving maximum strength, speed and endurance. *Journal of Sports Medicine and Physical Fitness, 44,* 208-217.

State Nurse Practice Act—Example: Florida State Nurse Practice Act. (2005). Retrieved May 30, 2009, from the Florida Department of Health Web site: http://www.doh.state.fl.us/mqa/nursing/info_PracticeAct.pdf

Steer, R. A., Beck, A. T., Riskind, J. H., & Brown, G. (1986). Differentiation of depressive disorders from generalized anxiety by the Beck Depression Inventory. *Journal of Clinical Psychology, 42*(3), 475-478.

Sternas, K. A., & Scharf, M. A. (2006). *A partnership model for community assessment, planning and evidence-based interventions, which promote health of high-risk populations.* Paper presented at the 17th International Nursing Research Congress Focusing on Evidence-Based Practice, July 22, 2006. Retrieved May 30, 2009, from http://stti.confex.com/stti/congrs06/techprogram/paper_30894.htm

Stolarczyk, L. M., Heyward, V. H., Van Loan, M. D., Hicks, V. L., Wilson, W. L., & Reano, L. M. (1997). The fatness-specific bioelectrical impedance analysis equations of Segal et al.: Are they generalizable and practical? *American Journal of Clinical Nutrition, 66,* 8-17.

Stoll, B. A. (2002). Upper abdominal obesity, insulin resistance and breast cancer risk. *International Journal of Obesity and Related Metabolic Disorders, 26*(6), 747-753.

Stone, A. A., & Neale, J. M. (1984). Effects of severe daily events on mood. *Journal of Personality and Social Psychology, 46*(1), 137-144.

Stotland, S. C., & Larocque, M. (2005). Early treatment response as a predictor of ongoing weight loss in obesity treatment. *British Journal of Health Psychology, 10*(Pt 4), 601-614.

Stout, J. R., et al. (1994). Validity of percent body fat estimation in males. *Medicine & Science in Sports & Exercise, 26,* 632.

Stout, J. R., et al. (1996). Validity of methods of estimating percent body fat in young women. *Journal of Strength and Conditioning Research, 10,* 25.

Stuifbergen, A. K., Becker, H., Blozis, S., Timmerman, G., & Kullberg, V. (2003). A randomized clinical trial of a wellness intervention for women with multiple sclerosis. *Archives of Physical Medicine Rehabilitation, 84,* 467-476.

Stunkard, A., Sorensen, T., & Hanis, C. (1984). An adoption study of human obesity. *New England Journal of Medicine, 314,* 193-198.

Sudano, I., Binggeli, C., Spieker, L., Luscher, T. F., Ruschitzka, F., & Noll, G. (2005). Cardiovascular effects of coffee: Is it a risk factor? *Progressive Cardiovascular Nursing, 20*(2), 65-69.

Sue, D. (1972). The role of relaxation in systematic desensitization. *Behavioral Research and Therapy, 10*(2), 153-158.

Swain, R. (1994). Target HR for the development of CV fitness. *Medicine & Science in Sports & Exercise, 26*(1), 112-116.

Talking about health and wellness with patients: Integrating health promotion and disease prevention in your practice [Book review]. (2001). *New England Journal of Medicine, 344*(26), 2032-2033.

Tanaka, H., Monahan, K. D., & Seals, D. R. (2001). Age-predicted maximal heart rate revisited. *Journal of the American College of Cardiology, 37*(1), 153-156.

Tarnopolsky, M. A., Atkinson, S. A., MacDougall, A., Phillips, C. S., & Schwarcz, H. (1992). Evaluation of protein requirements for trained strength athletes. *Journal of Applied Physiology, 73,* 1986-1995.

Tarnopolsky, M. A., Parise, G., Yardley, C. S., Ballantyne, S., Olatunji, S., & Phillips, S. M. (2001a). Creatine-dextrose and protein-dextrose induce similar strength gains during training. *Medicine & Science in Sports & Exercise, 33*(12), 2044-2052.

Tarnopolsky, M. A., Parise, G., Yardley, C. S., Ballantyne, S., Olatunji, S., & Phillips, S. M. (2001b). Effect of protein supplementation on strength, power and body composition changes in experienced resistance trained men. *Medicine & Science in Sports & Exercise, 37*(5), S45.

Taylor, J. D. (2007). The impact of a supervised strength and aerobic training program on muscular strength and aerobic capacity in individuals with type 2 diabetes. *Journal of Strength and Conditioning Research, 21*(3), 824.

Terlouw, T. J. A. (2007). Roots of physical medicine, physical therapy, and mechanotherapy in the Netherlands in the 19th century: A disputed area within the health care domain. *J Manual Manipulative Ther, 15,* E23-E41.

Testwell wellness inventory. (2004). National Wellness Institute. Retrieved August 8, 2004, from http://www.testwell.org/; Retrieved November 28, 2008, from http://www.nationalwellness.org/TestWell/index.htm

Thakar, R., & Stanton, S. (2000). Management of urinary incontinence in women. *British Medical Journal. 321*(7272), 1326-1331.

Thomas, A., Magran, T., Marcello, B., Moulton, C., Roberts, M., Rohle, D., et al. (2005). Effects of the Curves(r) fitness & weight loss program II: Resting energy expenditure. *Journal of the American Societies for Experimental Biology, LBA,* 55.

Thompson, P. D., Buchner, D., Pina, I. L., Balady, G. J., Williams, M. A., Marcus, B. H., et al. (2003). Exercise and physical activity in the prevention and treatment of atherosclerotic cardiovascular disease: A statement from the Council on Clinical Cardiology (Subcommittee on Exercise, Rehabilitation, and Prevention) and the Council on Nutrition, Physical Activity, and Metabolism (Subcommittee on Physical Activity). *Circulation, 107,* 3109-3116.

Three stages of burnout. (n.d.). Retrieved August 18, 2006, from http://72.14.209.104/search?q=cache:dF_3G-PpCYgJ:smhp.psych.ucla.edu/qf/burnout_qt/3stages.pdf+stages%2Bburnout&hl=en&gl=us&ct=clnk&cd=7

Three unique PTs and their specialized fitness programs. (1994, May). *Magazine of Physical Therapy.* Retrieved August 8, 2004, from http://www.ptjournal.org/pt_journal/May94.cfm

Tichet, J., Vol, S., & Balkau, B. (1993). Android fat distribution by age and sex: The waist–hip ratio. *Diabete et Metabolisme, 19,* 273-276.

Todd, M., Stevens, W., Wagner, C., & Cramer, C. (1998). Effect of single dose protein supplement on blood lactate concentrations after resistance exercise. *Medicine & Science in Sports & Exercise, 30*(5), S18.

Tokar, S. (2006, February). *Liver damage and increased heart attack risk caused by anabolic steroid use.* Retrieved May 30, 2009, from http://www.medicalnewstoday.com/articles/38069.php

Tonigan, J. S., Miller, W. R., & Schermer, C. (2002). Atheists, agnostics and Alcoholics Anonymous. *Journal of Studies on Alcohol and Drugs, 63*(5), 534-541.

TopEndSports.com. (2007a). *Balke Test Treadmill.* Retrieved May 30, 2009, from http://www.topendsports.com/testing/tests/balke.htm

TopEndSports.com. (2007b). *Bruce Protocol Stress Test.* Retrieved May 30, 2009, from http://www.topendsports.com/testing/tests/bruce.htm

Toth, M., Wolsko, PM., Foreman, J., Davis, R. B., Delbanco, T., Phillips, R. S., et al. (2007). A pilot study for a randomized, controlled trial on the effect of guided imagery in hospitalized medical patients. *Journal of Alternative Complementary Medicine, 13*(2), 194-197.

Toyoshima, H., Masuoka, N., Hashimoto, S., Otsuka, R., Sasaki, S., Tamakoshi, K., et al. (2009). Effect of the interaction between mental stress and eating pattern on body mass index gain in healthy Japanese mail workers. *Journal of Epidemiology, 19*(2), 88-93.

Travis, J. W. (n.d.). The illness wellness continuum. Retrieved May 13, 2006, from http://www.thewellspring.com/Pubs/iw_cont.html

Trephination, An Ancient Surgery. (n.d.). Retrieved February 10, 2009, from the University of Illinois at Chicago, Classes Web site: http://www.uic.edu/classes/osci/osci590/13_3%20Trephination%20An%20Ancient%20Surgery.htm

Trock, B. J., Lanza, E., & Greenwalk, P. (1990). High fiber diet and colon cancer: A critical review. *Progressive Clinical Biological Research, 46,* 145-157.

Trunk, D. (2006). UF experts: Decaffeinated coffee is not caffeine-free. *University of Florida News.* Retrieved February 10, 2009, from http://news.ufl.edu/2006/10/10/decaf/

TruthorFiction.com. (2008). *Coke vs water.* Retrieved February 28, 2009, from http://www.truthorfiction.com/rumors/w/watervscoke.htm

Tsa, A. G., & Wadden, T. A. (2005). Systemic review: An evaluation of major commercial weight loss program in the United States. *Annals of Internal Medicine, 142*(1), 56-66.

Tsang, W., & Hui-Chan, C. (2004). Effect of 4- and 8-wk intensive tai chi training on balance control in the elderly. *Medicine & Science in Sports & Exercise, 36,* 648-657.

Tsuritani, I., Honda, R., Noborisaka, Y., Ishida, M., Ishizaki, M., & Yamada, Y. (2002). Impact of obesity on musculoskeletal pain and difficulty of daily movements in Japanese middle-aged women. *Maturitas, 42*(1), 23-30.

Tucker, L. A., & Maxwell, K. (1992). Effects of weight training on the emotional well-being and body image of females: Predictors of greatest benefit. *American Journal of Health Promotion, 6*(5), 338-344, 371.

Two obesity self-report measures. (2004). *Nutrition Research Newsletter, 23*(2), 8-10.

Tymchuk, C. N., Barnard, R. J., Heber, D., & Aronson, W. J. (2001). Evidence of an inhibitory effect of diet and exercise on prostate cancer cell growth. *Journal of Urology, 166*(3), 1185-1189.

United States Department of Agriculture. (1992). *Food guide pyramid.* Retrieved May 30, 2009, from http://www.everydiet.org/food_pyramid_old.htm

United States Department of Agriculture. (2002). *Nutritive value of foods.* Retrieved May 30, 2009, from http://www.nal.usda.gov/fnic/foodcomp/Data/HG72/hg72_2002.pdf

United States Department of Agriculture. (2004). *Dietary reference intakes: An update.* Retrieved May 30, 2009, from http://ific.org/publications/other/driupdateom.cfm?renderforprint=1

United States Department of Agriculture. (2005a). *Dietary guidelines.* Retrieved February 20, 2009, from http://www.mypyramid.gov/guidelines/index.html

United States Department of Agriculture. (2005b). *Inside the pyramid.* Retrieved February 20, 2009, from http://www.mypyramid.gov/pyramid/meat.html

United States Department of Agriculture. (2008a). *About USDA.* Retrieved May 30, 2009, from http://www.usda.gov/wps/portal/!ut/p/_s.7_0_A/7_0_1OB/.cmd/ad/.ar/sa.retrievecontent/.c/6_2_1UH/.ce/7_2_5JN/.p/5_2_4TR/.d/0/_th/J_2_9D/_s.7_0_A/7_0_1OB?PC_7_2_5JN_navid=MISSION_STATEMENT&PC_7_2_5JN_navtype=RT&PC_7_2_5JN_parentnav=ABOUT_USDA#7_2_5JN

United States Department of Agriculture. (2008b). *Dietary guidance.* Retrieved May 30, 2009, from http://fnic.nal.usda.gov/nal_display/index.php?info_center=4&tax_level=3&tax_subject=256&topic_id=1342&level3_id=5142

United States Department of Agriculture. (2008c). *Inside the pyramid.* Retrieved May 30, 2009, from http://www.mypyramid.gov/pyramid/vegetables.html

United States Department of Agriculture. (2008d). *What counts as a cup of vegetables?* Retrieved May 30, 2009, from http://www.mypyramid.gov/pyramid/vegetables_counts.html#

United States Department of Agriculture. (2008e). *What foods are included in the milk, yogurt, and cheese (milk) group?* Retrieved May 30, 2009, from http://www.mypyramid.gov/pyramid/milk.html

United States Department of Agriculture. (2008f). *What foods are in the grain group?* Retrieved May 30, 2009, from http://www.mypyramid.gov/pyramid/grains.html

United States Department of Agriculture. (2008g). *What foods are in the vegetable group?* Retrieved May 30, 2009, from http://www.mypyramid.gov/pyramid/vegetables.html

United States Department of Agriculture. (2009). *MyPyramid.* Retrieved February 20, 2009, from http://www.mypyramid.gov/

United States Department of Agriculture and United States Department of Health and Human Services. (1992). *USDA's food guide pyramid.* Home and Garden Bulletin No. 249. Hyattsville, MD: Government Printing Office.

United States Department of Agriculture and United States Department of Health and Human Services. (1995). *Nutrition and your health: Dietary guidelines for Americans* (4th ed.). Home and Garden Bulletin No. 232. Hyattsville, MD: Government Printing Office.

United States Department of Agriculture and United States Department of Health and Human Services. (2005). Alcoholic beverages. In *Dietary Guidelines for Americans* (pp. 43-46). Washington, DC: U.S. Government Printing Office. Retrieved May 30, 2009, from http://www.health.gov/DIETARYGUIDELINES/dga2005/document/html/chapter9.htm

United States Department of Health and Human Services. (n.d.). *What are its goals?* Retrieved March 20, 2009, from http://www.healthypeople.gov/About/goals.htm

United States Department of Health and Human Services. (n.d.). *What is Healthy People 2010?* Retrieved March 20, 2009, from http://www.healthypeople.gov/About/whatis.htm

United States Department of Health and Human Services. (2000). *Healthy People 2010.* Washington, DC: U.S. Government Printing Office.

United States Department of Health and Human Services. (2004). *Physical activity and fitness.* Retrieved May 10, 2005, from http://www.healthypeople.gov/data/2010prog/focus22/-PhysicalFitnessPR.pdf

United States Department of Health and Human Services. (2006). *Overweight and obesity: At a glance.* Retrieved March 20, 2009, from http://www.surgeongeneral.gov/topics/obesity/calltoaction/fact_glance.htm

United States Department of Health and Human Services, Centers for Disease Control and Prevention. (2004). *2004 Surgeon General's Report: The health consequences of smoking.*

Retrieved February 20, 2009, from http://www.cdc.gov/tobacco/data_statistics/sgr/sgr_2004/highlights/3.htm

United States Department of Health and Human Services, Centers for Disease Control and Prevention, National Center for Chronic Disease Prevention and Health Promotion. (1996). *Physical activity and health: A report of the Surgeon General.* Atlanta, GA: U.S. Department of Health and Human Services.

Vaidva, V. (2006). Psychosocial aspects of obesity. *Advances in Psychosomatic Medicine, 27,* 73-85.

van Dalen, D. B. (1979). *Understanding educational research: An introduction* (4th ed.). New York: McGraw-Hill.

van der Kooy, K., Leenen, R., & Seidell, J. C. (1993). Waist–hip ratio is a poor predictor of changes in visceral fat. *American Journal of Clinical Nutrition, 57,* 327-333.

van der Watt, G., Laugharne, J., & Janca, A. (2008). Complementary and alternative medicine in the treatment of anxiety and depression. *Current Opinion in Psychiatry, 21*(1), 37-42.

van Horn, L. (1997). Fiber, lipids, and coronary heart disease. A statement for healthcare professionals from the Nutrition Committee, American Heart Association. *Circulation, 95,* 2701-2704.

van Mechelen, W., Hlobil, H., Kemper, H. C., Voorn, W. J., & de Jongh, H. R. (1993). *American Journal of Sports Medicine, 21*(5), 711-719.

Varady, K. A., Santosa, S., & Jones, P. J. H. (2007). Validation of hand-held bioelectrical impedance analysis with magnetic resonance imaging for the assessment of body composition in overweight women. *American Journal of Human Biology, 19,* 429-433. Abstract retrieved December 18, 2007, from http://www3.interscience.wiley.com/cgi-bin/abstract/114208438/ABSTRACT?CRETRY=1&SRETRY=0

The Vegetarian Society. (n.d.). *Information sheet.* Retrieved February 28, 2009, from http://www.vegsoc.org/info/whatis.html

Vehrs P., et al. (1998). Reliability and concurrent validity of Futrex and bioelectrical impedance. *International Journal of Sports Medicine, 19,* 560.

Velazquez, I., & Alter, B. P. (2004). Androgens and liver tumors: Fanconi's anemia and non-Fanconi's conditions. *American Journal of Hematology, 77*(3), 257-267.

Venes, D. (Ed.). (2001). *Taber's cyclopedic medical dictionary.* Philadelphia: F. A. Davis.

Verdens, G. (2001). *Best trent I hele verden?* [Norwegian]. Retrieved May 30, 2009, from http://www.vg.no/vg/sport/ski/vm97/0226best.html

Verstappen, F. T., Huppertz, R. M., & Snoeckx, L. H. (1982). Effect of training specificity on maximal treadmill and bicycle ergometer exercise. *International Journal of Sports Medicine, 3*(1), 43-46.

Vinai, P., Allison, K. C., Cardetti, S., Carpegna, G., Ferrato, N., Masante, D., et al. (2008). Psychopathology and treatment of night eating syndrome: A review. *Eating and Weight Disorders, 13*(2), 54-63.

Vincent, E. (2008). Dieters need flexibility and professional support to succeed. *Journal of the American Dietetic Association, 108*(4), 647-648.

VividSoft. (1999). *Aerobic fitness information.* Retrieved June 16, 2006, from http://www.aerobictest.com/FitnessNorms.htm#categories

Vogel, W. H. (1985). Coping, stress, stressors and health consequences. *Neuropsychobiology, 13*(3), 129-135.

Vogt, D. S., Rizvi, S. L., Shipherd, J. C., & Resick, P. A. (2008). Longitudinal investigation of reciprocal relationship between stress reactions and hardiness. *Personality and Social Psychological Bulletin, 34*(1):61-73.

Volkow, N. D. (2009). *Research report series: Anabolic steroid abuse.* Retrieved March 20, 2009, from the National Institute on Drug Abuse Web site: http://www.drugabuse.gov/PDF/RRSteroids.pdf

Vue, H., Degeneffe, D., & Reicks, M. (2008). Need states based on eating occasions experienced by midlife women. *Journal of Nutrition Education and Behavior, 40*(6), 378-384.

Wade, G. N., & Gray, J. M. (1979). Gonadal effects on food intake and adiposity: A metabolic hypothesis. *Physiology and Behavior, 22*, 583-593.

Waller, S. M., Vander Wal, J. S., Klurfeld, D. M., McBurney, M. I., Cho, S., Bijlani, S., et al. (2004). Evening ready-to-eat cereal consumption contributes to weight management. *Journal of American College of Nutrition, 23*(4), 316-321.

Walonick, D. (1997). *Survival statistics: Master statistical analysis techniques without pain.* Minneapolis: StatPac. Retrieved August 8, 2004, from http://www.statpac.com/statistics-book/basics.htm#VariabilityandError

Walsh, P. D. (2003). Lack of effect of a low-fat, high-fruit, -vegetable, and -fiber diet on serum prostate-specific antigen of men without prostate cancer: Results from a randomized trial. *Journal of Clinical Oncology, 20*(17), 3592-3598.

Waschbisch, A., Tallner, A., Pfeifer, K., & Mäurer, M. (2009, January 23). Multiple sclerosis and exercise: Effects of physical activity on the immune system [Epub ahead of print; German]. *Der Nervenarzt.*

Washburn, R. A., & Montoye, H. J. (1986). The assessment of physical activity by questionnaire. *American Journal of Epidemiology, 123*, 563-575.

Watanabe, E., Fukuda, S., Hara, H., Maeda, Y., Ohira, H., & Shirakawa, T. (2006). Differences in relaxation by means of guided imagery in a healthy community sample. *Alternative Therapies in Health and Medicine, 12*(2), 60-66.

Webb, P. (1981). Energy expenditure and fat-free mass in men and women. *American Journal of Clinical Nutrition, 34*(9), 1816-1826.

Weinstein, A. (2008). The joint effects of physical activity and body mass index on coronary heart disease in women. *Archives of Internal Medicine, 168*, 884-890.

Weisberg, M. B. (2008). 50 years of hypnosis in medicine and clinical health psychology: A synthesis of cultural crosscurrents. *American Journal of Clinical Hypnosis, 51*(1), 13-27.

Weiss, E. C., Galuska, D. A., Khan, L. K., Serdula, M. K. (2006). Weight control practices among U.S. adults, 2001–2002. *American Journal of Preventative Medicine, 31*(1), 18-24.

Weissinger, E., & Bandalos, D. (1995). Development, reliability and validity of a scale to measure intrinsic motivation in leisure. *Journal of Leisure Research, 27*, 379-400.

Wellness. (2008a). In *Dictionary.com unabridged (v. 1.1).* Retrieved August 8, 2008, from Dictionary.com Web site: http://dictionary.reference-.com/search?q=wellness

Wellness. (2008b). In *Merriam-Webster Online.* Retrieved October 30, 2008, from http://www.m-w.com/dictionary/wellness

Wellness Associates. (2009). *Key concept #1: The illness–wellness continuum revisited.* Retrieved February 13, 2009, from http://www.thewellspring.com/wellspring/introduction-to-wellness/357/key-concept-1-the-illnesswellness-continuum.cfm

Wellness center for people with disabilities opens. (2001, November). *Magazine of Physical Therapy, 9*(11), 14.

The Wellness Model. (n.d.). Retrieved February 15, 2009, from Illinois Wesleyan University Web site: http://www.iwu.edu/greek/current/officers/Wellness_Model.doc

Wellness quotes. (2006). Retrieved May 30, 2009, from http://thinkexist.com/quotes/mary_anne_radmacher/

Wendler, M. C. (2001, August). Triangulation using a meta-matrix. *Journal of Advanced Nursing, 35*(4), 521-526.

Wenley, R. M. (1899). Naturalism and agnosticism. *Science, 10*(247), 417-418. Citation retrieved May 30, 2009, from http://www.ncbi.nlm.nih.gov/pubmed/17751576

Westerterp, K. R. (2004). Diet induced thermogenesis. *Nutrition and Metabolism, 1,* 5. Retrieved May 30, 2009, from http://www.nutritionandmetabolism.com/content/1/1/5/abstract/

Whang, W., Manson, J. E., Hu, F. B., Chae, C. U., Rexrode, K. M., Willett, W. C., et al. (2006). Physical exertion, exercise, and sudden cardiac death in women. *JAMA, 295*, 1399-1403.

What is wellness? (n.d.). Retrieved May 30, 2009, from California State University Web site: http://www.csuchico.edu/wellness/whatis/environmental.shtml

Whelan, W. J. (2004). The wars of the carbohydrates: Part 3: Maltose. *IUBMB Life, 56*(10), 641.

White, J., Austin, K., Greer, B., St. John, N., & Panton, L. (1997). Effect of carbohydrate–protein supplement timing on exercise-induced muscle. *Medicine & Science in Sports & Exercise, 38*(5), S341.

White, L. J., & Dressendorfer, R. H. (2004). Exercise and multiple sclerosis. *Sports Medicine, 34*(15), 1077-1001.

Whitt, M. C., Levin, S., Ainsworth, B. E., & DuBose, K. D. (2003). Observations from the CDC: Evaluation of a two-part survey item to assess moderate physical activity: The cross-cultural activity participation study. *Journal of Women's Health, 12,* 203-212.

Whorton, J. C. (1988). Patient, heal thyself: Popular health reform movements as unorthodox medicine. In: Gevitz N, Ed. *Other Healers: Unorthodox Medicine in America.* Baltimore, MD: Johns Hopkins.

Willett, W. C. & Skerrett, P. J. (2005). *Eat, Drink, and Be Healthy.* New York: Free Press/Simon & Schuster.

Williams, D. M. (2008). Exercise, affect, and adherence: An integrated model and a case for self-paced exercise. *Journal Sport Exercise Physiology, 30*(5), 471-496.

Williams, M. A., Haskell, W. L., Ades, P. H., Amsterdam, E. A., Bittner, V., Franklin, B. A., et al. (2007). Resistance exercise in individuals with and without cardiovascular disease: 2007 update. *Circulation, 116,* 572-584.

Williams, S. R. (2001). *Basic nutrition and diet therapy.* St. Louis, MO: Mosby.

Wilmore, J. H., & Costill, D. L. (2005). *Physiology of Sport and Exercise* (3rd ed.). Champaign, IL: Human Kinetics.

Wilson, L. L., & Wilson, B. A. (1989). *Self-esteem and motivation.* Surry Hills, New South Wales: Australian College of Applied Physiology.

Wilson, P. W. (1998). Prediction of coronary heart disease using risk factor categories. *Circulation, 97*(18), 1837-1847.

Wilson, P. W. (2009). Risk scores for prediction of coronary heart disease: An update. *Endocrinology Metabolism Clinics of North America, 38*(1), 33-44.

Wing, R. R., & Phelan, S. (2005). Long-term weight loss maintenance. *American Journal of Clinical Nutrition, 82*(Suppl 1), 222S-225S.

Witmer, J. M., & Sweeney, T. J. (1992). A holistic model for wellness and prevention over the life span. *Journal of Counseling & Development, 71,* 140-148.

Wojciechowski, M. (2006a). The future of physical therapy education: APTA's education strategic plan. *Magazine of Physical Therapy, 14*(7), 54-59. Retrieved May 30, 2009, from http://www.apta.org/AM/Template.cfm?Section=Archives3&CONTENTID=33519&TEMPLATE=/CM/HTMLDisplay.cfm

Wojciechowski, M. (2006b). Giving back to the community. *Magazine of Physical Therapy, 14*(5). Retrieved May 30, 2009, from http://www.apta.org/AM/Template.cfm?Section=Archives3&CONTENTID=32601&TEMPLATE=/CM/HTMLDisplay.cfm

Wolever, T. M., & Jenkins, D. J. (1997). What is a high fiber diet? *Advanced Experimental Medical Biology, 427,* 35-42.

Wolf, S., Barnhart, H., & Ellison, G. (1997). The effect of tai chi quan and computerized balance training on postural stability in older subjects. *Physical Therapy, 7,* 371-385.

Wolf, S. L., & Binder-Macleod, S. A. (1983). Electromyographic biofeedback applications to the hemiplegic patient: Changes in upper extremity neuromuscular and functional status. *Physical Therapy, 63*(9), 1393-1402.

Wolf, S. L., Nacht, M., & Kelly, J. L. (1982). EMG feedback training during dynamic movement for low back pain patients. *Physical Therapy, 13,* 395-406.

Wolk, A. (1999). Long-term intake of dietary fiber and decreased risk of coronary heart disease among women. *JAMA, 281,* 1998.

Wolpe, J. (1961). The systematic desensitization treatment of neuroses. *Journal of Nervous and Mental Disorders, 132,* 189-203.

Wood, R. J. (2006a). *Fitness testing.* Retrieved March 20, 2009, from http://www.topendsports.com/testing/vo2norms.htm

Wood, R. J. (2006b). *Fitness testing glossary.* Retrieved March 20, 2009, from http://www.topendsports.com/testing/glossary.htm#M

Wood, R. J. (2006c). *Maximal oxygen consumption test.* Retrieved March 20, 2009, from http://www.topendsports.com/testing/tests/VO2max.htm

World Health Organization. (1947). Constitution of the World Health Organization. *Chronicle of the World Health Organization, 1*(1-2), 29-43.

World Health Organization. (1990). *Diet, nutrition, and the prevention of chronic diseases.* Geneva: World Health Organization.

World Health Organization. (2004). *About WHO.* Retrieved May 30, 2009, from http://www.who.int/about/en/

World Health Organization. (2009). *World Health Organization frequently asked questions.* Retrieved January 30, 2009, from http://www.who.int/suggestions/faq/en/index.html

Worldwide adherents of all religions by six continental areas, mid-1995. (n.d.). Retrieved May 30, 2009, from http://www.zpub.com/un/pope/relig.html

Wozniak, R. H. (1995). *Rene Descartes and the legacy of mind/body dualism.* Retrieved February 15, 2009, from http://serendip.brynmawr.edu/Mind/Descartes.html

Wyatt, H. R., Grunwald, G. K., Mosca, C. L., Klem, M. L., Wing, R. R., & Hill, J. O. (2002). Long-term weight loss and breakfast in subjects in the National Weight Control Registry. *Obesity Research, 10*(2), 78-82.

Xu, X., Hoebeke, J., & Björntorp, P. (1990). Progestin binds to the glucocorticoid receptor and mediates antiglucocorticoid effect in rat adipose precursor cells. *Journal of Steroid Biochemistry, 36,* 465-471.

Yamamoto, Y., Moore, R., Hess, H., Guo, G., Gonzalez, F., Korach, K., et al. (2006). Estrogen receptor alpha mediates 17alpha-ethynylestradiol causing hepatotoxicity. *Journal of Biological Chemistry, 281*(24), 16625-16631.

Yancey, A. K., Lewis, L. B., Sloane, D. C., Guinyard, J., Diamant, A. L., Nascimento, L. M., et al. (2004, March/April). Leading by example: A local health department-community collaboration to incorporate physical activity into organizational practice. *Journal of Public Health Management & Practice, 10*(1), 116-124.

Yanda, R. L. (1979). Biofeedback in pulmonary diseases. *West Journal Medicine, 131*(1), 49-50.

Ye, X. Q., Chen, W. Q., Lin, J. X., Wang, R. P., Zhang, Z. H., Yang, X., et al. (2008). Effect of social support on psychological-stress-induced anxiety and depressive symptoms in patients receiving peritoneal dialysis. *Journal of Psychosomatic Research, 65*(2), 157-164.

Yesalis, C. E., Kennedy, N. J., Kopstein, A. N., & Bahrke, M. S. (1993). Anabolic–androgenic steroid use in the United States. *JAMA, 270*(10), 1217-1221.

York, J. L., Welte, J., & Hirsch, J. (2003). Gender comparison of alcohol. *Journal Studies Alcohol, 64,* 790-802.

Young, T., Peppard, P. E., & Gottlieb, D. J. (2002). Epidemiology of obstructive sleep apnea: A population health perspective. *American Journal of Respiratory and Critical Care Medicine, 165*(9), 1217-1239.

Yu, M. W., Hsieh, H. H., & Pan, W. H. (1995). Vegetable consumption, serum retinol level, and risk of hepatocellular carcinoma. *Cancer Research, 55*(6), 1301-1305.

Zalewska-Pucha_a, J., Majda, A., Ga_uszka, A., & Kolonko, J. (2007). Health behaviour of students versus a sense of self-efficacy. *Advanced Medical Science, 52*(Suppl 1), 73-77.

Zeki, S. (2007). The neurobiology of love. *FEBS Letters, 581*(14), 2575-2579.

Zellner, D. A., Loaiza, S., Gonzalez, Z., Pita, J., Morales, J., Pecora, D., et al. (2006). Food selection changes under stress. *Physiology & Behavior, 87*(4), 789-793.

Zhao, L. J., Liu, Y., Liu, P., Hamilton, J., Recker, R., & Deng, H. (2007). Relationship of obesity with osteoporosis. *Journal of Clinical Endocrinological Metabolism, 92*(5), 1640-1646.

Ziedonis, D., Hitsman, B., Beckham, J. C., Zvolensky, M., Adler, L. E., Audrain-McGovern, J., et al. (2008). Tobacco use and cessation in psychiatric disorders: National Institute on Mental Health Report. *Nicotine and Tobacco Research, 10*(12), 1691-1715.

Zuckerman, P. (2005). Atheism: Contemporary rates and patterns. In M. Martin (Ed.), *The Cambridge companion to atheism.* Cambridge: Cambridge University Press.

Index